Outcome Measures in Trauma

Outcome Measures in Trauma

Edited by

P. B. Pynsent PhD
Research and Teaching Centre
Royal Orthopaedic Hospital
Birmingham

J. C. T. Fairbank MD, FRCS
Nuffield Orthopaedic Centre
Oxford

and

A. J. Carr ChM, FRCS
Nuffield Orthopaedic Centre
Oxford

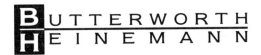

Butterworth-Heinemann Ltd
Linacre House, Jordan Hill, Oxford OX2 8DP

$\mathcal{R}$ A member of the Reed Elsevier plc group

OXFORD   LONDON   BOSTON
MUNICH   NEW DELHI   SINGAPORE   SYDNEY
TOKYO   TORONTO   WELLINGTON

First published 1994

© Butterworth-Heinemann Ltd 1994

British Library Cataloguing in Publication Data
Pynsent, P. B.
  Outcome Measures in Trauma
  I. Title
  617.1

ISBN 0 7506 1653 9

Library of Congress Cataloguing in Publication Data
Outcome measures in trauma/edited by P. Pynsent, J. Fairbank, A. Carr.
  p. cm.
Sequel to: Outcome measures in orthopaedics.
Includes bibliographical references and index.
ISBN 0 7506 1653 9
1. Wounds and injuries—Treatment—Evaluation. 2. Musculoskeletal
system—Wounds and injuries—Treatment—Evaluation. 3. Outcome
assessment (Medical care) I. Pynsent, P. B., 1945–   .
II. Fairbank, J. C. T., 1948–   . III. Carr, A. (Andrew)
IV. Outcome measures in orthopaedics.
[DNLM: 1. Wounds and Injuries. 2. Outcome Assessment (Health Care)—standards. WO
700 094 1994]
RD93.095 1994
617.1—dc20
DNLM/DLC   94-9397
for Library of Congress   CIP

Typeset by Keytec Typesetting Ltd, Bridport, Dorset
Printed in Great Britain at the University Press, Cambridge

Contents

Faculty

Union and Non-union of Fractures

Authors
  J. G. Andrew, FRCS, Hope Hospital, Eccles Old Road, Salford, Lancs.
  P. R. Kay, FRCS, Hope Hospital, Eccles Old Road, Salford, Lancs.

Osteoarthritic Risks of Intra-articular Fractures

Authors
  S. G. Gregg-Smith, FRCS, Nuffield Orthopaedic Centre, Headington, Oxford.
  S. H. White, FRCS, Nuffield Orthopaedic Centre, Headington, Oxford.

Growth Plate Injuries

Author
  D. M. Eastwood, FRCS, Royal Free Hospital, London.
Group Chairman
  M. Saleh, FRCS, Northern General Hospital, Herries Road, Sheffield.
Group members
  P. Alderman, FRCS, Cardiff Royal Infirmary, Cardiff.
  C. F. Bradish, FRCS, Royal Orthopaedic Hospital, Northfield, Birmingham.
  M. Burton, Northern General Hospital, Sheffield.
  A. T. Cross, FRCS, Sunderland District Hospital, Sunderland, Tyne & Wear.
  A. F. G. Groom, FRCS, Kings College Hospital, London.
  S. Kendall, FRCS, John Radcliffe Hospital, Headington, Oxford.
  J. J. L. Plewes, FRCS, The General Hospital, Birmingham.
  W. J. Ribbans, FRCS, Royal Free Hospital, London.
  D. Riley, FRCS, Pontefract General Infirmary, Pontefract, West Yorkshire.
  K. M. Willett, FRCS, John Radcliffe Hospital, Headington, Oxford.

Trauma Scores

Author
  C. A. Pailthorpe, FRCS, Cambridge Military Hospital, Aldershot.

Complications in the Treatment of Musculoskeletal Trauma

Author
  S. Frostick, FRCS, University Hospital, Queen's Medical Centre, Nottingham.
  J. B. Hunter, FRCS, University Hospital, Queen's Medical Centre, Nottingham

Peripheral Nerve Injuries

Author
  D. Marsh, FRCS, Hope Hospital, Salford, Lancs.

Vascular Trauma

Authors
  N. C. Hickey, FRCS, Worcester Royal Infirmary.
  M. Simms, FRCS, Selly Oak Hospital, Birmingham.
Group Chairman
  R. J. Cherry, FRCS, Birmingham Heartlands Hospital, Birmingham.
Group members
  D. A. Boot, MChOrth, FRCS, Warrington District Hospital, Warrington.
  J. P. Bull, CBE, MD, FRCP, Burns Research Group, Birmingham Accident Hospital, Birmingham.
  R. Fitzpatrick, PhD, Department of Public Health & Primary Care, Radcliffe Infirmary, Oxford.
  D. Griffiths, Royal Infirmary, Hartshill, Stoke-on-Trent.
  J. Hutchinson, Department of Orthopaedics, Medical School, University of Aberdeen, Forester Hill, Aberdeen.
  D. H. A. Jones, FRCS, Ysbyty Gwynedd, Bangor, Gwynedd.
  S. Matthews, FRCS, John Radcliffe Hospital, Headington, Oxford.
  A. Phipps, FRCS, Pinderfields General Hospital, Wakefield, W. Yorks.
  M. Woodford, North Western Injury Research Centre, Hope Hospital, Salford, Lancs.

The Shoulder and Humerus

Author
  C. A. Pailthorpe, FRCS, Cambridge Military Hospital, Aldershot.

The Elbow and Forearm

Author
D. M. Williamson, FRCS, Princess Margaret Hospital, Swindon.
Group Chairman
A. J. Carr, ChM, FRCS, Nuffield Orthopaedic Centre, Headington, Oxford.
Group members
C. J. K. Bulstrode, FRCS, Nuffield Orthopaedic Centre, Headington, Oxford.
N. D. Citron, MChir, FRCS, St Helier Hospital, Carshalton, Surrey.
P. B. Pynsent, PhD, Royal Orthopaedic Hospital, Northfield, Birmingham.

The Wrist

Author
J. Dias, FRCS, The Royal Infirmary, Leicester.

Hand and Flexor Tendon Injury

Authors
C. Kelly, FRCS, North Staffordshire Royal Infirmary, Stoke-on-Trent.
A. Macey, FRCS, Sligo General Hospital, The Mall, Sligo, Eire.
Group Chairman
P. J. Mulligan, FRCS, Royal Orthopaedic Hospital, Northfield, Birmingham.
Group members
P. D. Burge, FRCS, Nuffield Orthopaedic Centre, Headington, Oxford.
P. R. Stuart, FRCS, Newcastle General Hospital, Newcastle upon Tyne.
P. J. F. Wade, FRCS, Coventry & Warwickshire Hospital, Coventry.

Spine and Spinal Cord Injury

Author
P. Sett, MS, FRCS (Ed), FRCS(SN), Mersey Regional Spinal Injuries Centre, Southport and Formby District General Hospital, Southport, Merseyside.

The Pelvis and Acetabulum

Author
R. B. C. Treacy, FRCS, Royal Orthopaedic Hospital, Northfield, Birmingham.

Group Chairman

J. C. T. Fairbank, MD, FRCS, Nuffield Orthopaedic Centre, Heading-ton, Oxford.

Group members

M. E. Blakemore, FRCS, Coventry & Warwickshire Hospital, Coventry.

M. A. Foy, FRCS, Princess Alexandra Hospital, RAF Wroughton, Swindon, Wilts.

H. Frost, MCSP, Nuffield Orthopaedic Centre, Headington, Oxford.

C. G. Greenough, MD, FRCS, Middlesbrough General Hospital, Middlesbrough, Cleveland.

S. J. Krikler, BSc, PhD, FRCS(Ed), Royal Orthopaedic Hospital, Northfield, Birmingham.

A. M. C. Thomas, FRCS, Royal Orthopaedic Hospital, Northfield, Birmingham.

A. G. Thompson, FRCS, Royal Orthopaedic Hospital, Northfield, Birmingham.

K. M. Willett, FRCS, John Radcliffe Hospital, Oxford.

Femoral Head and Neck Fractures

Authors

D. A. Macdonald, FRCS, St James's University Hospital, Leeds.

S. Calder, FRCS, The General Infirmary, Leeds.

Femoral and Tibial Shaft Fractures

Authors

E. F. Wheelwright, FRCS, Orthopaedic Trauma Unit, Glasgow Royal Infirmary, Glasgow.

Group Chairman

G. C. Bannister, MChOrth, FRCS, Southmead Hospital, Westbury on Trym, Bristol.

Group members

J. S. Albert, FRCS, Norfolk and Norwich Hospital, Norwich.

I. A. Bacarese-Hamilton, FRCS, Chelsea Westminster Hospital, London.

M. F. Brown, FRCS, Department of Orthopaedics, Hammersmith Hospital, London.

M. I. Goodwin, FRCS, Royal United Hospital, Bath.

W. Harper, FRCS, Glenfield General Hospital, Leicester.

J. O'Dowd, FRCS, Queen Mary's Hospital for Sick Children, Carshal-ton, Surrey.

C. Withey, Department of Public Health Medicine, UMDS, St Thomas' Hospital, London.

The Knee

Author
D. R. Bickerstaff, MD, FRCS, FRCS (Ed), Royal Hallamshire Hospital, Sheffield.

The Ankle

Author
A. H. R. W. Simpson, DM, FRCS, Nuffield Orthopaedic Centre, Headington, Oxford.

The Foot

Author
D. O'Doherty, MD, FRCS (Ed), Cardiff Royal Infirmary, Cardiff.
Group Chairmen
G. Bentley, FRCS, Royal National Orthopaedic Hospital, Stanmore, Middx.
O. N. Tubbs, FRCS, The General Hospital, Birmingham.
Group members
A. M. Davies, FRCR, Royal Orthopaedic Hospital, Northfield, Birmingham.
D. Learmonth, FRCS, Birmingham Accident Hospital, Birmingham.
R. W. Morris, PhD, Department of Public Health and Primary Care, Royal Free Hospital School of Medicine, London.

Pain Measurement

Authors
A. R. Jadad, MD, ICRF, Building, Churchill Hospital, Oxford.
H. J. McQuay, DM, ICRF Building, Churchill Hospital, Oxford.

Head Injuries

Authors
T. A. D. Cadoux-Hudson, FRCS, Frenchay Hospital Trust, Bristol.
R. S. C. Kerr, BSc, MS, FRCS, Radcliffe Infirmary NHS Trust, Oxford.

Thoracic and Cardiac Trauma

Authors
S. W. H. Kendall, BSc, MBBS, FRCS (Ed), John Radcliffe Hospital, Oxford.
S. Westaby, BSc, MS, FRCS, John Radcliffe Hospital, Oxford.

Abdominal Trauma

Author
P. J. Clarke, FRCS, John Radcliffe Hospital, Oxford.

The Urogenital Tract

Authors
J. M. T. Perkins, FRCS, Churchill Hospital, Oxford.
D. Cranston, DPhil, FRCS, Churchill Hospital, Oxford.

Burns

Author
A. Phipps, FRCS, Pinderfields General Hospital, Wakefield, W. Yorks.

Missile and Gunshot Wounds

Author
S. J. E. Matthews, FRCS, RAMC, Queen Elizabeth Military Hospital, Woolwich.

Preface

Outcome is defined as a visible or practical result (*Oxford English Dictionary*). Outcome measures play an important rôle in medical practice. They should provide the basis for both clinical audit and research. However they are a topic that has been addressed by few clinicians. The principal object of this book is to provide references to sources of instruments and techniques used for outcome measurement in trauma, and to advise on the optimum choice of instrument. It will become clear to any student of this topic that it is not an easy subject and there remain many areas without adequate outcome measures. This work is a sequel to a volume on outcome measures in orthopaedics (Pynsent *et al.*, 1993). There are inevitably areas where these two books overlap.

The text is primarily aimed at medical staff in trauma centres and accident and emergency departments. The book may also be of value to metrologists, research nurses and others involved in clinical research into trauma. There is a medicolegal dimension to this topic. Outcome measures are vital to the setting of standards of care and their measurement, as well as in the assessment of injury severity. This is of relevance to both lawyers and clinicians in this area, who will find in this book a reference to the most appropriate outcome measures for their purpose. The setting of standards of care and the assessment of the quality of care is also of concern to doctors in public health medicine, purchasers and government. It is important for the clinician to maintain an interest in this field, not least to ensure that managers are receiving accurate and relevant clinical information about his or her activities.

We expect that most users of this book will be specialists in the area of musculoskeletal trauma but we have invited contributions on other aspects of trauma. These non-musculoskeletal areas are of considerable relevance to the overall management of the polytrauma patient. Measurement of the outcome of these injuries is a vital, though neglected area of practice.

The British Paediatric Association Outcome Measures Working Group (British Paediatric Association, 1992) has presented a number of definitions: a *Health Status Measurement* is a direct measure of some aspect of health in which improvement is sought, whether or not its relationship to any intervention, social or environmental circumstance is understood. An example is infant mortality rate. An *Outcome Measurement* is a subtype of health status measurement where changes in the measure are known (or at least believed) to be largely attributable to a health service intervention. An example, in the field of paediatrics, is life expectancy for people with cystic fibrosis. An *Implied Outcome Measurement* is an indirect indicator of health which can be used as a valid proxy for an outcome measurement. Examples are immunisation coverage, and coverage of a screening programme of proven effectiveness. In our view the health status measurement may also be described as 'functional status measurement' and a 'quality of life measure'. These measurements can be made without necessarily seeking improvement.

In general, many of the outcome measures in trauma practice are based on scoring systems. Most of these systems are poorly validated. Newcomers to the field will experience difficulties not only in finding the available instruments, but also in making an informed choice as to the most appropriate for their purpose. This book is designed to help in making such a choice. We have tried to be descriptive as well as proscriptive. Often there are differences between the requirements of outcome measures for audit as opposed to clinical research. In most cases there is a pay-off between the demands of speed, efficiency and acceptability to both doctor and patient, and the demands of precision and specificity. In our opinion some instruments are so complex that they have become impossible to use. Where possible, we would like to indicate where apparently clear-cut measures of outcome (e.g. union of a fractured tibia) may be vulnerable to confounding factors, such as clinical judgement, age or intercurrent illness. An instrument should be quick, simple to use, reliable, specific to the question being investigated, cost-effective and applicable. In most cases this ideal instrument does not exist although many measures have come into general use without meeting these criteria.

In this book we have tried to indicate areas where there are deficiencies in the currently available instruments. These may represent avenues for future research. We would expect the pragmatic reader should be content with the best available instrument but, if dissatisfied, an innovator should be stimulated to develop new systems for the future. Streiner and Norman (1989) provide invaluable advice on how this may be achieved. An area which has not been addressed is the question of who should do the measurements in research. It is sometimes possible to have a research nurse or an independent observer to fulfil this important task. In practice, it is usually the surgeon who is obliged to perform the measurements. Whoever performs this task will introduce their own biases. A North American view on general outcome measures can be found in Spilker (1990); these should be only used in the UK with some circumspection.

Outcome measures may be broadly distinguished into those used to measure the doctor's assessment and those used to measure the patient's own assessment of their problem. In most cases it is appropriate to record both types of outcome. The latter are widely used by health economists, managers and politicians. As these two approaches are likely to be measuring different factors, it is our opinion that they should normally be presented as separate outcomes. The problems and advantages of these two groups of measurement should be addressed in the text. The more we have investigated this field, the more we have become convinced of the value of patient-based measures. In the past these have been dismissed as too unreliable for serious consideration by clinical investigators, in fact these assessments tend to follow the main indication for the original intervention closely. These are often termed health status, functional status or quality of life measures, as mentioned already.

We have found the World Health Organisation's (1986) definitions of impairment, disability and handicap of considerable value. Impairment is a demonstrable anatomical loss or damage, such as the loss of range of movement of a joint. Disability is the functional limitation caused by an impairment, which interferes with something a patient wishes to or must achieve. Handicap depends on the environment. For example a patient confined to a wheelchair may be fully mobile on the level, but be completely immobilised by a flight of stairs.

The measurement of complications is not strictly speaking an outcome measure. However, complications are commonly the major component of review in clinical audit, as it is currently practised in the UK. They may be of importance in clinical trials and are routinely reported in most retrospective reviews of a condition and its treatment.

This book has been prepared in a somewhat unconventional fashion. The chapters were the subject of a 2-day meeting held at the Royal Orthopaedic Hospital, Birmingham in February, 1993. This meeting followed the Dahlem principle (Dixon, 1987), where small working groups of clinicians and other experts reviewed each contribution in detail. Where appropriate, the working group's comments and recommendations have been added to the end of each chapter under the heading of 'Group discussions'.

This book is one of the first devoted to this topic. It is appropriate for us to reflect on the direction the subject of outcome measures is going. We have aimed to report the currently available systems and to recommend 'best buys'. This has highlighted many deficiencies in the currently available instruments and illustrates the considerable scope for improvement in their quality. Defining techniques of measurement, who does them and, most importantly, reliability, are usually not described. With the increasing cost of health care, the development of effective outcome measures is crucial in defining both benefits and the costs of treatment.

Jeremy Fairbank, Andrew Carr, Paul Pynsent

References

British Paediatric Association (1992) *Outcome Measurements for Child Health*. London: British Paediatric Association

Dixon B (1987) Scientifically speaking. *Br. Med. J.*; **294**: 1424

Pynsent PB, Fairbank JCT, Carr AJ (1993) *Outcome Measures in Orthopaedics*. Oxford: Butterworth Heinemann

Spilker B (1990) *Quality of Life Assessments in Clinical Trials*. New York: Raven Press

Streiner DL, Norman GR (1989) *Health Measurement Scales: a practical guide to their development and use*. Oxford: Oxford Medical Publications

World Health Organisation (1986) *International Classification of Impairments, Disabilities and Handicaps*. Geneva: WHO

Acknowledgements

We are grateful to Smith & Nephew Richards for their generous sponsorship of the review meeting held at the Royal Orthopaedic Hospital, Birmingham. Our thanks are also due to Mrs Sheila Sellars of Butterworth-Heinemann for her interest and enthusiastic support in the production of this volume.

We are all indebted to Ann Weaver for her contribution to the collation and preparation of the manuscripts. Also, we acknowledge that her organisational ability ensured the smooth running of the Birmingham meeting.

Chapter 1

Trauma scores

C. A. Pailthorpe

Introduction

Accurate audit of patient data is now mandatory and the analysis of such data is becoming increasingly sophisticated. In the field of trauma the methodologies generated to assess outcome are well established. They are important in not only the assessment of patient care and quality assurance, but also in the promotion of regional trauma centres. Several systems have been devised to assess trauma outcome. This chapter aims to describe the principal trauma scales in current use and their evolution into outcome predictors of survival and mortality.

Definition

Outcome from trauma can be defined in several ways but is usually considered in terms of survival or death (Krischer, 1976; Cayten and Evans, 1979). It can refer to the extent of disability and functional recovery (Jennett and Boyd, 1975) and the length of stay in hospital (Semmlow and Cone, 1976; Fetter, 1984). Outcome is being incorporated into a broader reflection of health care evaluation allowing the performance of a trauma unit to be assessed (Champion *et al.*, 1992; Crawford, 1991; Grevitt *et al.*, 1991) and the comparison of individual institutions (Boyd, 1987).

Development of scoring systems

A variety of systems have been developed, some of which relate purely to injury severity, some to physiological parameters which allow triage of patients and some a combination of both. It is not the purpose of the author to catalogue a chronological list of the different scoring systems. The interested reader is directed to the further reading list at the end of the chapter. There are, however, certain key systems that should be considered and these will be discussed.

Anatomical scoring systems

The Abbreviated Injury Scale (AIS) (Committee on Medical Aspects of Automotive Safety, 1971; American Association for Automotive Medicine, 1985) provided the first universally accepted method for rating the severity of tissue damage caused from vehicle injuries.

It is anatomically based and categorises the injuries into regions of the body and attributes a severity rating score of one to six from minor to unsurvivable (Table 1.1). The early system did not incorporate scores for penetrating injuries but this was rectified in the 1985 revision (AIS-85). The AIS has limitations particularly in respect to multiple injuries as it is not possible to apply linear mathematical calculations to the scores to obtain an overall severity score (Baker *et al.*, 1974).

The AIS is, however, the basis of the Injury Severity Score (ISS) (Baker *et al.*, 1974). This system was devised in an attempt to assess the overall severity of multiple injuries and give a method for comparing mortality in groups of injured patients. It is based on the AIS and divides the body into six regions (Table 1.2). Each region injured is scored using the AIS and the ISS is calculated by adding together the squares of the highest AIS rating for each of the three most severely injured body regions.

Thus the maximum ISS is 75 calculated from $5^2 + 5^2 + 5^2$. If any one of the body regions is rated as AIS-6 the ISS is automatically defined as 75. Several studies have confirmed that the ISS relates well to mortality and length of hospital stay (Semmlow and Cone, 1976; Bull, 1977).

Accurate anatomical rating demands precise identification of the extent of injury. This may only be available retrospectively from autopsy (Harviel *et al.*, 1989) but operation and investigation results should be utilised.

None of the above systems incorporated a factor for age. Bull in 1975 highlighted (from a purely anatomical aspect) that mortality from major trauma increased with age and by using probit analysis, produced a 'lethal dose' injury severity score for 50% of patients (LD_{50}). Thus, the LD_{50} for the patients in his study was an ISS of 40 for ages 15–44, 29 for ages 45–64 and 20 for ages 65 and older.

Table 1.1 The Abbreviated Injury Score

AIS code	Description
1	Minor
2	Moderate
3	Serious
4	Severe
5	Critical
6	Unsurvivable

Table 1.2 Body regions used in the Injury Severity Score

1	Head and neck
2	Face
3	Chest
4	Abdomen/pelvis
5	Extremities/pelvic girdle
6	Body surface

Physiological scoring systems

Physiological scoring systems have been used in the early triage of patients to identify those patients requiring more intensive treatment. The Glasgow Coma Scale (GCS) (Teasdale and Jennett, 1974) has been widely accepted as the fundamental scoring system for the assessment of the central nervous system in patients with head injuries. The Triage Index (Champion et al., 1980) assesses injury severity and is based on a series of functional variables measuring dysfunction in the respiratory, cardiovascular and central nervous systems. It was modified to include systolic blood pressure (SBP) and respiratory rate (RR) producing the Trauma Score (TS) (Appendix 1.1) (Champion et al., 1981).

The Trauma Score has been used as a predictor of survival by determining the probability of survival (P_s) for each value of the TS (Figure 1.1) (Champion et al., 1981).

The TS has been used mainly as triage tool in the field to decide where to send casualties. In the USA casualties with a TS of 13 or less are taken to a Level 1 Trauma Centre. However, there are deficiencies in this system, particularly in the estimation of 'capillary refill' and 'respiratory expansion' at night. It was for this reason that the system was further modified by Champion in 1989, leaving out capillary refill and respiratory expansion (Table 1.3). The Revised Trauma Score (RTS) is based on data from the Major Trauma Outcome Study (MTOS) (an outcome evaluation study organised through the Committee on Trauma of the American College of Surgeons, Champion, 1990). Unlike the TS the RTS results in non-integer values ranging from 0 to 8.

Walker and Duncan (1967) described a recursive technique in estimating regression coefficients. Using this regression analysis of the MTOS data, weighting coefficients for the GCS, SBP and RR have been produced. The resultant coefficient will depend on the database used for analysis.

Thus the Revised Trauma Score can be calculated by using the following formula:

$$RTS = 0.9368(GCS \text{ coded value}) + 0.7326(SBP \text{ coded value})$$

$$+ 0.2908(RR \text{ coded value})$$

The TS is deficient in its predictive capability for serious head injuries in that a patient with a GCS of 3 and normal SBP and RR would have a TS of 12 and a survival probability of 0.83 (Figure 1.1). This is clearly inappropriate scoring. The RTS with its weighting coefficients derived

Table 1.3 The Revised Trauma Score, modifications made by Champion et al., 1984

Glasgow Coma Score	Systolic blood pressure (mmHg)	Respiratory rate (min)	Coded value
13–15	> 89	10–29	4
9–12	76–89	> 29	3
6–8	50–75	6–9	2
4–5	1–49	1–5	1
3	0	0	0

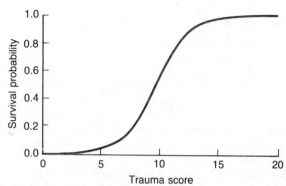

Figure 1.1 The Trauma Score plotted against probability of survival to show the form of function

from MTOS data will give a significantly better prediction of outcome. As an example consider,

RTS = 0.9368(GCS = 0) + 0.7326(SBP = 4) + 0.2908(RR = 4)

RTS = 0 + 2.9304 + 1.1632

RTS = 4.0936

The survival probability (P_s) of a patient with a RTS of 4.0 is 0.605 (Figure 1.2), which is substantially lower than that predicted by the TS.

Physiological scoring systems have been developed to assess the outcome of intensive care patients and the most widely used is the APACHE system (**A**cute **P**hysiology **a**nd **C**hronic **H**ealth **E**valuation). First described in 1981 by Knaus *et al.* it was revised to APACHE II in 1985 (Knaus *et al.*, 1985). A software package is now available in the USA to permit the use of APACHE III (recently modified from APACHE II). APACHE is a scoring system that aims to predict the individual prognosis of patients, to classify them into sets of increasing mortality, to assess the nursing requirement and to allow comparison of one intensive care unit with another. It is more useful in assessing a group of patients rather than an individual. APACHE II uses a score based upon the initial values of 12 routine physiological measurements together with previous health

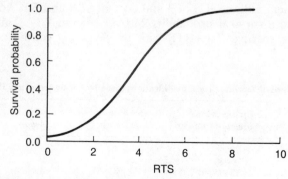

Figure 1.2 The form of survival probability (P_s) curve for the Revised Trauma Score

status to determine a general measure of the severity of the disease. An increasing score (0–71) correlates with increasing mortality. Using daily APACHE II scores Chang *et al.* (1988) showed that the predictive power of the scores was increased fourfold, however, Vassar *et al.* (1992) has recently reported that the APACHE system significantly overestimated mortality in the lower ranges of predicted risk and underestimated mortality in the higher ranges. Vassar has introduced another outcome system for ICU patients, a 24-hour ICU point system, based upon neurological, pulmonary and cardiovascular indices. It was compared to both APACHE II and TRISS (see below) and performed well.

Other physiologically based scoring systems for ITU patients include the Respiratory Index (RI) (Golfarb *et al.*, 1975) which is a measure of the respiratory status of the patient and reflects the level of hypoxia. It is derived from the following equation:

$$RI = \frac{P(AaDO_2)}{PaO_2}$$

where

$P(AaDO_2)$ = alveolar − arterial oxygen difference

PaO_2 = arterial partial pressure of oxygen

The Therapeutic Intervention Scoring System (Cullen *et al.*, 1974) provides a measure of ITU patient resource utilisation. The Simplified Acute Physiology Score (Le Gall *et al.*, 1984) is used in France and elsewhere in Europe.

Combined anatomical and physiological scoring systems

In the 1980s a methodology utilising both the TS and the ISS was developed (Boyd *et al.*, 1987). This incorporated the **TR**auma score, **ISS** (TRISS) and a weighted coefficient for age. Initially the TS was used but has now been superseded by the RTS. TRISS methodology produces a probability of survival (P_s) based on the following formula:

$$P_s = \frac{1}{1 + e^{-b}}$$

where

$b = b_0 + b_1(\text{RTS}) + b_2(\text{ISS}) + b_3(A)$

e = constant − the base of Napierian logarithms approximately equal to 2.718282

A = 0 if the patient's age is 54 years or less, or 1 if over 54 years

$b_{0...3}$ are coefficients derived from Walker–Duncan regression analysis (Walker and Duncan, 1967) applied to the MTOS data and at present this is based on the RTS and AIS-85. Values for both blunt and penetrating injuries have been determined (Table 1.4).

Evaluation of trauma care is best accomplished by assessing both anatomical and physiological indices. A three-step approach has been devel-

Table 1.4 Revised coefficients for blunt and penetrating injuries

	b_0	b_1	b_2	b_3
Blunt	−1.2470	0.9544	−0.0768	−1.9052
Penetrating	−0.6029	1.1430	−0.1516	−2.6676

oped (Champion *et al.*, 1983) that provides a qualitative and quantitative assessment of patient severity and outcome.

The first step is a method called PRE (derived from **PRE**liminary), it identifies those patients whose outcome was unexpected, whether it be death or survival. If a graph is plotted of RTS against ISS a scatter diagram is produced (Figure 1.3).

Survivals and deaths are indicated by the Ls and Ds respectively. The diagonal line indicates the 50% chance of survival, so a patient whose point is above the line has less than a 50% chance of surviving. Those survivors whose points are above the line and those deaths that are below the line can then be identified and reviewed. When used in this manner the 50% isobar allows comparison of each patient's outcome against a predicted expectation based on thousands of patients' data. However, it is important to recognise that for a given probability of survival, e.g. $P_s = 0.67$, there will be an inevitable mortality, i.e. one in three. Thus it is more appropriate to consider that those survivors above the line survived in an area of high mortality, and conversely those deaths below the line died in an expected high survival area. The term 'unexpected outcome' is frequently used in this context, but it should be used circumspectly.

The second method, the State Transition Screen (STS), is a series of concepts which attempt to identify those patients who are expected to die but who improve before dying and those that are expected to survive but who go through a period of deterioration before ultimately surviving. These concepts including the Global Score, the Morbidity Transition and the Minimum Morbidity have not gained universal use.

The third method is called DEF (from **DEF**initive) and is a statistical comparison of trauma care between institutions. The institution's own study results can be compared against a baseline population with

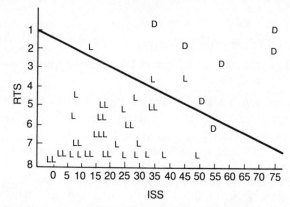

Figure 1.3 Sample pre-chart using Injury Severity Score and the Revised Trauma Score

'expected' results. The DEF methodology will take account of variations in the patient severity mix.

The z statistic was described by Flora in 1978 for the comparison of a 'test' institution with a 'standard' institution. It will highlight the differences between the predicted number of deaths for a unit against the actual number. It is derived from the following formula:-

$$z = \frac{D - \sum_{i=1}^{n} Q_i}{\sqrt{\sum_{i=1}^{n} P_i Q_i}}$$

where

D = actual number of deaths

$Q_i = (1 - P_i)$, the predicted probability of death for patient i

$\sum Q_i$ = predicted number of deaths

P_i = predicted Ps for patient i (from baseline norm)

An example of calculating the z statistic is given in Table 1.5. Using the above formula mortality is studied, however, the formula can be used to assess the predicted survival as follows:

$$z = \frac{S - \sum_{i=1}^{n} P_i}{\sqrt{\sum_{i=1}^{n} P_i Q_i}}$$

where

S = actual number of survivors

P_i = predicted P_s for patient i (from baseline norm)

Table 1.5 An example of using the z statistic

Patient number	Lived/died	P_i	Q_i	$P_i Q_i$
1	L	0.997	0.003	0.00299
2	L	0.994	0.006	0.00596
3	L	0.992	0.008	0.00794
4	D	0.049	0.951	0.04660
5	L	0.938	0.062	0.05816
6	L	0.673	0.327	0.22007
7	L	0.800	0.200	0.16000
8	L	0.134	0.866	0.11604
9	D	0.004	0.996	0.00398
10	D	0.287	0.713	0.20463
$n = 10$	$D = 3$	$\Sigma P_i = 5.686$	$\Sigma Q_i = 4.132$	$\Sigma P_i Q_i = 0.82637$

Applying these values to the formula, z can be calculated thus:

$$z = \frac{(3 - 4.132)}{\sqrt{0.82637}}$$

$$z = \frac{-1.132}{0.909}$$

$$z = -1.24$$

$\sum P_i$ = predicted number of survivors (from baseline norm)

Q_i = probability of death $(1 - P_i)$.

The z statistic can be either positive or negative, depending on whether the number of survivors in the test population, is greater or less than that predicted by TRISS from the baseline population. Absolute values of z greater than 1.96 are statistically significant ($p < 0.05$) and if this result occurs suggests that the test institution's care is significantly different from the care expected in the baseline population. Caution must be taken in interpreting these results too literally. Cottington *et al.* (1989) have shown that it is erroneous to conclude that a non-significant z statistic means that there is no difference between the observed and expected survival in the study group. The sample size may be too small to show a statistically significant difference and there may be considerable variation in the severity mix. The limitations in the TRISS indices have been highlighted by Krischer (1976) who showed that mortality is not a strictly increasing function of the ISS.

A further score, W has been utilised by the MTOS in the USA to quantify the clinical significance of the difference between the actual (A) and the expected (E) number of survivors. The latter are derived from the z statistic.

$$W = \frac{100(A - E)}{N}$$

where

N = the number of patient's in the unit's sample.

Thus for units with a significantly negative z score, W will reflect the decrease in the number of survivors per 100 patients treated compared with the expected norm. Some studies use the number of survivors to derive the z statistic and a positive result is the desired one, however if mortality is studied then a negative result would be expected. It is important to recognise which method has been used to avoid confusion.

An M statistic has been used to measure the injury severity match between the test and baseline patient groups. Values range from zero to one and the closer to one the better the match of injury severity. The M statistic is derived from the comparison of the probability of survival (P_s) of the test group and the baseline. The P_s is divided into six increments and the fraction of patients in each is represented by $f_{1...6}$ for the baseline set and $g_{1...6}$ for the test set. The smaller of the two values f_n or g_n equals s_n. The sum of the six s_n gives the M statistic. An example is given in Figure 1.4. However, as proposed the M statistic is unreliable since several different disparities can produce the same value.

Paediatric scoring systems

The Paediatric Trauma Score (PTS) was developed by Tepas *et al.* in 1988 in response to the requirement for a specific trauma score for children. It is based upon six physiological and anatomical factors and produces a score which reflects those children at increased risk of mortality and morbidity (Table 1.6).

P_s range	Fraction of patients within study cohort (g)	P_s Range baseline subset (f)
0.96–1.00	0.842	0.828
0.91–0.95	0.053	0.045
0.76–0.90	0.052	0.044
0.51–0.75	0.00	0.029
0.26–0.50	0.043	0.017
0.00–0.25	0.010	0.036

thus $M = s1 + s2 + s3 + s4 + s5 + s6$
$M = 0.0828 + 0.045 + 0.044 + 0.017 + 0.010$
$M = 0.944$

Figure 1.4 Example of calculating the M statistic

If a proper sized BP cuff is not available, the BP can be assessed by assigning:

$+2$ – pulse palpable a wrist

$+1$ – pulse palpable at groin

-1 – no pulse palpable

Limitations of the outcome systems

With the intensive research into the different scoring systems it has become clear that there are definite limitations in the comparison of groups of injured patients with respect to case mix and injury severity. It has been shown that there is considerable heterogeneity within ISS cohorts (Copes *et al.*, 1988; Cayten *et al.*, 1991). As the ISS is derived from the highest AIS scores from the body regions injured, the severity of injuries within one body region (e.g. within the abdomen) can be underestimated. There is, also, an assumption that the AIS scores have been assigned consistently throughout the body regions. The ISS is dependent upon an accurate anatomical diagnosis which may not be available on admission and the recording of the RTS frequently does not relate to the time of injury.

There is wide variation in mortality rates within the major subdivisions

Table 1.6 Paediatric Trauma Score devised by Tepas *et al*.

Component	Category		
	+2	+1	−1
Size of child (kg)	> 20	10–20	< 10
Airway	Normal	Maintainable	Unmaintainable
Systolic BP	> 90 mmHg	50–90 mmHg	< 50 mmHg
CNS	Awake	Obtunded/LOC	Coma/decerebrate
Skeletal	None	Closed fractures	Open/multiple fractures
Cutaneous	None	Minor	Major/penetrating

Sun (PTS) ⎯⎯⎯⎯⎯⎯⎯⎯⎯⎯⎯
Reproduced from Tepas *et al.*, 1988.

of the categories of blunt and penetrating injuries and there is an inability of the TRISS method to predict the survival rates of patients suffering injuries from low falls (e.g. elderly females with isolated hip fractures). Cayten recommends that these patients are excluded from analyses using the TRISS methodology; this has recently been confirmed by Yates *et al.* (1992) in the MTOS (UK) study.

Recent developments

The Major Trauma Outcome Study (MTOS) is well established in the USA to collect and analyse data from Trauma Centres around the country. MTOS (UK) has been initiated and aims to improve the quality of information obtained concerning the management of severely injured patients. It is centrally collating the physiological and anatomical data of injured patients at the scene of the accident, during transportation to the hospital and at all stages during the hospital stay and allows anonymous comparison of the performance of Trauma Units. The preliminary analysis has been published (Yates *et al.*, 1992) and has confirmed that reduced revised trauma scores and increased injury severity score are associated with greater mortality. It identified differences between the standard of care of blunt injuries in the UK compared to the USA but not the cause. There were difficulties in data collection making examination of some aspects of the trauma care impossible but modifications of the system have been introduced and further analysis continues. Because of the variation in case mix between the USA and the UK, the comparison of TRISS using USA weightings on UK data is flawed. With increased UK data collection, UK TRISS weightings can be formulated allowing better interpretation of predicted versus observed results.

The search continues for a better quantitative characterisation of injury to allow better integration with the physiological scoring systems and thus produce more accurate patient outcome. To this end, Champion *et al.* (1990a) have proposed a new characterisation of injury termed ASCOT (**A** **S**everity **C**haracterisation **O**f **T**rauma). The main limitations with ISS are the failure to account for multiple injuries in one region and to give equal weighting to each of the six body regions (e.g. a severe head injury has the same value as a severe skin injury). Thus Champion suggests using an Anatomical Profile (AP) which is a summary score for all serious injuries to one region (Table 1.7) and gives greater weights to injuries in certain parts of the body.

ASCOT incorporates AIS-85 and ICD-9-CM codes (International Classification of Diseases, 1977, 9th Revision, Clinical Modification). Utilising MTOS data from 1982 to 1988, model weighting coefficients were derived using the Walker–Duncan method. The probability of survival could then be estimated using the formula below:

$$P_s = \frac{1}{1 + e^{-k}}$$

where $k = k_1 + k_2G + k_3S + k_4R + k_5A + k_6B + k_7C + k_8\text{Age}*$

$G = GCS$

Table 1.7 The injury assignments to Anatomical Profile components

Component	Injury	AIS Severity	ISS Body Regions	ICD-9-CM Codes
A	Head/brain	3–5	1	800,801,803,850–854
	Spinal cord	3–5	1,3,4	806,950,952,953
B	Thoracic	3–5	3	807,839.61/.71,860–862, 901
	Front of neck	3–5	1	807.5/.6,874,900
C	Abdomen/pelvis	3–5	4	863–868,902
	Spine w/o cord	3	1,3,4	805,839
	Pelvic fracture	4–5	5	808,839.42/.52/.69/.79
	Femoral artery	4–5	5	904.0/.1
	Crush above knee	4–5	5	928.00/.01,928.8
	Amputation above knee	4–5	5	897.2/.3/.6/.7
	Popliteal artery	4	5	904.41
D	Face	1–4	2	802,830
	All others	1–2	1–6	—

Reproduced from Champion *et al.*, 1990a.

$$S = SBP$$

$$R = RR$$

D has been excluded as it was found not to influence predictions. Patient age (Age*) is more precisely modelled than in TRISS (Table 1.8).

ASCOT results were compared to those derived from TRISS and were found to provide better discrimination for patients with penetrating injuries but only modest improvement for those with blunt injuries. Overall there was improved sensitivity and predictive reliability over TRISS. Anatomical profile appears to give a more accurate method of characterising injury by maintaining separate scores by body region and including AIS scores for all serious injuries within a region, but, inevitably it remains dependent upon accurate coding of the injury. The first independent validation of ASCOT was undertaken by Markle *et al.* (1992) using a different trauma registry. They conclude that the relatively small gain in predictive accuracy of ASCOT over TRISS is largely offset by its intricacy and increased computer processing requirements. Neither index was found to provide good statistical agreement between predicted and actual outcomes for either blunt or penetrating injury patients.

Participation in the MTOS schemes, in which a selected group of trained coders are used to code all injuries, may result in a better overall

Table 1.8 The patient age characterisation utilised by the ASCOT system

Age	Ages (yr)
0	0–54
1	55–64
2	65–74
3	75–84
4	> 85

analysis. However, no statistical analysis of injury severity can produce perfect predictions and clinical acumen will remain an essential component of quality assurance. There will always be some variation in care between institutions, especially when factors such as the number of elderly patients with fractured hips are considered and, also, the influence of pre-injury disease (MacKenzie *et al.*, 1989).

Peer review is being used to assess differences within and between institutions (Collopy *et al.*, 1992; Davis *et al.*, 1992; Karmy-Jones *et al.*, 1992). Using TRISS methodology cases of unexpected outcome can be identified and then subjected to scrutiny. Errors in patient management can be detected (Davis *et al.*, 1992), leading to improvements in patient care. Within an institution this has been shown to be highly effective in improving patient care over several years (Champion *et al.*, 1992).

Conclusions

Increasingly the 'audit' of an institution's work is becoming an integral part of that work. The requirement for accurate data collection is mandatory and will increase the workload within a unit. Precise coding of the data is required and this may be best performed within MTOS. The evaluation of the performances of individual units may produce results divergent from the 'norm' and it is important that this statistical comparison should incorporate corrections for the variation in case severity mix and sample size. Used as a 'total hospital scoring system' the methodology can pick out patients whose deaths may have been preventable and highlight those that survived, then peer review will allow more realistic interpretation.

The statistical methodology described above is inherently retrospective and it should not be used for assessing the prognosis of an individual patient during treatment. It is completely dependent upon accurate coding and this information may not be apparent during the treatment phase of a patient and may be difficult to achieve (Zoltie and de Dombal, 1993). The limitations of ISS and TRISS stimulated the development of ASCOT which appears to improve sensitivity and predictive reliability but with some loss of simplicity. MTOS is promoting further research into severity indices and their interpretation for the purposes of quality assurance and this should lead to better patient care and outcome.

References

American Association for Automotive Medicine (1985) *The Abbreviated Injury Scale (AIS)*, 1985 revision. Des Plaines, Illinois

Baker SP, O'Neill B, Haddon W, Long WB (1974) The Injury Severity Score: a method for describing patients with multiple injuries and evaluating emergency care. *J. Trauma*; **14**: 187–196

Benzer A, Mitterschiffthaler G, Marosi M, Luef G, Puhringer F, De-la-Renotiere K, Lehner H, Schmutzhard E (1991) Prediction of non-survival after trauma: Innsbruck coma scale. *Lancet*; **338**: 977–978

Boyd CR, Tolson MA, Copes WS (1987) Evaluating trauma care: The TRISS Method. *J. Trauma*; **27**: 370–378

Bull JP (1977) Measures of severity of injury. *Injury*; **9**: 184–187

Cayten CG, Evans W (1979) Severity Indices and their implications for emergency medical services research and evaluation. *J. Trauma*; **19**: 98–102

Cayten CG, Stahl WM, Murphy JG, Agarwal N, Byrne DW (1991) Limitations of the TRISS method for inter-hospital comparisons: a multi-hospital study. *J. Trauma*; **31**: 471–482

Champion HR, Sacco WJ, Carnazzo AJ, Copes WS, Fouty WJ (1981) Trauma score. *Crit. Care Med.*; **9**: 672–676

Champion HR, Sacco WJ, Copes WS, Gann DS, Genarelli TA, Flanagen ME (1989) A revision of the trauma score. *J. Trauma*; **29**: 623–629

Champion HR, Sacco WJ, Hunt TK (1983) Trauma severity scoring to predict mortality. *World J. Surg.*; **7**: 4–11

Champion HR, Sacco WJ, Hannon DS, Lepper RL, Atzinger ES, Copes WS, Prall RH (1980) Assessment of injury severity: the Triage Index. *Crit. Care Med.*; **8**: 201–208

Champion HR, Sacco WJ, Copes WS (1992) Improvement in outcome from trauma center care. *Arch. Surg.*; **127**: 333–338

Champion HR, Copes WS, Sacco WJ, Lawnick MM, Bain LW, Gann DS, Genarelli TA, Mackenzie E, Schwaitzberg S (1990a) A new characterization of injury severity. *J. Trauma*; **30**: 539–546

Champion HR, Copes WS, Sacco WJ, Lawnick MM, Keast SL, Bain LW, Flanagan ME, Frey CF (1990b) The Major Trauma Outcome Study: establishing national norms for trauma care. *J. Trauma*; **30**: 1356–1365

Chang RWS, Jacobs S, Lee B, Pace N (1988) Predicting deaths among intensive care unit patients. *Crit. Care Med.*; **16**: 34–42

Collopy BT, Tulloh BR, Rennie GC, Fink RLW, Rush JH, Trinca GW (1992) Correlation between injury severity scores and subjective ratings of injury severity: a basis for trauma audit. *Injury*; **23**: 489–492

Committee on Medical Aspects of Automotive Safety (1971) Rating the Severity of Tissue Damage: I. The Abbreviated Scale. *JAMA*; **215**: 277–280

Committee on Medical Aspects of Automotive Safety (1972) Rating the Severity of Tissue Damage: II. The Comprehensive Scale. *JAMA*; **220**: 717–720

Copes WS, Lawnick M, Champion HR, Sacco WJ (1988a) A comparison of abbreviated injury scale 1980 and 1985 versions. *J. Trauma*; **28**: 78–85

Copes WS, Champion HR, Sacco WJ, Lawnick MM, Keast SL, Bain LW (1988b) The injury severity score revisited. *J. Trauma*; **28**: 69–76

Cottington EM, Shufflebarger CM, Townsend R (1989) The power of the Z statistic: implications for trauma research and quality assurance review. *J. Trauma*; **29**: 1500–1509

Crawford R (1991) Trauma audit: experience in north-east Scotland. *Br. J. Surg.*; **78**: 1362–1366

Cullen DJ, Civetta JM, Briggs BA, Ferrara LC (1974) Therapeutic intervention scoring system: a method for quantitative comparison of patient care. *Crit. Care Med.*; **2**: 57–60

Davis JW, Hoyt DB, McArdle MS, Mackersie RC, Eastman AB, Virgilio RW. Cooper G, Hammill F and Lynch FP (1992) An analysis of errors causing morbidity and mortality in a Trauma System: a guide for quality improvement. *J. Trauma*; **22**: 660–665

Fetter RB (1984) Diagnosis related groups: the product of the hospital. *Clin. Res.*; **32**: 336–340

Flora JD (1978) A method for comparing survival of burn patients to a standard survival curve. *J. Trauma*; **18**: 701–705

Goldfarb MA, Ciurej TF, McAslan TC, Sacco WJ, Weinstein MA, Cowley RA (1975) Tracking respiratory therapy in the trauma patient. *Am. J. Surg.*; **129**: 255–258

Grevitt MP, Muhiudeen HA, Griffiths C (1991) Trauma care in a military hospital. *J. R. Army Med. Corps*; **137**: 131–135

Harviel JD, Landsman I, Greenberg A, Copes WS, Flanagan ME, Champion HR (1989) The effect of autopsy on injury severity and survival probability calculations. *J. Trauma*; **29**: 766–773

International Classification of Diseases (1977) 9th revision, Clinical Modification. Ann Arbor, MI: Edwards Brothers

Jennett B, Bond M (1975) Assessment of outcome after severe brain damage. *Lancet*; i: 481–484

Karmy-Jones R, Copes WS, Champion HR, Weigelt J, Shackford S, Launick M, Rozycki SS, Hollingsworth-Fridland P, Klein J (1992) Results of multi-institutional outcome assessment: results of peer review of TRISS-designated unexpected outcomes. *J. Trauma*: **32**: 196–203

Knaus WA, Zimmerman JE, Wagner DP, Draper EA, Lawrence DE (1981) APACHE – acute physiology and chronic health evaluation: a physiologically based classification system. *Crit. Care Med.*; **9**: 591–597

Knaus WA, Draper EA, Wagner DP, Zimmerman JE (1985) APACHE II: a severity of disease classification system. *Crit. Care Med.*; **13**: 818–829

Krischer JP (1976) Indexes of Severity: underlying concepts. *Health Serv. Res.*; **11**: 143–157

Le Gall JR, Loirat P, Alperovitch A, Glaser P, Granthil C, Mathieu D, Mercier P, Thomas R, Villers D (1984) A simplified acute physiology score for ICU patients. *Crit. Care Med.*; **12**: 975–977

MacKenzie EJ, Morris JA, Edelstein SL (1989) Effect of pre-existing disease on length of hospital stay in trauma patients. *J. Trauma*; **29**: 757–765

Markle J, Cayten CG, Byrne DW, Murphy JG (1992) Comparison between TRISS and ASCOT methods in controlling for injury severity. *J. Trauma*; **33**: 326–332

Semmlow JL, Cone R (1976) Utility of the Injury Severity Score: a confirmation. *Health Serv. Res.*; **11**: 45–51

Teasdale G, Jennet B (1974) Assessment of coma and impaired consciousness. *Lancet*; ii: 81–84

Tepas JJ, Ramenofsky ML, Mollitt DL, Gans BM, DiScala C (1988) The pediatric trauma score as a predictor of injury severity: an objective assessment. *J. Trauma*; **28**: 425–429

Vassar MJ, Wilkerson CL, Duran PJ, Perry CA, Holcroft JW (1992) Comparison of APACHE II, TRISS, and a proposed 24-hour ICU point system for prediction of outcome in ICU trauma patients. *J. Trauma*; **32**: 490–499

Walker SH, Duncan DB (1967) Estimation of the probability of an event as a function of several independent variables. *Biometrika*; **54**: 167–179

Yates DW, Woodford M, Hollis S (1992) Preliminary analysis of the care of injured patients in 33 British hospitals: first report of the United Kingdom major trauma outcome study. *Br. Med. J.*; **305**: 737–740

Zoltiie N, de Dombal (1993) The hit and miss of ISS and TRISS. *Br. Med. J.*; **307**: 906–909

Further general reading

Baker SP, O'Neill B (1976) The Injury Severity Score: an update. *J. Trauma*; **16**: 882–885

Barancik JI, Chatterjee BF (1981) Methodological considerations in the use of the Abbreviated Injury Scale in trauma epidemiology. *J. Trauma*; **21**: 627–631

Boyd DR, Lowe JL, Baker RJ, Nyhus LM (1973) Trauma registry: new computer method for multifactorial evaluation of a major health problem. *JAMA*; **223**: 423–428

Boyd CR, Corse KM, Campbell RC (1989) Emergency interhospital transport of the major trauma patient: air versus ground. *J. Trauma*; **29**: 789–794

Bull JP (1982) Injury severity scoring systems. *Injury*; **14**: 2–6

Cales RH (1986) Injury severity determination: requirements, approaches and applications. *Ann. Emerg. Med.*; **15**: 1427–1433

Champion HR (1982) Field triage of trauma patients: editorial. *Ann. Emerg. Med.*; **11**: 160–161

Champion HR, Sacco WJ (1982) Measurement of patient illness severity. *Crit. Care Med.*; **10**: 552–553

Champion HR, Sacco WJ, Carnazzo AJ, Copes WS, Fouty WJ (1981) Trauma Score. *Crit. Care Med.*; **9**: 672–676

Civil ID, Schwab CW (1988) The abbreviated injury scale, 1985 revision: a condensed chart for clinical use. *J. Trauma*; **28**: 87–90

Copes WS, Champion HR, Sacco WJ, Lawnick MM, Gann DS, Gennarelli T, Mackenzie E, Schwaitzberg (1990) Progress in characterizing anatomic injury. *J. Trauma*; **30**: 1200–1207

Dragsted L, Jorgensen J, Jensen NH, Bonsing E, Jacobsen E, Knaus WA, Qvist J (1989) Interhospital comparisons of patient outcome from intensive care: importance of lead-time bias. *Crit. Care Med.*; **17**: 418–422

Dykes EH, Spence LJ, Bohn DJ, Wesson DE (1989) Evaluation of pediatric care in Ontario. *J. Trauma*; **29**: 724–729

Eastham JN, Steinwachs DM, Mackenzie EJ (1991) Trauma care reimbursement: comparison of DRGs to an injury severity-based payment system. *J. Trauma*; **31**: 210–216

Eichelberger MR, Mangubat EA, Sacco WS, Bowman LM, Lowenstein AD (1988) Comparative outcomes of children and adults suffering blunt trauma. *J. Trauma*; **28**: 430–434

Goris RJA, Gimbrere JSF, Niekerk JLM, Schoots FJ, Booy LHD (1982) Early osteosynthesis and prophylactic mechanical ventilation in the multi-trauma patient. *J. Trauma*; **22**: 895–902

Gormican SP (1982) CRAMS scale: field triage of trauma victims. *Ann. Emerg. Med.*; **11**: 132–135

Greenspan L, McLellan BA, Greig H (1985) Abbreviated injury scale and injury severity scoring: a scoring chart. *J. Trauma*; **25**: 60–64

Haddon W (1973) Energy damage and the ten countermeasure strategies. *J. Trauma*; **13**: 321–331

Hershman MJ, Cheadle WG, Kuftinec D, Polk HC, George CD (1988) An outcome predictive score for sepsis and death following injury. *Injury*; **19**: 263–266

Hoyt DB, Shackford SR, McGill T, Mackenzie R, Davis J, Hansborough J (1989) The impact of in-house surgeons and operating room resuscitation on outcome of traumatic injuries. *Arch. Surg.*; **124**: 906–910

Kondziolka D, Schwartz ML, Walters BC, McNeill I (1989) The Sunnybrook neurotrauma assessment record: improving trauma data collection. *J. Trauma*; **29**: 730–735

Krischer JP (1979) Indexes of Severity: conceptual development. *Health Serv. Res.*; **14**: 56–67

McLellan BA, Koch JP, Wortzman D, Rogers C, Szalai J, Williams D (1988) *Early Identification of the High Risk Patient Using the Estimated Injury Severity Score and Age.* 32nd Annual Proceedings: Association for the Advancement of Automotive Medicine, Seattle, Washington, pp. 173–185

Moylan JA, Detmer DE, Rose J, Schultz R (1976) Evaluation of the quality of hospital care for major trauma. *J. Trauma*; **16**: 517–523

Nayduch DA, Moylan J, Rutledge R, Baker CC, Meredith W, Thomason M, Cunningham PG, Oller D, Azizkhan RG, Mason T (1991) Comparison of the ability of adult and pediatric trauma scores to predict pediatric outcome following major trauma. *J. Trauma*; **31**: 452–457

Pal J, Brown R, Fleiszer D (1989) The value of the Glasgow Coma Scale and Injury Severity Score: predicting outcome in multiple trauma patients with head injury. *J. Trauma*; **29**: 746–748

Parrillo JE (1991) Research in critical care medicine: present status of critical care investigation. *Crit. Care Med.*; **19**: 569–577

Rhodes M, Brader A, Lucke J, Gillott A (1989) Direct transport to the operating room for resuscitation of trauma patients. *J. Trauma*; **29**: 907–915

Rocca B, Martin C, Viviand X, Bidet PF, Saint-Gilles HL, Chevalier A (1989) Comparison of four severity scores in patients with head trauma. *J. Trauma*; **29**: 299–305

Sacco WJ, Jameson JW, Copes WS, Lawnick MM, Keast SL, Champion HR (1988) Progress toward a new injury severity characterization: severity profiles. *Comput. Biol. Med.*; **18**: 419–429

Smith EJ, Ward AJ, Smith D (1990) Trauma scoring methods. *Br. J. Hosp. Med.*; **44**: 115–118

Tepas JJ, Ramenofsky ML, Mollitt DL, Gans BM, DiScala C (1988) The Paediatric Trauma Score as a predictor of injury severity: an objective assessment. *J. Trauma*; **28**: 425–429

Trunkey DD, Siegel J, Baker SP, Gennarelli TA (1983) Panel: current status of trauma severity indices. *J. Trauma*; **23**: 185–201

Waller JA, Payne SR, McClallen JM (1989) Trauma centers and DRGs – Inherent conflict?. *J. Trauma*; **29**: 617–622

Young JC, Macioce DP, Young WW (1990) Identifying injuries and trauma severity in large databases. *J. Trauma*; **30**: 1220–1226

Appendix 1.1 The Trauma score of Champion *et al*.

Trauma score	Value	Points	Score
A. Respiratory rate	10–24	4	
Number of respirations in 15 sec multiply by four	25–35	3	
	> 35	2	
	< 10	1	
	0	0	A. ____
B. Respiratory effort			
Shallow – markedly decreased chest movement or air exchange	Normal		
Retractive – use of accessory muscles or intercostal retraction	Shallow or retractive		B. ____
C. Systolic blood pressure	> 90	4	
Systolic cuff pressure – either arm-auscultate or palpate	70–90	3	
	50–69	2	
	< 50	1	
	0	0	C. ____
D. Capillary refill			
Normal – forehead, lip mucosa or nail bed colour refill in 2 sec	Normal	2	
Delayed – more than 2 sec of capillary refill	Delayed	1	
None – no capillary refill	None	0	D. ____

E. Glasgow Coma Scale		Total GCS Points	Score
1. Eye opening		14–15	5
Spontaneous	____ 4	11–13	4
To voice	____ 3	8–10	3
To pain	____ 2	5–7	2
None	____ 1	3–4	1	E. ____

2. Verbal response
Orientated ____ 5
Confused ____ 4
Inappropriate words ____ 3
Incomprehensible words ____ 2
None ____ 1

3. Motor response
Obeys commands ____ 6
Purposeful movement (pain) ____ 5
Withdraw (pain) ____ 4
Flexion (pain) ____ 3   Trauma score

Extension (pain) ____ 2   (Total points
None ____ 1   A + B + C + D + E)

Total GCS Points (1 + 2 + 3) ____

Reproduced from Champion *et al*., 1981.

Chapter 2

Pain measurement

A. R. Jadad and H. J. McQuay

Trauma is always associated with pain and pain relief should be one of the main priorities of patient management. However, pain measurement is rarely part of the initial assessment and treatment of injured patients. Pain is a multidimensional personal experience and as such it cannot be measured reliably by objective physical tests. This explains in part why the measurement of pain is so underused as a clinical tool.

Although subjective measures are often underestimated, it is clear that pain can be measured reliably and most methods available can be applied under most clinical circumstances with remarkably cheap, quick, sensitive and reproducible results. Those methods have been developed and validated in the research field where they have been used to determine and compare the efficacy of new and established analgesic interventions either in the acute or in the chronic pain setting.

This chapter describes the most relevant methods for the measurement of pain due to trauma and focuses on their characteristics and limitations. Our aim is to give elements to health professionals involved in the care of trauma patients to assess pain reliably and to use the information to determine the effectiveness of treatments and to ensure that patients are given the best therapeutic options.

Methods for pain measurement

Pain can be measured with scales, questionnaires or with indirect methods. The scales are usually simple and consume little time. The questionnaires are more complex, demand more time and usually look at more than one dimension of the pain experience. The indirect methods are not very accurate but they are used as substitutes for scales and questionnaires when it is not possible to obtain the patient's own report of pain.

Rating scales

Pain scales are probably the simplest way to measure pain. They can only analyse one dimension at a time, usually pain intensity or relief. In increasing order of complexity the most widely used scales are binary, categorical and visual analogue (VAS).

Binary scales

They are very simple and are designed to produce only a yes/no answer to a question that usually includes a cut-off point. For instance, to measure pain relief the patient is asked: 'Is your pain more than half relieved?' These scales were included in clinical trials and validated more than 30 years ago (Lasagna and Beecher, 1954; Beecher, 1957) and it has been shown that they provide reliable information that correlates satisfactorily with more complex methods. Their main limitation is the poor discriminatory power. Patients are forced to choose from only two states and it is impossible to identify differences between treatments whose effects elicit the same answer. The effects of two different drugs might be indistinguishable even if one of them produced complete pain relief and the other only 60% when administered to the same patient or population of patients. Therefore, binary scales are of no value in clinical trials designed to detect differences between treatments but they might be very useful to monitor the clinical response of patients to analgesic interventions in casualty units.

Categorical verbal rating scales

These are also known as categorical scales and are the oldest of the standard methods for pain measurement (Keele, 1948). The patient is given a list of descriptors and is asked to choose the word which is most appropriate to reflect the magnitude of a pain dimension.

The most popular categorical scale measures pain intensity and includes four categories: none, mild, moderate and severe. A good alternative or complement is a categorical scale to measure relief. In this case, five categories are frequently used: none, slight, moderate, good and complete paediatric visual analogue scale. The assessment of relief is more complex and sensitive than the assessment of pain intensity because to give a report the patient has to make a judgement on the analgesic action and side-effects (McQuay, 1990). Nevertheless, as the patient has to remember the baseline level of pain to measure relief, the accuracy of the results can be affected if the assessment is done in confused patients with memory impairment.

When these scales are used as outcome measures in clinical trials, it is common to give numerical scores to the verbal categories by using successive integers (Table 2.1). Although the linearity of the categories is controversial, several studies on healthy volunteers and patients have compared numerical scores from categorical scales with simultaneous measurements from visual analogue scales (see below) using cross-modality matching techniques and good correlation has been shown, especially with relief scales (Scott and Huskisson, 1976; Wallenstein et al., 1980; Littman et al., 1985).

The main advantage of these scales is their simplicity and quick scoring and their discriminative power is definitely higher than for binary scales.

Table 2.1 Categorical verbal rating scales

Pain intensity	Pain relief
Severe 3	Complete 4
Moderate 2	Good 3
Slight 1	Moderate 2
None 0	Slight 1
	None 0

On the other hand, they can be scored even by patients with eye injuries or unable to write because of lesions in the upper limbs.

The main criticism of these scales is that the number of descriptors is insufficient and that it limits and forces the patient to choose particular categories.

Visual analogue scales

Visual analogue scales are usually 10-cm lines whose ends are labelled with extreme descriptions of a dimension (Figure 2.1). Subjects are asked to mark the line at a point corresponding to the magnitude of the dimension which is being measured (Huskisson, 1974). The magnitude of the dimension generally increases from left to right. The scores are obtained by measuring the distance between the end which represents the minimal magnitude of the dimension and the patient's mark, and they are expressed in millimetres (centimetres when longer scales are used).

The scales can be straight or curvilinear, vertical or horizontal, continuous or graded, but it seems that to achieve maximal sensitivity they must be administered as straight, horizontal and ungraded lines (Sriwatanakul et al., 1982). The advantages of the visual analogue scales are that they are relatively simple, quick to score, do not involve imprecise descriptive terms and provide many points from which to choose. Disadvantages are that they require both more concentration than the categorical scales and visual and motor coordination, which may be lacking in patients with head trauma, eye injury or lesions of the upper extremities.

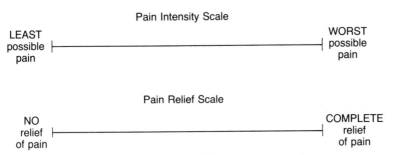

Figure 2.1 Visual analogue scales

Verbal numerical scales

This group of scales combines the advantages of the categorical and visual analogue scales. Patients are asked to express numerically the magnitude of the dimension under study, pain relief or intensity. The assessment of pain can be performed in patients with vision and/or motor impairment with almost no restriction on the number of scoring steps. There have been very few attempts to validate these scales but at least there is evidence for good correlation between a 11-point scale for pain intensity and a conventional 10-cm unmarked horizontal visual analogue scale (Murphy *et al.*, 1988).

Other scales and measures

SUMMARY SCORES

When pain is measured at multiple points, it is possible to combine the scores at the different assessment times to obtain scores that summarise the analgesic response. The most important derived scores are the Summed Pain Intensity Difference (SPID) and the Total Pain Relief (TOTPAR). The SPID is the sum of the differences between the baseline score for pain intensity (from any scale) and the values obtained at each measurement time during the relevant period of time. The TOTPAR is much simpler. It is the sum of all the pain relief scores obtained after the intervention.

These two calculations are estimates of the area under the time–effect curve of the analgesic intervention and reflect the magnitude of the analgesic response. Unfortunately, they do not provide information about the onset or duration of the pharmacological effect (Max and Laska, 1991).

GLOBAL SCORES

These scales are used as a complement to the others. Originally, they were numerical scales (Calimlim *et al.*, 1977). The patients were asked to judge and rate the effect of the intervention by giving a number from 1 (poor effect) to 5 (excellent). We use global scales as part of research trials but we find it easier for the patients to understand and score as a categorical scale. We ask the patient to qualify the treatment as poor, fair, good, very good or excellent and we allocate numerical values from 0 to 5 only for analytical purposes.

PAEDIATRIC SCALES

Conventional visual analogue scales have been modified in such a way that pain can be measured reliably in children from 4 years of age. The simplest method uses a set of poker chips (usually four) and the child is asked to indicate how many 'pieces of hurt' he or she feels. Another method that can be used from the same age is a set of faces (pictures or photographs) with expressions progressing from very sad to very happy (Figure 2.2). For children older than 7 years of age, pain has been

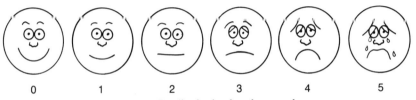

Figure 2.2 Paediatric visual analogue scale

measured reliably with a graphic representation of a thermometer with a numerical scale (McGrath *et al.*, 1986). Unfortunately, there are no validated scales to measure pain in children younger than 4 years of age and even less in newborns and infants.

Questionnaires

The main advantage of questionnaires is that they allow multidimensional measurement of pain. The McGill Pain Questionnaire (MPQ) has been validated extensively and measures the sensory, affective and evaluative aspects of pain. It contains 78 descriptors divided into 20 subgroups. Another valid and reliable alternative to the MPQ is the Wisconsin Brief Pain Questionnaire (Daut *et al.*, 1983). This instrument focuses on pain intensity, relief, site, walking, sleeping and effects of pain in relations with other people, enjoyment of life and mood. It can be self-administered and therefore it is regarded as the cheapest and least time-consuming of the questionnaires. However, even the Wisconsin Brief Pain Questionnaire takes much longer to score than the other scales and therefore questionnaires have very limited use for the assessment of pain after trauma.

Indirect methods for pain assessment

Physiological and behavioural methods

The assessment of pain with scales is not possible in preverbal children, in patients with head trauma and/or under artificial ventilation in intensive therapy units. In those cases, it would be desirable to have objective pain measures. Unfortunately, there is no way to assess someone's pain reliably by measuring changes in blood, urine or in neurophysiological tests. Attempts to identify exclusive pain behaviours have failed. Probably the most reliable use of behaviour is to rule out pain in children. It could be assumed that a child is not in pain if he/she is quiet. However, this is not applicable in very ill children or in patients under heavy sedation or mechanical ventilation. Needless to say, visual analogue scales scored by parents (Martin, 1982) or health professionals are of very questionable validity.

Vital signs share some of the problems of behavioural measures. Elevations of blood pressure, pulse, respiratory rate and skin temperature are well-known responses to acute pain. Unfortunately they are associated with other conditions that could be present after trauma such as anxiety or infections. As with behaviour, normal vital signs could be used to rule out pain, provided that the patient is not under treatment with beta-blockers.

The failure of simple vital sign measurement to assess pain has moti-vated the use of more complex and high technology methods such as measurement of adrenocortical activity, skin conductance and resistance, electroencephalogram and evoked potentials. These measures have very limited clinical use as they are not only non-specific and expensive, but usually very time consuming (Chapman *et al.*, 1985; McGrath, 1989).

Colours and drawings

Several attempts have been made to measure pain by asking the patients, usually very young children, to represent their pain with drawings or colours. Further research to determine their validity and reliability is necessary.

Analgesic consumption and time to next analgesic (TNA)

The number of doses of analgesic requested by the patient (analgesic consumption) and the time between an intervention and the first request of an analgesic dose (Time to Next Analgesic or TNA), can provide indirect estimates of analgesic efficacy. They have been used effectively in research trials (McQuay *et al.*, 1980; Moore *et al.*, 1984), but under normal clinical conditions their results can be affected by so many factors such as patterns of analgesic prescription and number of nurses in the wards, that they should not be used as an alternative to more reliable scales.

Measuring pain efficiently

For accurate results, the methods for pain measurement must be selected and administered appropriately.

The selection of the *method* depends mainly on the condition of the *patient*. As the severity of the trauma increases, the number of methods that can be used to measure pain decreases. However, only in a small group of patients is it impossible to measure pain reliably. This group includes very young children, patients with severe anxiety, moderate to severe head trauma, aphasia, mental retardation, heavy sedation or mechanical ventilation.

Once the appropriate method has been selected, the selection of the *dimension(s)* depends on the *objective* of the measurement. If the object-ive of the measurement is to determine the state of pain, pain intensity scales are more appropriate than pain relief scales. Once an analgesic intervention has been made, pain relief scales become more relevant to monitor the analgesic response. When the aim of the measurement is to assess the efficacy of an intervention or to compare treatments for research purposes, both dimensions should be measured with multiple scales. The use of multiple scales allows the observer to question the patient again when incompatible scores are obtained for the same dimension.

The selection of appropriate methods and dimensions is not enough to guarantee optimum results. The person in charge of the measurements plays an important role in determining the accuracy and reliability of the measurements. In analgesic studies, for instance, the measurements should be performed by the same person and under ideal conditions that person should be a research nurse with adequate training in techniques for pain assessment. For clinical or audit purposes, casualty and ward nurses should be in charge of the assessments. They should be trained in how to measure pain and include pain measurement, storing the scores with the other usual measurements (blood pressure, temperature, etc.).

There should be agreement as to whether current or typical pain is to be measured. If current, the patients must report what he/she is feeling at the time of the assessment. If typical, the report should be a summary of the pain experience during a definite period of time. Typical pain is less precise than current pain, but may be more appropriate to assess inter-mittent pains or analgesic effects that could be shorter than the assess-ment periods. Current and typical pain assessments are not exclusive and could be used simultaneously. The same conditions, however, must be reproduced at each assessment time.

Multiple pains must be evaluated separately and the frequency of the measurements must be modified according to the characteristics of the analgesic intervention.

Conclusions

Trauma is always associated with pain and adequate pain relief should be one of the main priorities of treatment. Although pain measurement can be remarkably quick, cheap, simple and reliable, it has been sadly neglected in clinical practice and very little information is available on its use as an outcome measure.

Every health professional should know how to assess pain reliably and pain should be measured systematically as part of the management of any patient with trauma to ensure that unnecessary suffering is avoided.

References

Beecher HK (1957) The measurement of pain. *Pharmacol. Rev.*; **9**: 59–210

Calimlim JF, Wardell WM, Davis HT, Lasagna L, Gillies AJ (1977) Analgesic efficacy of an orally administered combination of pentazocine and aspirin with observations on the use and statistical efficiency of GLOBAL subjective efficacy ratings. *Clin. Pharmacol. Ther.*; **21**: 34–43

Chapman CR, Casey KL, Dubner R, Foley KM, Gracely RH, Reading AE (1985) Pain measurement: an overview. *Pain*; **22**: 1–31

Daut RL, Cleeland CS, Flanery RC (1983) Development of the Wisconsin brief pain questionnaire to assess pain in cancer and other diseases. *Pain*; **17**: 197–210

Huskisson EC (1974) Measurement of pain. *Lancet*; **ii**: 1127–1131

Keele KD (1948) The pain chart. *Lancet*; **ii**: 6–8

Lasagna L, Beecher HK (1954) The optimal dose of morphine. *JAMA*; **156**: 230–234

Littman GS, Walker BR, Schneider BE (1985) Reassessment of verbal and visual analogue ratings in analgesic studies. *Clin. Pharmacol. Ther.*; **38**: 16–23

Martin LVH (1982) Postoperative analgesia after circumcision in children. *Br. J. Anaesth.*; **54**: 1263–1266

Max MB, Laska EM (1991) Single-dose analgesic comparisons. In Max MB, Porternoy RK and Laska EM (eds) *Advances in Pain Research and Therapy*, vol. 18. New York: Raven, pp. 55–95

McGrath PA (1989) Evaluating a child's pain. *J. Pain Symptom Manag.*; **4**: 198–214

McGrath PA, Cunningham SJ, Goodman JT, Unruh A (1986) The clinical measurement of pain in children: a review. *Clin. J. Pain*; **1**: 221–227

McQuay HJ, Bullingham RES, Evans PJD (1980) Demand analgesia to assess pain relief from epidural opiates. *Lancet*; **i**: 768–769

McQuay HJ (1990) Assessment of pain, and effectiveness of treatment. In: Hopkins A, Costain D (eds) *Measuring the Outcomes of Medical Care*. London: Royal College of Physicians, pp. 43–57

Moore RA, Paterson GMC, Bullingham RES, Allen MC, Baldwin D, McQuay HJ (1984) A controlled comparison of intrathecal cinchocaine with intrathecal cinchocaine and morphine: clinical effects and plasma morphine concentrations. *Br. J. Anaesth.*; **56**: 837–841

Murphy DF, McDonald A, Power C, Unwin A, MacSullivan R (1988) Measurement of pain: a comparison of the visual with a nonvisual analogue scale. *Clin. J. Pain*; **3**: 197–199

Scott J, Huskisson EC (1976) Graphic representation of pain. *Pain*; **2**: 175–184

Sriwatanakul K, Kelvie W, Lasagna L (1982) The quantification of pain: an analysis of words used to describe pain and analgesia in clinical trials. *Clin. Pharmacol. Ther.*; **32**: 143–148

Wallenstein SL, Heidrich G, Kaiko R, Houde RW (1980) Clinical evaluation of mild analgesics: the measurement of clinical pain. *Br. J. Clin. Pharmacol.*; **10**: 319S–327S

Chapter 3

Head injuries

T. A. D. Cadoux-Hudson and R. S. C. Kerr

Introduction

The development of repeatable and reliable head injury outcome scores has proved to be a considerable challenge. Head injuries can be caused by a wide range of insults and result in a variety of functional or visible results (outcomes). Premorbid personality, mechanism of injury (Goldsmith and Ommaya, 1984) and pathophysiological response of the central nervous system (Adams *et al.*, 1982; Genneralli, 1986) are some factors influencing the diversity of outcome. Not surprisingly, the development of outcome scores has not received as much attention as the clinical management of the acute injury. However, the standardisation of outcome scores is essential for research into more effective and efficient acute and long-term care.

The prediction of outcome, stimulated by the desire to know what the future will bring, has attracted more interest than the accurate measure of the result (Genneralli *et al.*, 1982). In no other human system is the creation and testing of outcome scores more difficult than that of the central nervous system. Outcome scores to date have concentrated on measuring social handicap such as level of dependence and ability to work. Functional impairment and relevant disability have been largely ignored. The ideal outcome score should include both subjective and objective assessments which can be reliably and repeatably carried out.

The incidence of head injury in peace time remains high with 200–300 per 100000 of population being admitted to hospital (Anderson and McLaurin, 1980; Jennett and McMillan, 1981) and many more being seen in the casualty department (Jennett and Teasdale, 1981). The head-injured patient tends to be male with only minor functional impairment (Miller and Jones, 1985). Only a small percentage of patients (5%) are comatosed, with as many as 50% of these requiring surgery. Road traffic accidents remain the commonest cause of severe head injury, and are frequently associated with injuries of other systems (Miller *et al.*, 1978), particularly skeletal (lower limbs 45%, upper limbs 23%) (London, 1963). The development of rapid transfer to specialist trauma centres will, hopefully, increase the survivors of severe injury, increasing the head-injured population and the demand for rehabilitation.

Head injury is the leading cause of death in persons under 40 years

(Selecki *et al.*, 1977). Morbidity remains a serious sequelae with some 37 000 severely and 17 000 moderately disabled patients surviving per year in the USA. A single traumatic event on one individual may have long-term emotional and financial effects on both the family and society.

The premorbid CNS structure, function and personality are important factors when measuring the outcome after injury. Variations in the scalp and skull thickness and shape will alter the result of sharp or blunt injury (Gurdjian, 1972). Age will also vary the degree of bony, dural and soft tissue damage, secondary complications (Galbraith, 1973) and recovery. Previous head injury or primary cerebral atrophy may make a minor head injury a devastating event. The 'punch-drunk' syndrome of boxers is an example of the cumulative effect of multiple minor to moderate injuries (Potter, 1958; Roberts, 1969). The premorbid personality may have profound influence on the rehabilitation phase and affect outcome.

Trauma to the skull and scalp may be sharp (often penetrating) or blunt, typically as a result of a road traffic accident, blow to the head or fall. Penetrating injuries will damage neuronal structures directly. Devastating focal or generalised functional loss may result and the outcome be predictable. However the small depressed compound skull fracture from a golf club injury in a young child may result in life-long epilepsy, but have a 'good outcome' by functional measure.

The mechanism of blunt injury to the cranium will have differing effects on the scalp, skull and soft tissue (Becker and Povlishock, 1985). The effect of these forces to the skull is similar to any bony structure; closed or compound, simple or comminuted and displaced (depressed). Scalp lacerations can lead to a loss of large quantities of blood (up to or more than 50% of circulating volume). The resulting hypotension and poor perfusion of the moderately injured brain could result in a poor outcome. A skull fracture requires considerable force but is not always associated with CNS damage, reflecting its protective role. Despite this observation, a head-injured patient with a skull fracture is at greater risk of developing secondary complications (e.g. extradural haematoma) and a poor outcome if left untreated.

CNS soft tissue damage may be focal (cortical contusions or intracranial haematoma) or diffuse (widespread functional or neuronal disruption). The soft tissue damage may be coup or contra-coup causing multiple centres of focal damage, with serious functional consequences on the outcome. The normal response to tissue damage involves an inflammatory response, alteration in blood flow, capillary dynamics and cellular biochemistry, leading to brain swelling (Cooper, 1987). Diffuse axonal injury may be mixed with areas of focal damage and petechial haemorrhages.

Spinal injuries, damage to the cranial nerves and pituitary gland are associated with head injury and will alter the final outcome. These additional injuries will worsen the outcome of head injury despite effective and efficient care.

Simple physical relationships, such as the volume and pressure curve, though pertinent become inadequate when disruption in blood flow auto-regulation, changes in capillary permeability and neurotransmitter biochemistry are added in to the equation.

Outcome measures

Accurate outcome measures help in developing more effective clinical management and treatment of head injury, and form the basis of prognosis and public health management (Langfitt, 1978). Several outcome measures have been proposed for the assessment of head injury, ranging from the widely accepted Glasgow Outcome Scale (GOS) (Jennett and Bond, 1975) through to the more complex systems such as Disability Rating Scale (DRS) (Rappaport et al., 1982, 1989). Any scoring system weighs simplicity and efficiency against complexity, inefficiency and increased error for the gain of more information. Important variables in addition to scoring system are:

- The interviewer, trained and experienced for the task.
- The informant, the patient and carer.
- The medium, direct interview rather than telephone or postal questionnaire.

These variables should be recorded when the information is gathered. Patients tend to have overoptimistic opinions of their abilities; relatives and carers tend to be inconsistent particularly over the telephone (Maas et al., 1983). Clinicians should refer to written definitions prior to recording a score.

Mortality can be used as a crude but definite measure of outcome. Mortality for severe head injuries remains at between 40% and 50% (Miller and Jones, 1985), falling to 2–5% for moderate and less than 1% for minor head injury. Mortality may be due to primary (neuronal damage and associated petechial haemorrhages) or secondary (haematoma, swelling, infection or epilepsy) damage (Miller, 1982). However, the head injury may not be instrumental in the cause of death. Post-mortem examination will increase accuracy in identifying the cause of death and separating primary from secondary damage (Clifton et al., 1981). Histopathological studies will help in interpreting changes in death rates. Improvement in acute head injury care need not always be associated with significant drops in mortality rates (Graham et al., 1989). Comparisons of death rates in severe and moderate head injuries between two cohorts (1970 ± 2, 1981 ± 1) showed mortality rates of approximately 50% at 6 months. Histopathological examination revealed a reduction in damage to the cerebral cortex at the arterial boundary zones, in comparison with earlier cohort, possibly as a result of better intensive care. The increase in diffuse ischaemic and neuronal damage was a result of increased initial survival (acute resuscitation) from more severe road traffic accidents. These diverging trends maintained the overall mortality at approximately 50%.

The International Trauma Coma Data Bank requires the patient to be in a comatose state, Glasgow Coma Scale (GSC) 7/8 or below (Teasdale and Jennett, 1974), at 6 hours for inclusion into a severe head injury study. Despite this strict entry criteria large variations in mortality exist, from 33% to 51% (Jennett et al., 1979; Bowers and Marshall, 1980; Miller et al., 1981; Genneralli et al., 1982; Levati et al., 1982). Large variations in mortality rates suggest that other factors such as time of transfer, type of injury and care prior to referral to the neurosurgical unit are as important as acute clinical care in an intensive care unit.

The GOS was devised by Jennett and Bond (Jennett and Bond, 1975) with the specific intention of assessing survival, social integration and level of care for daily living rather than looking specifically at impairment, disability or handicap. The scale contains five exclusive levels (Table 3.1).

The scale has been expanded to eight points, splitting the last three categories into better and worse levels (Jennett *et al.*, 1981). The repeatability of the GOS in the 5- and 8-point forms have been tested for inter-rater agreement (Maas *et al.*, 1983). Seventeen patients were tested by four clinicians by direct interview. Disagreement occurred in four patients by 1 point on the 5-point scale (23%), and in 10 patients (59%) using the 8-point version. Intra-observer disagreement was also high (19%) on assessment of recorded data by the same physician. These findings suggest that the 5-point scale is more reliable and repeatable than the 8-point version when assessing care needed for daily living. The

Table 3.1 Glasgow Outcome Scale (5-point version)

1. *Death;*
   Due to head injury usually within 48 hours

2. *Persistent vegetative state;*
   Criterion
      cycles of sleep and waking
      eye opening
      unresponsive to commands
      speechless
      no meaningful psychomotor interaction with the environment
   Progress after injury (Braakman et al., 1988)
   1 month: 10% of all severe head injuries
   1 year: 51% will die
                  10% remain PVS
                  26% improved, severely disabled
                  10% improved, moderately disabled
                     (all under 40 years of age)

3. *Severe disability*: conscious but disabled
   Criterion
      dependent on others for daily living due to neuropsychological or physical disability

4. *Moderate disability*:
   independent in daily living
   live and work in sheltered environment
   physical disabilities such as: hemiparesis
                                   aphasia
                                   impaired memory
                                   altered personality

5. *Good recovery*:
   resume normal lifestyle
   return to work
   may still have minor neurobehavioural/neurophysical sequelae

timing of assessment after injury is also important. GOS assessments are usually performed at 1 year after injury. However, 60% of the moderate or good recovery groups assessed at 1 year will have reached this level by 3 months and 90% by 6 months (Jennett *et al.*, 1977). Severely disabled patients at 3 months were unlikely to improve by GOS scoring. Cognitive and motor skills can continue to improve for many years after injury (Prigatano *et al.*, 1984; Stern *et al.*, 1986). These observations and the desire for more subtle levels of outcome to be recorded have stimulated the development of other scoring systems (Evans *et al.*, 1976; Storer and Zeigler, 1976; Smith *et al.*, 1979; Carey and Posavac, 1982) as well as acceptance of disability (Melamed *et al.*, 1992).

The Disability Rating Scale (Rappaport *et al.*, 1982) is a 30-point scale in which 30 is death, 0 is no impairment (Figure 3.1). Areas scored include eye opening, verbal response, motor response, cognitive ability in feeding, toileting, grooming, dependence on others and employability. The reliability and repeatability (Gouvier *et al.*, 1987) has been tested with low inter-rater variation. The DRS has been compared to the GOS as a measure of progress and found to be more sensitive (71% improved by DRS; 31% by GOS) (Hall *et al.*, 1985) due to the extensive questionnaire.

The Glasgow Assessment Schedule (Livingstone and Livingstone, 1985) assesses 40 specific areas (Figure 3.2). The schedule is problem orientated, and also identifies areas for rehabilitation effort. The schedule has not been independently assessed but has good reliability (Kappa coefficient greater than 0.7). Other assessment scales include the Storer–Zeigler Scale (Storer and Zeigler, 1976) and Levels of Cognitive Functioning Scale. General neuropsychological testing which includes Barthel score (Figure 3.2) (Lincoln and Leadbitter, 1979), Mini-mental State Scores (Commenges *et al.*, 1992), Weschler Memory Scale (Sheridan *et al.*, 1988) and the Minnesota Multiphasic Personality Inventory (Bornstein *et al.*, 1989) can also be used.

Many rehabilitation units will have specific scoring systems for motor, speech and ambulatory skills. These can be viewed as measures of progress rather than outcome scores and have not been tested for reliability and repeatability.

Outcome scores all rely on assessing social function and handicap rather than measuring impairment and disability by subjective means. However, during the course of the recovery several clinical factors and investigations are known to be significant objective assessors of the eventual outcome and could become important parts of scoring systems. Currently they tend to be used as predictors of outcome (Myles Gibson and Stephenson, 1989), with varying degrees of success (MacPherson *et al.*, 1992).

The physical condition of the patients prior to injury will affect the outcome. Anatomical anomalies at birth such as the size of the tentorial hiatus and cerebrospinal fluid spaces will affect the response of the brain to injury. Existing CNS disorders such as previous head injury, cerebrovascular events or hydrocephalus will make minor head injury more serious and the recovery slower.

Age remains the greatest influence on outcome, with mortality and

DISABILITY RATING (DR) SCALE●

Name _____ Sex ____ Birthdate _____ Brain Injury Date _____

Cause of Injury: _____ MVA/MCA* _____ Head Trauma** _____ Infection _____ Stroke _____ Anoxia

_____ Development (Congenital) _____ Degenerative _____ Metabolic _____ Drowning

_____ Other (Specify) _____

*MVA = Motor Vehicle Accident; MCA = Motorcycle Accident. *Circle one.*

**Gun shot, blunt instrument, blow to head, fall, etc.

DATE OF RATING

CATEGORY	ITEM▲								
Arousability	Eye Opening[1]								
Awareness and	Communication Ability[2]†								
Responsibility●●	Motor Response[3]								
Cognitive Ability for	Feeding[4]								
Self Care	Toileting[4]								
Activities	Grooming[4]								
Dependence on Others●●●	Level of Functioning[5]								
Psychosocial Adaptability	"Employability"[6]								
COMMENTS:	**Total**								

[1]Eye Opening

0 Spontaneous
1 To Speech
2 To Pain
3 None

[2]Communication Ability†
Either Verbal: Writing or Letter Board:
or Sign (viz, eye blink, head nod. etc.)

0 Oriented
1 Confused
2 Inappropriate
3 Incomprehensible
4 None

[3]Best Motor Resp.

0 Obeying
1 Localizing
2 Withdrawing
3 Flexing
4 Extending
5 None

[4]Cognitive Ability for Feeding,
Toileting, Grooming (Does patient
know how and when? Ignore motor
disability.)

0 Compete
1 Partial
2 Minimal
3 None

† In presence of tracheostomy (place T next to score): for voice or speech dysfunction (place D next to score if there is a dysarthria, dysphonia, voice paralysis, aphasia, apraxia, etc.)

[5]Level of Functioning
(Consider both physical &
cognitive disability)

0 Completely independent
1 Independent in special environment
2 Mildly dependent   – (a)
3 Moderately dependent – (b)
4 Markedly dependent   – (c)
5 Totally dependent   – (d)

a   needs limited assistance (non-resident helper)
b   needs moderate assistance (person in home)
c   needs assistance with all major activities at all times
d   24-hour nursing care required

[6]"Employability"
(As a full time worker,
homeworker or student)

0 Not restricted
1 Selected jobs, competitive
2 Sheltered workshop.
    non-competitive
3 Not employable

Disability Categories

Total DR Score	Level of Disability
0	None
1	Mild
2–3	Partial
4–6	Moderate
7–11	Moderately severe
12–16	Severe
17–21	Extremely severe
22–24	Vegetative state
25–29	Extreme vegetative state
30	Death

●Rappaport et al. Disability Rating Scale for Severe Head Trauma Patients: Coma To Community. Arch Phys Med Rehab. 63:118–123, 1982
▲ See over for item definitions
Revised 8/87
●●Modified from Teasdale, Jennett, Lancet 2:81–83, 1974
●●●Modified from Scranton et al. Arch Phys Med Rehab. 51:1–21, 1970

ITEM DEFINITIONS

Eye opening

0—SPONTANEOUS: eyes open with sleep/wake rhythms indicating active arousal mechanisms; does not assume awareness.

1—TO SPEECH AND/OR SENSORY STIMULATION: a response to any verbal approach, whether spoken or shouted, not necessarily the command to open the eyes. Also, response to touch, mild pressure.

2—TO PAIN: tested by a painful stimulus.[1]

3—NONE: no eye opening even to painful stimulation.

Best communication ability (if patient cannot use voice because of tracheostomy or is aphasic or dysarthric or has vocal cord paralysis or voice dysfunction then estimate patient's best response and enter note under comments.)

0—ORIENTED: implies awareness of self and the environment. Patient able to tell you a) who he is; b) where he is; c) why he is there; d) year; e) seasonl f) month; g) day; h) time of day.

1—CONFUSED: attention can be held and patient responds to questions but responses are delayed and/or indicate varying degrees of disorientation and confusion.

2—INAPPROPRIATE: intelligible articulation but speech is used only in an exclamatory or random way (such as shouting and swearing); no sustained communication exchange is possible.

3—INCOMPREHENSIBLE: moaning, groaning or sounds without recognizable words; no consistent communication signs.

4—NONE: no sounds or communications signs from patient.

Best motor response

0—OBEYING: obeying commands to move finger on best side. If no response or not suitable try another command such as "move lips," "blink eyes," etc. Do not include grasp or other reflex responses.

1—LOCALIZING: a painful stimulus[1] at more than one site causes a limb to move (even slightly) in an attempt to remove it. It is a deliberate motor act to move away from or remove the source of noxious stimulation. If there is doubt as to whether withdrawal or localization has occured after 3 or 4 painful stimulations rate as localization.

2—WITHDRAWING: any generalized movement away from a noxious stimulus that is more than a simple reflex response.

3—FLEXING: painful stimulation results in either flexion at the elbow, rapid withdrawal with abduction of the shoulder or a slow withdrawal with adduction of the shoulder. If there is confusion between flexing and withdrawing, then use pin prick on hands, then face.

4—EXTENDING: painful stimulation results in extension of the limb.

5—NONE: no response can be elicited. Usually associated with hypotonia. Exclude spinal transection as an explanation of lack of response; be satisfied that an adequate stimulus has been applied.

Cognitive ability for feeding, toileting and grooming.

Rate each of the three functions separately. For each function answer the question, does the patient show *awareness of how and when* to perform each specified activity. *Ignore motor disabilities* that interfere with carrying out a function. (This is rated under level of Functioning described below.) Rate best response for toileting based on bowel and bladder behavior. Grooming refers to bathing, washing, brushing of teeth, shaving, combing or brushing of hair and dressing.

0—COMPLETE: *continuously shows awareness that he knows how* to feed, toilet or groom self and can convey unambiguous information that he *knows when* this activity should occur.

1—PARTIAL: *intermittently shows awareness that he knows how* to feed, toilet or groom self and/or can intermittently convey reasonably clearly information that he *knows when* the activity should occur.

2—MINIMAL: shows *questionable or infrequent awareness that he knows in a primitive way how* to feed, toilet or groom self and/or shows infrequently by certain signs, sounds or activites that he *vaguely aware when* the activity should occur.

3—NONE: *shows virtually no awareness at any time* that he knows how to feed, toilet or groom self and *cannot convey information by signs, sounds, or activity that he knows when* the activity should occur.

Level of functioning

0—COMPLETELY INDEPENDENT: able to live as he wishes, requiring no restriction due to physical, mental, emotional or social problems.

1—INDEPENDENT IN SPECIAL ENVIRONMENT: capable of functioning independently when needed requirements are met (mechanical aids).

2—MILDLY DEPENDENT: able to care for most of own needs but requires limited assistance due to physical, cognitive and/or emotional problems (e.g., needs nonresident helper).

3—MODERATELY DEPENDENT: able to care for self partially but needs another person at all times.

4—MARKEDLY DEPENDENT: needs help with all major activities and the assistance of another person at all times.

5—TOTALLY DEPENDENT: not able to assist in own care and requires 24-hours nursing care.

"Employability"

The psychosocial adaptability or "employability" item takes into account overall cognitive and physical ability to be an employee, homemaker or student. This determination should take into account considerations such as the following:

1. able to understand, remember and follow instructions; 2. can plan and carry out tasks at least at the level of an office clerk or in simple routine, repetitive industrial situations or can do school assignments: 3. ability to remain oriented, relevant and appropriate in work and other psychosocial situations; 4. ability to get to and from work or shopping centers using private or public transportation effectively; 5. ability to deal with number concepts; 6; ability to make purchases and handle simple money exchange problems; 7. ability to keep track of time schedules and appointments.

0—NOT RESTRICTED: can compete in the open market for a relatively wide range of jobs commensurate with existing skills: or can initiate, plan, execute and assume responsibilites associated with homemaking; or can understand and carry out most age relevant school assignments.

1—SELECTED JOBS, COMPETITIVE: can compete in a limited job market for a relatively narrow range of jobs because of limitations of the type described above and/or because of some physical limitations; or can initiate, plan, execute and assume many but not all responsibilities associated with homemaking: or can understand and carry out many but not all school assignments.

2—SHELTERED WORKSHOP, NON-COMPETITIVE: cannot compete successfully in job market because of limitations described above and/or because of moderate or severe physical limitations; or cannot without major assistance initate, plan, execute and assume responsibilities for homemaking; or cannot understand and carry out even relatively simple school assignments without assistance.

3—NOT EMPLOYABLE: completely unemployable because of extreme psychosocial limitations of the type described above; or completely unable to initate, plan, execute and assume any responsibilities associated with homemaking; or cannot understand or carry out any school assignments.

Instructions: Place date of rating at top of column. Place appropriate rating next to each of the eight items listed. Add eight ratings to obtain total DR score.

---

[1]*Standard painful stimulus is the application of pressure across index fingernail of best side with wood of a pencil; for quadriplegics pinch nose tip and rate as 0, 1, 2 or 5.*

Figure 3.1 Disability Rating Scale

BARTHEL ASSESSMENT

NAME...

		pre ad. level	Date			
Feeding	Independent	2				
	Needs help	1				
	Dependent	0				
Grooming	Independent	1				
	Dependent	0				
Bowels	Fully continent	2				
	Occasional accident	1				
	Incontinent	0				
Bladder	Fully continent	2				
	Occasional accident	1				
	Incontinent	0				
Dressing	Independent	2				
	Needs help	1				
	Dependent	0				
Chair/bed transfer	Independent	3				
	Minimal help	2				
	Able to sit	1				
	Dependent	0				
Toilet	Independent	2				
	Needs help	1				
	Dependent	0				
Mobility	Independent walking	3				
	Minimal help	2				
	Independent in w/chair	1				
	Immobile	0				
Stairs	Independent	2				
	Needs help	1				
	Unable	0				
Bathing	Independent	1				
	Dependent	0				
	TOTAL BARTHEL SCORE					

AIDS AND EQUIPMENT

WHEELCHAIR

PRESSURE CUSHION

OTHER SEATING ADAPTATION

PERCEPTUAL/COGNITIVE PROBLEMS

Figure 3.2 Barthel assessment

morbidity increasing with age (Lucroon *et al.*, 1988; Michaud *et al.*, 1992). Some reports have suggested higher mortality in the under 5 years group whilst others have reported a lower rate (Raimondi and Hirschauer, 1984). Whether ageing represents an inability of CNS tissue to repair following injury or is a reflection of disease in other systems is not clear (Miller *et al.*, 1977). The higher incidence of intracranial haematoma has been suggested as a cause of poor outcome in the older age group (Becker *et al.*, 1977).

The actual mechanism of injury could be expected to influence outcome. The intensity and direction are obvious factors. Despite this there is no significant difference in the outcome between road traffic accidents, with the higher incidence of direct axonal injury from shearing forces, and falls, with the higher incidence of intracranial haematoma. However penetrating injuries such as gunshot wounds have a direct relation to these mechanical factors, immediate mortality (60%) and discharge from hospital (15%) (Kaufman *et al.*, 1983); important factors are calibre, velocity, direction, self-infliction and neurological status on admission.

Physical deficits as a result of severe head injury are common and affect all levels of CNS function. Despite this up to 26% of these patients may have no physical disability (Jennett *et al.*, 1981) with the neuropsychological impairment being the greater cause of handicap. Cerebral hemisphere dysfunction (59%) includes hemiparesis (49%), dysphasia (29%) and homonymous hemianopia (5%). Interestingly hemiparesis is more common (60% risk) if there is no haematoma.

Cranial nerve dysfunction (32%) is also a common impairment with optic nerve damage present in 13% of severe head injury and 5% overall. Other cranial nerve palsies occur (9%) and may also be troublesome. Post-traumatic epilepsy (15% risk) may complicate head injury, being more common with intracranial haematoma (21%) but still present without intracranial haematoma (5%). Ataxia (9%) may force the patient to travel in a wheelchair, causing significant handicap.

The Glasgow Coma Scale (GCS; Teasdale and Jennett, 1974) is a crude but effective measure of the global functional loss before and after resuscitation and prior to definitive treatment. This scale assesses coma as a range, with minor head injury being scored at between 13 and 15, moderate (9–12) and severe (3–8) concentrating on speech, motor function and eye opening. The GCS is a measure of the general neurological status of the patient, with motor function being the most sensitive. The normal response to pain, semipurposeful withdrawal, and abnormal 'decorticate' flexion response have been separated by a point on the scale and has now been amended to include this. Eye opening is a useful indicator in the first 72 hours, and verbal response usually heralds an end to coma. Post-traumatic amnesia (PTA), the time taken for continuous memory to return, correlates well with outcome (Russell and Smith, 1961) and is usually three times longer than the period of coma. Post-traumatic amnesia of less than 1 hour represents a mild head injury; more than 1 hour to 24 hours, a moderate injury. The length of PTA will increase with age (Carlsson *et al.*, 1968).

Both assessment of coma (GCS) and duration of post-traumatic amnesia (Russell and Smith, 1961; Ommaya and Genneralli, 1974) are measures of global CNS response to injury. When combined they correlate closely with eventual outcome (Bishara *et al.*, 1992). Post-traumatic amnesia is a retrospective measure and could be included in an outcome score.

Head-injured patients with an intracranial haematoma causing a mass effect have twice the mortality rate (40%) of those without (23%). Those with a haematoma are admitted in a poorer neurological state and have a worse outcome (good recovery 29% compared to 40%) (Narayan *et al.*, 1981).The type of intracranial mass is important. Extradural haematoma will fare better than subdural and intracerebral worst of all (Stuart *et al.*, 1983). If the extradural haematoma is treated promptly the mortality can be expected to be near zero (Bricolo and Pasut, 1984) with moderate and good outcome at 89%, unlike subdural haematoma where mortality remains between 30% and 50% despite early evacuation (Seelig *et al.*, 1981).

Secondary insults to the injured brain will cause an increase in mortality, worsen morbidity and cause a poor outcome, particularly systemic hypotension and respiratory failure. The respiratory function may be compromised by central dysfunction, as well as direct injury to the lungs from aspiration of vomitus and neurogenic pulmonary insufficiency. In these patients the long-term outcome was found to correlate to the degree of arteriovenous shunting (Frost *et al.*, 1979). Multiple injuries will also increase mortality (30–50%) (Braakman *et al.*, 1980).

Bilaterally fixed pupils are associated with a 80–90% mortality and closely correlate with abnormal brain stem evoked potentials reflecting brain stem damage (Greenberg *et al.*, 1977). Short duration of coma is associated with a better outcome. Poor outcomes increase if coma last more than 2 weeks.

Postconcussional syndrome, including headaches, dizziness and various 'nervous disorders' remains common after head injury and may affect outcome in a disproportionate manner (20% at long-term follow-up) (Cartlidge, 1978), with gradual resolution over 2 years.

Plain radiography will demonstrate fractures to the skull vault and cervical spine. Skull vault fractures have a significant association with extradural haematomas, particularly if the level of consciousness is depressed (1:6). Fractures to the cervical spine are associated with increased risk of cord damage and poor outcome.

Computed tomography (CT) scanning has greatly improved the clinical management of head injury. In severe head injury a 'normal' CT scan is associated with a better outcome despite a low GCS score, reflecting the poor outcome of those with an intracerebral haematoma and mass effect. The degree of hemisphere swelling can also be assessed, and unilateral swelling (with midline shift greater than 8 mm) correlates with clinical findings and poor outcome (Clifton *et al.*, 1980). Magnetic resonance imaging (MRI) has the ability to assess brain swelling in response to head injury and has been used to predict and assess outcome (Wilson *et al.*, 1988). If the intracranial pressure is raised more than 40 mmHg for long periods of time and there is an inappropriate blood pressure response, there is an increased mortality and poor outcome (Johnston *et al.*, 1970).

Whilst the standard electroencephalogram (EEG) has not been useful in assessing brain injury, evoked potentials, though difficult to carry out in the electrically hostile environment of the ward or intensive care unit, are useful. The presence of increased latency and loss of signal correlates with overall outcome and specific neurological deficits (Greenberg et al., 1977). However, the evoked potential data alone or in part (sensory vs brain stem auditory) can be confusing with poor correlation with outcome (Anderson et al., 1983).

Biochemical indices have been used to predict and assess outcome. Particular attention has focused on creatine kinase BB isoenzyme (Cooper et al., 1983), neurone specific enolase (Daubaerschmidt et al., 1983) and CSF lactate (Bakay and Ward, 1983; Bourguigat et al., 1983). There is often a rise in these biochemical markers, but there is poor correlation with outcome. The level of CSF cyclic AMP serum myelin basic protein is, however, a good predictor of outcome (Thomas et al., 1979).

Conclusions

The Glasgow Outcome Scale remains the most commonly used outcome scoring system and represents the 'rough and ready' type, recording the 'social' handicap but not scoring the impairment or disability in detail. The advantage and disadvantages have been discussed. Outcome scores as early as 12 hours from injury can be made (Myles Gibson and Stephenson, 1989) with 100% prediction of mortality in 15% of the cases. These scores can be made more accurate by the addition of further clinical data such as post-traumatic amnesia (PTA) and investigative measures, such as imaging and electrophysiological tests.

More complex scoring systems have been used but little information exists about their reliability and repeatability, particularly when carried out by independent groups. Such studies are underway. With the financial pressures being put on health care worldwide and the increasing evidence that long-term rehabilitation will improve outcome from head injury, there is a need for a robust scoring system which will include general and specific neurological impairment scores. Current outcome scores are heavily reliant on subjective assessments which inevitably have the large margins of error seen in the GOS. One way of resolving this is to broaden the categories; a 5-point scale appears more reliable than an 8-point but with a loss of sensitivity. Objective measures should help in reducing errors and maintain sensitivity such as imaging and electrophysiology. However we are always reminded of the patient with a minor head injury and severe postconcussional headache who views their outcome as poor and the hemiparetic patient who feels 'lucky to be alive' and achieving a good outcome.

References

Adams JH, Graham DI, Murray LS, Scott G (1982) Diffuse axonal injury due to nonmissile head injury in humans: an analysis of 45 cases. Ann. Neurol.; 12: 557–563

Anderson DC, Colombo F, Nertempi P, Benedtti A (1983) Cognitive outcome in early indices of severity of head injury. *J. Neurosurg.*; **59**: 751–761

Anderson DW, McLaurin RL (1980) The national head and spinal cord injury survey. *J. Neurosurg.*; **53**: suppl. S1

Bakay RA, Ward AA (1983) Enzymatic changes in serum and cerebrospinal fluid in neurological injury. *J. Neurosurg.*; **58**: 27–37

Becker DP, Povlishock JT (1985) *Central Nervous System Trauma Research Status Report.* NIH, National Institute of Neurological and Communicative Disorders and Stroke

Becker DP, Miller JD, Ward JD, Greenberg RP, Young HF, Sakalas R (1977) The outcome from severe head injury with early diagnosis and intensive management. *J. Neurosurg.*; **47**: 491–502

Bishara SN, Partridge FM, Codfrey PD, Knight RG (1992) Post-traumatic amnesia and Glasgow Coma Scale related to outcome in survivors in a consecutive series of patients with severe closed-head injury. *Brain Injury*; **6**: 373–380

Bourguigat S, Albert A, Ferard G, Tulsane PA, Kempf J, Metais R (1983) Prognostic value of combined data on enzymes and inflammation markers in plasma in cases of severe head injury. *Clin. Chem.*; **29**: 1904–1907

Bornstein RA, Miller HB, Van Schoor ST (1989) Neuropsychological deficit and emotional disturbance in head-injured patients. *J. Neurosurg.*; **70**: 509–513

Bowers SA, Marshall LF (1980) Outcome in 200 consecutive cases of severe head injury treated in San Diego county: a prospective study. *Neurosurgery*; **6**: 237–242

Braakman R, Gelpke GJ, Habbema JD, Maas AIR, Minderhoud JM (1980) Systematic selection of prognostic features in patients with severe head injury. *Neurosurgery*; **6**: 362–370

Braakman R, Jennett B, Minderhoud JM (1988) Prognosis of the post-traumatic vegetative state. *Acta Neurochir. (Wein)*; **95**: 49–52

Bricolo AP, Pasut LM (1984) Extradural haematoma: toward zero mortality: a prospective study. *Neurosurgery*; **14**: 8–12

Carey RG, Posavac EJ (1982) Rehabilitation programme evaluation using the revised Level of Rehabilitation Scale (LORS-11). *Arch. Phys. Med. Rehabil.*; **63**: 367–370

Carlsson CA, von Essen C, Lofgren J (1968) Factors affecting the clinical course of patients with severe head trauma. Part 1: Influence of biological factors. Part 2: Significance of post-traumatic coma. *J. Neurosurg.*; **29**: 242–251

Cartlidge NEF (1978) Post-concussional syndrome. *Scot. Med. J.*; **23**: 103

Clifton GL, Grossman RG, Makela ME *et al.* (1980) Neurological course and correlated computer tomography findings after closed head injury. *J. Neurosurg.*; **52**: 611–624

Clifton GL, McCormick WL, Grossman RG (1981) Neurophathology of early and late deaths after head injury. *J. Neurosurg.*; **58**: 309–313

Commenges D, Gagnon M, Letenneur L, Dartigues JF, Barberger-Gateav P, Salmon R (1992) Improving screening for dementia in the elderly using mini-mental state examination sub-scores, Benton's visual retention test and Isaac's set test. *Epidemiology*; **3**: 185–188

Cooper PR (1987) *Head Injury.* Baltimore: Williams and Wilkins

Cooper PR, Chalif DJ, Ramsey JF, Moore RJ (1983) Radiommunoassay of the brain type isoenzyme of creatine phosphokinase (CK-BBB): a new diagnostic tool in the evaluation of patients with head injury. *J. Neurosurg.*; **12**: 536–541

Daubaerschmidt R, Marangos PJ, Zinsmeyer J, Bender V, Klages G, Gross J (1983) Severe head trauma and the changes of concentration of neuron-specific enolase in plasma and in cerebro-spinal fluid. *Clin. Chim. Acta.*; **131**: 165–170

Evans CD, Bull CPI, Devonport MJ *et al.* (1976) Rehabilitation of brain-damaged survivor. *Injury*; **8**: 80–97

Frost EAM, Arancibia CU, Shulman K (1979) Pulmonary shunt as a prognostic indicator in head injury. *J. Neurosurg.*; **50**: 768–772

Galbraith SL (1973) Age distribution of extradural haemorrhage without skull fracture. *Lancet*; **i**: 1217–1218

Genneralli TA (1986) Mechanisms and pathophysiology of cerebral contusion. *J. Head Trauma Rehabil.*; **1**: 23–29

Genneralli TA, Spielman GM, Langfitt TW *et al*. (1982) Influence of the type of intracranial lesion on the outcome of severe head injury: a multicentre study using a new classification system. *J. Neurosurg.*; **56**: 26–32

Goldsmith W, Ommaya AK (1984) Head and neck injury criteria and tolerance levels. In: Aldman B, Champon A (eds) *The Biomechanics of Impact Trauma*. Amsterdam: Elsevier, pp. 149–187

Gouvier WD, Blanton PD, La Porit KK *et al*. (1987) Reliability and validity of the disability rating scale and levels of cognitive functioning scale in monitoring recovery from severe head injury. *Arch. Phys. Med. Rehabil.*; **68**: 94–97

Graham DI, Ford I, Adams JH, Doyle D *et al*. (1989) Ischaemic brain damage is still common in fatal non-missile head injury. *J. Neurol. Neurosurg. Psychiatry*; **52**: 346–350

Greenberg RP, Becker DP, Miller JD, Mayer DJ (1977) Evaluation of brain function in severe human head trauma with multimodality evoked potentials. Part II: Localisation of brain dysfunction and correlation with post-traumatic neurological conditions. *J. Neurosurg.*; **47**: 163–177

Gurdjian ES (1972) Recent advances in the study of the mechanisms of impact injury of the head: A summary. *Clin. Neurosurg.*; **19**: 1–42

Hall K, Cope DN, Rappaport M (1985) Glasgow outcome scale and disability rating scale comparative usefulness in following recovery in traumatic head injury. *Arch. Phys. Med. Rehabil.*; **66**: 35–37

Jennett B, Bond M (1975) Assessment of outcome after severe brain damage. *Lancet*; **i**: 480–484

Jennett B, McMillan R (1981) Epidemiology of head injury. *Br. Med. J.*; **282**: 101

Jennett B, Teasdale G (1981) *Management of Head Injuries*. Philadelphia: Davies.

Jennett B, Teasdale G, Galbraith S *et al*. (1977) Severe head injuries in three countries. *J. Neurol. Neurosurg. Psychiatry*; **40**: 291–298

Jennett B, Teasdale G, Braakman R, Minderhoud J, Heiden J, Kurze T (1979) Prognosis of patients with severe head injury. *Neurosurgery*; **4**: 283–289

Jennett B, Snoek J, Bond MR, Brooks N (1981) Disability after severe head injury: observations on the use of the Glasgow outcome scale. *J. Neurol. Neurosurg. Psychiatry*; **44**: 285–293

Johnston IH, Johnston JA, Jennett WB (1970) Intracranial pressures following head injury. *Lancet*; **ii**: 433–436

Kaufman HH, Loyola WP, Makela ME, Frankowski RF *et al*. (1983) Civilian gunshot wounds: the limit of salvageability. *Acta Neurochir.*; **67**: 115–125

Langfitt TW (1978) Measuring outcome from head injuries. *J. Neurosurg.*; **48**: 673–678

Levati A, Farina ML, Vecchi G, Rossanda M, Marrubini MB (1982) Prognosis of severe head injuries. *J. Neurosurg.*; **57**: 779–783

Lincoln N, Leadbitter D (1979) Assessment of motor function in stroke patients. *Physiotherapy*; **65**: 48–52

Livingstone MG, Livingstone HM (1985) The Glasgow assessment schedule: clinical and research assessment of head injury outcome. *Int. Rehabil. Med.*; **7**: 145–149

London PS (1963) Survival after serious injury. *Proc. R. Soc. Med.*; **56**: 821–823

Luerssen TG, Klauber MR, Marshall LF (1988) Outcome from head injury related to patient's age. *J. Neurosurg.*; **68**: 409–416

Maas AIR, Braakman R, Schoutin HJA, Minderhoud JM, Van Zombren AH (1983) Agreement between physicians on assessment of outcome following severe head injury. *J. Neurosurg.*; **58**: 321–325

MacPherson V, Sullivan SJ, Lambert J (1992) Prediction of motor status 3 and 6 months post severe traumatic brain injury: a preliminary study. *Brain Injury*; **6**: 489–498

Melamed S, Groswasser Z, Stern M (1992) Acceptance of disability, work involvement and subjective rehabiltation status of traumatic brain-injured (TBI) patients. *Brain Injury*; **6**: 233–243

Michaud LJ, Rivara FP, Grady MS, Reay DT (1992) Predictors of survival and severity of disability after severe brain injury in children. *Neurosurgery*; **31**: 254–264

Miller JD (1982) Physiology of trauma. *Clin. Neurosurg.*; **29**: 103–120

Miller JD, Jones PA (1985) The work of a regional head injury service. *Lancet*; **i**: 1141–1144

Miller JD, Becker DP, Ward JD, Sullivan HG, Adams WE, Rosner MJ (1977) Significance of intracranial hypertension in severe head injury. *J. Neurosurg.*; **47**: 503–516

Miller JD, Sweet RC, Narayan R, Becker DP (1978) Early insults to the injured brain. *JAMA*; **240**: 439–442

Miller JD, Butterworth JF, Gudeman SK *et al*. (1981) Further experience in the management of severe head injury. *J. Neurosurg.*; **54**: 289–299

Myles Gibson R, Stephenson GC (1989) Aggressive management of severe closed head trauma: time for reappraisal. *Lancet*; **ii**: 369–370

Narayan RK, Greenberg RP, Miller JD *et al*. (1981) Improved confidence of outcome in severe head injury. *J. Neurosurg.*; **54**: 751–762

Ommaya AK, Genneralli TA (1974) Cerebral concussion and traumatic unconsciousness: correlation of experimental and clinical observations on blunt head injury. *Brain*; **97**: 633–654

Potter J (1958) Footballer's amnesia. *J. Neurol. Neurosurg. Psychiatry*; **21**: 67–68

Prigatano GP, Pordace DJ, Zeiner HK *et al*. (1984) Neuropsychological rehabilitation after closed head injury in young adults. *J. Neurol. Neurosurg. Psychiatry*; **47**: 505–513

Raimondi AJ, Hirschauer J (1984) Head injury in the infant and toddler: coma scoring and outcome scale. *Child's Brain*; **11**: 12–35

Rappaport M, Hall KM, Hopkins HK, Belleza T, Cope N (1982) Disability rating scale for severe head trauma: coma to community. *Arch. Phys. Med. Rehabil.*; **63**: 118–123

Rappaport M, Herrero-Backe C, Rappaport ML, Winterfield KM (1989) Head injury outcome up to 10 years later. *Arch. Phys. Med. Rehabil.*; **70**: 885

Roberts AH (1969) *Brain Damage in Boxers: a study of the prevalence of traumatic encephalopathy among professional boxers*. London: Pitman.

Russell WR, Smith A (1961) Post traumatic amnesia in closed head injury. *Arch. Neurol.*; **5**: 4–17

Seelig JM, Becker DP, Miller JD, Greenberg RP, Ward JD, Choi SC (1981) Traumatic acute subdural haematoma. Major mortality reduction in comatose patients treated within four hours. *N. Engl. J. Med.*; **304**: 1511–1518

Selecki BR, Ring IT, Simpson DA, Vanderfield GK, Sewell MF (1977) Trauma to the central and peripheral nervous systems: an overview of mortality, morbidity and costs, NSW. *Aust. N.Z. J. Surg.*; **52**: 93–98

Sheridan PH, Sato S, Foster N, Bruno G, Cox C, Fedio P, Chase TN (1988) Relation of EEG alpha background to parietal lore function in Alzheimer's disease as measured by position emmision tomography and psychometry. *Neurology*; **38**: 747–750

Smith RM, Fields FR, Lennox J *et al*. (1979) Functional scale of recovery from severe head trauma. *Clin. Neuropsychol.*; **1**: 48–50

Stern JM, Groswasser Z, Alis R *et al*. (1986) Day centre experience in rehabilitation of craniocerebral injured patients. *Scand. J. Rehabil. Med. Suppl.*; **12**: 53–58

Storer SL, Zeigler HE (1976) Head injury in children and teenagers: functional recovery correlated with duration of coma. *Arch. Phys. Med. Rehabil.*; **57**: 201–205

Stuart GG, Merry GS, Smith JA, Yelland JDN (1983) Severe head injury managed without intracranial pressure monitoring. *J. Neurosurg.*; **59**: 601–605

Teasdale G, Jennett B (1974) Assessment of coma and impaired consciousness. A practical scale. *Lancet*; **ii**: 81–84

Thomas DGT, Rabow L, Teasdale G (1979) Serum myelin basic protein, clinical responsiveness and outcome of severe head injury. *Acta Neurochir. (Suppl.)*; **28**: 93

Wilson JTL, Wiedman KD, Hadley DM, Condon B, Teasdale G, Brooks DN (1988) Early and late magnetic resonance imagining and neuropsychological outcome after head injury. *J. Neurol. Neurosurg. Psychiatry*; **51**: 391–396

Chapter 4

Thoracic and cardiac trauma

S. W. H. Kendall and S. Westaby

Introduction

Injuries to the thorax are a major contribution to the morbidity and mortality resulting from trauma. These injuries may result from penetrating, blunt or explosive trauma. Penetrating injuries are usually due to gunshot or stab wounds whereas blunt trauma is usually a result of a road traffic accident. In recent times body armour worn by military personnel and the police now converts penetrating missile injuries into a form of blunt trauma. In the USA 25% of deaths from road accidents are related to chest trauma and in a further 25% of deaths thoracic trauma was a major contributing factor (Cicero and Mattox, 1989). Experience of cardiothoracic trauma varies greatly; in South Africa there is a vast experience in stab injuries whereas in the USA the common penetrating wound to the chest is a gunshot. With the malignant expansion of mechanised transport blunt trauma to the chest is commonly encountered worldwide. Many patients with intrathoracic injury die at the site of the incident and those who reach an accident and emergency department are a self-selected group who should survive with early and intelligent medical intervention (Beck, 1926). However, this does not include emergency thoracotomy in the casualty where the occasional survivor is usually disabled due to cerebral hypoxia. Management of cardiothoracic trauma depends largely on the presence of trained surgeons and appropriate technical resources, such as the availability of autotransfusion and cardiopulmonary bypass equipment. These essentials are not widely available in the UK and this significantly affects the outcome since most cardiothoracic trauma cannot be appropriately dealt with.

Successful surgical intervention in thoracic trauma has developed in the past 30 years. Theodore Billroth advised against operations on the heart in his 1882 surgical text book and further commented that 'the surgeon who should attempt to suture a wound of the heart would lose the respect of his colleagues' (Cohn, 1972). In 1896 Rehn performed the first successful laceration of the right ventricle (Rhen, 1987) but despite subsequent advances there were still surgeons such as Blalock and Ravitch in the 1940s advocating repeated pericardiocentesis for cardiac trauma (Blalock and Ravitch, 1943). Surgery now has an established rôle for cardiothoracic injuries (Hood, 1983).

Frequently trauma to the thorax results in more than one organ being involved. However for the purpose of looking at outcome measures each 'organ' can be considered separately. Outcome measures will be discussed in relation to trauma of the heart, great vessels, lungs and major airways, oesophagus, chest wall and diaphragm resulting from blunt, penetrating or explosive trauma. The great majority of chest injuries do not require operative treatment apart from chest drain insertion. Where necessary surgery for thoracic trauma usually involves the control of haemorrhage and repair of blood vessels and airways. Usually the outcome is either successful or fatal but there is middle ground in the conservative and surgical management of thoracic trauma where other outcome measures are important.

Chest wall and diaphragmatic injury

Chest wall injury occurs in 40% of non-penetrating wounds of the chest (Naughton et al., 1989). Rib fractures are more common in the elderly patient and the third to ninth ribs are most commonly affected (Crawford et al., 1979). Pathological fractures should always be considered where the degree of injury is disproportionally large to the force of injury. Fracture of the upper and lower two ribs is often associated with visceral trauma and in all rib fractures there may be damage to the underlying lung and/or the intercostal bundle. Treatment of this condition is supportive with analgesia and physiotherapy.

Outcome measure of rib fracture should be confined to subjective relief of pain. Three months after the injury the patient should be free from pain. Persistent pain can be due to costochondral separation or development of intercostal neuroma; these may be treated surgically. Flail chest is a combination of multiple rib fractures and, usually, contusion to the underlying lung (Symbas et al., 1980). Outcome measures for flail chest would involve a combination of measures for pulmonary and rib injury. However there are a significant number of patients with flail chest who, after all their injuries have healed, continue to have disability with chest pain, dyspnoea and impairment of pulmonary function (Sawyers et al., 1975).

Fracture of the sternum is a much more common injury with road traffic accidents. Sternal fractures are occasionally associated with unstable spinal fractures. This injury is strongly associated with cardiac, pulmonary, aortic or large airway damage. Sternal fractures when undisplaced require supportive treatment only but when displaced open reduction and fixation is required. They usually heal well with minimal or no residual deformity and the morbidity and mortality associated with this injury is due to associated visceral injuries.

Between 2% and 7% of patients with major chest trauma are found to have diaphragmatic injury (Kirsh et al., 1976). The majority of patients are diagnosed correctly at admission to hospital but 10% will be diagnosed late (ranging from hours to years) following injury (Kinsella and Johnstrud, 1947). Usually the diagnosis is reached at emergency laparotomy but the late diagnosis is more often made on chest X-ray. There is a preponderance in the literature of reports of injuries to the left hemi-diaphragm with a radial tear. However some studies have suggested right hemidiaphragmatic rupture is just as common but that the diagnosis is often missed (Asfaw and Arbulu, 1977). Diagnosis may be confirmed with any one of a variety of tests: ultrasound study, CT scan, pneumo-peritoneum, barium study, nuclear liver scan or thoracoscopy. Once the diagnosis is established the defect should immediately be repaired to prevent herniation and strangulation of the gastrointestinal tract. Chronic traumatic diaphragmatic hernia is defined when diagnosis is made at least 1 month from the time of injury.

Outcome measures for this injury will depend on the timing of surgery and the extent of diaphragm injury. In patients with early repair subject-ive review will be relevant in regard to respiratory and gastrointestinal symptoms. Objective review can be performed including studies already described following lung trauma studying respiratory function. Anatom-ical studies can utilise plain radiography and CT scanning. Specific object-ive testing for diaphragmatic function is difficult; an impression may be made from ultrasound screening, or from the 'sniff' test monitored with fluoroscopy. Patients with chronic traumatic diaphragmatic hernia are initially likely to have low scores for outcome due to symptoms and poor diaphragmatic function. The outcome measure should improve following surgery with minimal long-term disability.

Injury to the lungs and major airways

Pulmonary injury is usually managed conservatively with intercostal tube drainage. This intervention is sufficient to deal with air and/or blood in the pleural cavity. Only with persistent bleeding or major air leaks is immediate thoracotomy necessary. This is true for both penetrating and blunt trauma and full recovery is expected. Lung contusion and adult respiratory distress syndrome are managed with medical support of the patient often necessitating mechanical ventilation. Occasionally late thoracotomy is indicated for persistent cavities or empyema.

Eighty per cent of major airway trauma occurs within 3 cm of the carina (Beal and Oreskovich, 1985) and, until modern times, these were rare and fatal injuries. Since 1960 with increased motorised transport and improvements in the transfer and treatment of such patients experience has greatly increased. Tracheobronchial injury with a substantial air leak resulting in inadequate ventilation requires immediate direct repair. Small defects in the trachea or bronchial injury with minor air leaks may be treated conservatively; bronchial stenosis can occur as a consequence of this injury. There is rarely a need to resect lung tissue except in late repairs where the distal lung may not re-expand.

As with cardiac injuries, victims of trauma to the lungs and major airways either die or make a full recovery with no residual respiratory impairment (Pomerantz et al., 1968). Respiration may be assessed by both subjective and objective methods. Subjective methods include the patients' and clinicians' assessment of functional ability with particular regard to employment and leisure. Objective measures should include respiratory function tests as a baseline and at follow-up. Although pre-trauma measurements will not be available, predicted values based on the patient's height and weight may be used for comparison. These tests can also be used to construct flow loops in the diagnosis of major airway stenosis. Arterial blood gas analysis is useful in the compromised patient or the patient with pre-existing lung disease. Radioisotope scans will reveal ventilation-perfusion defects and, where necessary, bronchoscopy should be utilised if abnormal tracheobronchial anatomy is suspected.

Cardiac injury

The incidence of blunt trauma to the heart is underestimated. The compulsory wearing of safety belts in motor vehicles has increased the incidence of trauma to the sternum and consequently the right ventricle beneath it. This cardiac trauma is often asymptomatic and only diagnosed by electrocardiograms, cardiac enzymes and echocardiography. The morbidity from this form of injury is extremely varied; from mild contusion with complete recovery to a large infarcted territory causing death.

The majority of blunt cardiac trauma may be managed conservatively with a small percentage requiring delayed surgery for injuries such as valve rupture or traumatic ventricular septal defects. Very occasionally blunt cardiac trauma requires immediate pericardiocentesis and sternotomy for rupture of a cardiac chamber. Temporary but potentially fatal dysrhythmias are common in blunt cardiac trauma, varying from unifocal ventricular ectopics to complete heart block. These are usually transient but occasionally persist due to damaged myocardium (Table 4.1). Therefore outcome measures following blunt cardiac trauma must take account of the amount of myocardium affected and whether surgical intervention was necessary.

Penetrating trauma of the heart is often fatal at the site of injury (Rasmussen et al., 1986). Successful resuscitation depends on the presence of a blood pressure on arrival at the hospital (Conn et al., 1963). Due to anterior placement of the right ventricle and right atrium these chambers are most commonly affected. Release of cardiac tamponade and repair of the defect is relatively straightforward and can usually be achieved without cardiopulmonary bypass. In these injuries little myocardium is lost and complete recovery expected. Missile injuries in civilian practice tend to be low velocity bullets whereas in the military the injuries are high velocity. The amount of disruption and amount of myocardium lost will be more varied than with simple stab wounds.

Penetrating trauma most commonly occurs in the 20–30-year age-group whereas blunt trauma has a much wider age distribution. When assessing

Table 4.1 Dysrhythmias due to cardiac trauma

1. Supraventricular tachycardia secondary to pericardial effusion
2. Ventricular ectopics or tachycardia secondary to myocardial contusion/coronary occlusion
3. Ventricular fibrillation
4. Partial or complete heart block

outcome, the pretrauma cardiac status is important as the elderly victim is likely to have ischaemic heart disease which will significantly affect their outcome.

In cardiac trauma the most important outcome measure is whether the patient is alive. Most patients who survive return to full activity but a small number of subjects require further objective assessment to investigate cardiac impairment. These investigations may reveal a surgically correctable defect or injury requiring medication.

Cardiac trauma commonly results in immediate death. In the survivors, subjective and objective criteria may be used. Subjective criteria relate to the patient's perception of their exercise ability pre- and post-trauma and the ability to return to work without limitations to any desired activity. Objective criteria may include the routine measures employed in cardiology. The New York Health Association scoring system gives a rough guide to a patient's health status (Table 4.2).

An exercise tolerance test will provide an accurate measure of a patient's ability. This is standardised by the Bruce protocol where exercise is performed on a treadmill with gradual increase in speed and gradient. Twenty-four hour Holter monitoring may be indicated where patients are suspected of dysrhythmias. Echocardiography is another non-invasive method to assess cardiac function. This will show competency of the cardiac valves, presence of traumatic intracardiac shunts (25% of patients following penetrating wound) and also give an impression of right and left ventricular function (Table 4.3).

Where there is doubt regarding ventricular function then more invasive investigation is required. Isotope studies are minimally invasive and give accurate information; left ventricular ejection fraction measured using an ECG gated radionuclide ventriculogram (MUGA scan) and a radio-nuclide myocardial perfusion scan (MIBI scan) will reveal perfusion defects in the myocardium. Rarely is right-heart catheterisation with thermodilution techniques (Swan Ganz) necessary for post-traumatic assessment. Where there is suspicion of damage to the coronary vasculature then left-heart catheterisation with coronary angiography is necessary at which time left ventriculography may also be performed.

Table 4.2 New York Health Association Health Status

Class I	No limitation of physical activity
Class II	Slight limitation; symptoms brought on by more than ordinary physical activity
Class III	Marked limitation; symptoms on less than ordinary activity
Class IV	Symptoms present even at rest and without physical activity

Table 4.3 Residual defects after recovery from cardiac injury

1. Ventricular/atrial scar with dysrhythmia
2. Ventricular septal defect
3. Mitral/aortic/tricuspid valve insufficiency
4. Coronary artery fistula
5. Aorto-pulmonary fistula
6. False aneurysm of cardiac chamber or vessel

Injury to the great vessels

Injury to the great vessels may result from penetrating or blunt trauma. The commonest aetiology is penetrating trauma but blunt trauma often affects the descending thoracic aorta, innominate artery, pulmonary veins and the vena cavae. The descending thoracic aorta is transected immediately distal to the origin of the left subclavian artery as a result of rapid deceleration; survival depends on the formation of a false aneurysm followed by surgical repair. Between 70% and 90% of patients undergoing surgery survive with a 2–5% incidence of paraplegia (Schaal *et al.*, 1979). The occurrence of the latter complication is reduced when either the 'cross-clamp' time is below 30 minutes or, if longer, satisfactory temporary vascular shunts are used to maintain perfusion of the spinal cord.

Injury to the main pulmonary artery and its branches have a high mortality prior to hospital admission. In the situation of hilar injury, surgery may have to proceed to pneumonectomy. Injuries to the vena cava have a high incidence of associated organ trauma and thus have a 60% mortality. Repair can be straightforward though inferior vena cava injuries often require cardiopulmonary bypass to control bleeding with cannulation of the abdominal inferior vena cava. The management of injuries to the great vessels involves surgical correction of the vessel. Therefore the initial outcome measure of patients that have survived to surgery is alive or dead. Survivors usually make a full recovery. In a small number of patients the surgical repair will result in physical impairment, and there is rarely a problem at the site of repair. The 2% incidence of paraplegia with repair of the descending thoracic aorta means that it is important to have preoperative documentation of peripheral neurology in case paraplegia occurred at the time of the trauma. Where lung resection is necessary, as in the control of hilar bleeding, then lung function should be assessed (see below). At the site of surgical correction local problems such as stenosis, false aneurysm, arteriovenous fistula and infection may develop, especially with the use of synthetic grafts. Hypertension due to disruption of the baroreceptors from the lumen is a common complication following surgery to the aorta. The patient can also suffer prolonged disability from the thoracotomy wound. A possible scheme for measuring outcome is summarised in Table 4.4.

Oesophageal injury

Oesophageal injury may result from direct penetrating trauma or generalised blunt trauma to the thorax or abdomen. This injury is usually overlooked at the initial assessment and is only subsequently diagnosed when the patient has been stabilised. Radiocontrast studies are the usual method of diagnosis but flexible oesophagoscopy may be used intraoperatively if the injury is found during the thoracotomy procedure. Once diagnosed the injury should be repaired without delay (Symbas *et al.*, 1986). Primary repair is preferable, although occasionally cervical oesophagostomy and a feeding gastrostomy may be necessary. This requires

Table 4.4 Outcome measure following injury to the great vessels

1. Alive/dead presurgery
2. Alive/dead postsurgery
3. Postsurgery; full recovery/disability
4. Disability:
    Permanent (paraplegia/loss of lung)
    Intermediate (hypertension)
    Temporary (local problem, i.e. wound/anastomosis)

delayed reconstruction with colonic or gastric conduit. The results depend on the site of injury, other injuries and the degree of local contamination (Meads *et al.*, 1977). Outcome measures for oesophageal injury are subjective and objective. Subjective measures will be the ability to swallow all foods normally, with no increase in reflux compared to pretraumatic status. Objective measures may be divided into anatomical and functional measures. Anatomical studies will involve radio-opaque contrast studies and oesophagoscopy. Functional studies may be divided into three areas: a cine-barium test demonstrating oesophageal motility; ambulatory pH monitoring to show frequency of gastric reflux, and isotope studies to show the volume of gastric reflux. In patients who have undergone reconstruction with colonic or gastric interposition these objective tests are less relevant and subjective evaluation coupled with an assessment of any aspiration from reflux is preferable.

References

Asfaw I, Arbulu A (1977) Penetrating wounds of the pericardium and heart. *Surg. Clin. North Am.*; **17**: 230

Beal SL, Oresksovich MR (1985) The unchanged mortality of flail chest injuries. *Am. J. Surg.*; **150**: 324

Beck CS (1926) Wounds of the heart. The technic of suture. *Arch. Surg.*; **13**: 205

Blalock A, Ravitch MM (1943) A consideration of the non-operative treatment of cardiac tamponade resulting from wounds of the heart. *Surgery.*; **14**: 157

Cicero J, Mattox KL (1989) Epidemiology of chest trauma. *Surg. Clin. North Am.*; **69**: 15–19

Cohn R (1972) Non-penetrating wounds of the lungs and bronchi. *Surg. Clin. North Am.*; **52**: 585

Conn HJ, Hardy JD, Fain WR (1963) Thoracic trauma: analysis of 1022 cases. *J. Trauma*; **3**: 22

Crawford ES, Palamara AE, Salem SE (1979) Aortic aneurysms. *Surg. Clin. North Am.*; **59**: 597

Hood RM (1983) Trauma to the chest. In Sabiston DC, Spencer FG (eds) *Gibbons Surgery of the Chest*. Philadelphia: Saunders, p. 299

Kinsella TJ, Johnstrud LW (1947) Traumatic rupture of the bronchus. *J. Thorac. Surg.*; **16**: 571

Kirs MM, Orringer MB, Behrendt DM (1976) Management of tracheobronchial disruption secondary to non-penetrating trauma. *Ann. Thorac. Surg.*; **22**: 93

Meacs CE, Carroll SE, Pitt DF (1977) Traumatic rupture of the right hemi-diaphragm. *J. Trauma*; **17**: 797

Naughton MJ, Brissie RM, Bessey PQ, Laws HL (1989) Denography of penetrating cardiac trauma. *Ann. Surg.*; **209**: 676–683

Pomerantz RM, Rodgers BM, Sabiston DC (1968) Traumatic diaphragmatic hernia. *Surgery*; **64**: 529

Rasmussen OV, Brynitz S, Struve-Christensen E (1986) Thoracic injuries. *Scand. J. Thorac. Cardiovasc. Surg.*; **20**: 71

Rhen LIX (1987) Ueber penetrirende ilerzwunden und herznaht. *Archiv. Klin. Chirurg.*; **55**: 315

Sawyers JL, Lane CE, Foster JH (1975) Oesophageal perforation. *Ann. Thorac. Surg.*; **19**: 233

Schaal MA, Fischer RP, Perry JF Jr (1979) The unchanged mortality of flail chest injuries. *J. Trauma*; **19**: 492

Symbas PN, Hatcher CR Jr, Vlassis SE (1980) Oesophageal gunshot injuries. *Ann. Surg.*; **191**: 703

Symbas PN, Vlassis SE, Hatcher CR Jr (1986) Blunt and penetrating diaphragmatic injuries with or without herniation of organs into the chest. *Ann. Thorac. Surg.*; **42**: 158

Chapter 5

Abdominal trauma

P. J. Clarke

Introduction

Intra-abdominal injury is an important cause of mortality and morbidity in the patient with multiple injuries. Careful evaluation and frequent re-evaluation of the patient is necessary, and prompt appropriate surgical intervention should follow the diagnosis of visceral damage in order to minimise the potentially serious sequelae which result from missed injuries.

A knowledge of the mechanism of trauma, if available, often yields important information. The injury patterns associated with blunt or penetrating trauma are different, and the management of an injury which may have caused damage to multiple intra-abdominal organs differs from that which is deemed likely to result in trauma to an isolated organ.

Assessment of the patient and the need for laparotomy may be made solely on clinical grounds, with or without the assistance of diagnostic peritoneal lavage, or may be aided by radiological techniques, such as abdominal X-rays, CT and ultrasound scanning. It cannot be overstressed that an initial clinical assessment of the abdomen may not reveal the presence of serious intra-abdominal pathology and thus assessment should be repeated as frequently as the clinical condition of the patient dictates.

Currently the assessment of outcome after abdominal trauma is poorly measured and the available data generally relate to survival. The aim of this chapter is to discuss available outcome measures for damage to each of the individual intra-abdominal viscera, with comments as appropriate.

Spleen

The spleen is commonly damaged in blunt abdominal trauma, especially in the presence of fractures to the left lower ribs. Delayed rupture of the spleen is said to occur when the clinical signs develop after a period of at least 48 hours. This phenomenon is generally believed to result from capsular tearing from the expansion of a subcapsular haematoma. Damage results in bleeding and the physical signs will be dictated by the amount of blood loss. The diagnosis is usually clinical, sometimes with the aid of diagnostic peritoneal lavage. Ultrasound scanning and CT are of use in the patient who remains stable after initial resuscitation in order to assess the degree of damage to the spleen. Such assessment can be used as a guide to the likelihood both of re-bleeding and the success of spleen-conserving surgery. Non-operative management of isolated splenic trauma is well established in specialised centres, especially those with a predominantly paediatric census. Operative management is dictated by the degree of splenic trauma and includes splenectomy, partial splenectomy and splenic repair techniques (splenorraphy). Complications of such repairs are few although the reported series are small. True failures seem rare, the majority represent inadequate assessment of splenic damage at the time of laparotomy, missed injuries or overambitious attempts to repair severely damaged spleens (Splenic Injury Study Group, 1987; Ghosh *et al.*, 1988).

Complications following splenic trauma and available outcome measures

Transient thrombocytosis

A transient thrombocytosis is common following splenectomy, putting the patient at an increased risk of developing a deep venous thrombosis and pulmonary embolism. The platelet count should be monitored carefully in the early postoperative period and aspirin therapy (150 mg per day) should be instituted in the short term if the count increases over $1000 \times 10^9 \, 1^{-1}$.

Overwhelming postsplenectomy infection (OPSI)

This syndrome comprises fulminant bacteraemia, frequent absence of a septic focus, coma, shock, consumptive coagulopathy and adrenal haemorrhage. It is usually associated with infection with *Streptococcus pneumoniae*, and less commonly with *Neisseria meningitidis*, *Escherichia coli* and *Haemophilus influenzae*. The overall incidence after splenectomy for trauma is between 1% and 2% but the incidence is consistently higher in the paediatric age groups (Sherman, 1980). It most commonly occurs within 3 years of the operation (Franke and Neu, 1981) and the mortality rate varies between 25% and 75% in the reported series (Sherman, 1980). In order to avoid this potentially fatal complication, it behoves the surgeon to preserve the spleen if at all possible. It has been estimated that 25–30 g of tissue is needed for protection against OPSI. Residual functioning of splenic tissue may be detected after trauma even if a splenectomy has been performed as a result of either splenosis or the presence of splenunculi. The implantation of diced splenic cubes into the omentum and other intra-abdominal sites has also been described and claims have been made that this decreases the incidence of OPSI but the reports are limited (Patel *et al.*, 1981).

If a splenectomy is unavoidable, vaccination is available to the pneumococcus, *H. influenzae* and the meningococcus. In the trauma victim this has to be given postoperatively, although the antibody levels which are achieved are less than 50% of those which occur if vaccination is given in the presence of an intact spleen. The role of prophylactic antibiotics is somewhat controversial but most centres would give an antibiotic to cover the pneumococcus for the short peri- and postoperative period and then advise the patient to have penicillin available at home for the treatment of upper respiratory tract infections. Children are frequently treated continuously with penicillin until puberty is reached.

Following spleen-preserving surgery splenic scintiscanning will demonstrate the presence of splenic tissue but this does not necessarily reflect normal function. Sophisticated techniques are described which can be used to assess splenic phagocytic activity, to measure the red cell pool and to assess the rôle of the spleen in platelet kinetics, but these tests have little place in the assessment of outcome following trauma surgery.

Liver

After the spleen, the liver is the organ most commonly injured following blunt abdominal trauma. Damage can also occur as a result of penetrating trauma to the upper abdomen or lower chest. The physical signs will depend on the degree of trauma and the amount of intraperitoneal blood loss. Accurate ultrasonography and CT assessment of the patient has resulted in approximately 30% of patients with isolated hepatic injury being managed without an operation. The overall mortality rate for all liver trauma is between 10% and 15%. The main cause of death is uncontrolled haemorrhage which usually follows severe trauma, although relatively trivial injuries can result in surprisingly severe damage. In 85% of liver injuries the bleeding either stops spontaneously or can be readily managed by conventional haemostatic techniques. The degree of surgical intervention will depend on the extent of the trauma and the experience of the operating surgeon. Operative measures will include selective arterial ligation distal to the gastroduodenal artery, debridement of ischaemic areas, hepatic repair or formal hepatectomy of one or more lobes. If definitive surgery is not feasible, packing has been shown to be useful, especially in patients with a coagulopathy and those requiring transfer to a tertiary centre. However in this group with severe injuries the mortality rate approaches 50%, with hypothermia and coagulopathies compounding the damage caused by continuing blood loss.

Complications following hepatic trauma and available outcome measures

Assessment of liver function

Standard serum 'liver function tests' are useful for assessment of liver damage rather than synthetic function. However, these tests can be used as predictors of outcome following major hepatic trauma. Hepatic transaminase levels are commonly elevated after trauma but have been shown to return to within normal limits within 40 days in both survivors and in those who subsequently die from their trauma. In contrast the level of alkaline phosphatase gradually increases in those patients who die. The elevation of serum bilirubin is less marked in survivors, with an eight-fold elevation at 10 days post-trauma in 80% of those patients who die. Total plasma protein falls immediately postinjury but has been shown to recover in those patients who are likely to survive. Serum cholesterol levels gradually increase after injury in survivors but a rapid fall to below $2.5 \, \text{mmol} \, 1^{-1}$ has been noted in those patients who die, reflecting the state of hepatic lipid metabolism. Liver function tests after 5 years following severe trauma are generally all within the normal ranges (Kaku, 1987).

Hepatic abscess

An abscess may develop within an area of damaged liver at any time from several days to several months following trauma. The symptoms and signs are pain, fever and abdominal tenderness.

Sterile haematoma

This presents with more subtle symptoms and signs and commonly needs no further treatment unless haemorrhage occurs.

Haemobilia

Haemobilia may occur at any time after liver trauma but if delayed is usually secondary to the formation of an abscess or a traumatic cyst. Late complications are rare if recovery in the first month after the injury has been straightforward (Olsen, 1982).

Stomach

Injury to the stomach is usually as a result of penetrating trauma to the upper abdomen or lower chest. The diagnosis of a full thickness laceration is usually made on clinical grounds with signs of peritonitis and radiological evidence of intraperitoneal air. Simple lacerations can be repaired without the need for resection but more serious damage may be judged at the time of surgery to require gastrectomy.

Complications of gastrectomy, and hence assessment of outcome following this procedure, have been well documented for peptic ulcer disease. There are no specific problems related to gastrectomy for trauma in cases of isolated gastric damage. In general terms, the complications following partial gastrectomy are few, but with more radical resections 5–10% of patients will develop severe intractible symptoms, leading to chronic ill health and malnutrition. These problems are considered below.

Complications following radical gastric surgery and available outcome measures

Diminution in gastric volume

A decrease in gastric capacity results initially in the need for smaller meals. This improves over a period of months in the postoperative period. Endoscopy will ascertain the exact anatomy and the size of the gastric reservoir.

Dumping syndromes (early and late)

These result from transient hypovolaemia and rebound hypoglycaemia respectively. The patient experiences symptoms of faintness, sweating, pallor and tachycardia. A provocative test consists of an oral challenge of 150 ml of 50% glucose solution, which precipitates symptoms and is accompanied by a fall in plasma volume (Le Quesne *et al.*, 1960). This test is rarely necessary as the diagnosis is primarily made on clinical grounds.

Bilary reflux

In this case, the patient experiences bilious vomiting. Endoscopy will reveal the presence of duodenogastric reflux of bile and the severity of any associated gastritis. Scanning with technetium-labelled imido-diacetic acid derivatives (HIDA) before and after intravenous cholecystokinin has been used as a non-invasive method for the detection and quantification of the duodenogastric reflux (Mackie *et al.*, 1982). This test is not routinely performed unless further surgery is planned.

Blind loop syndrome (after a Polya-gastrectomy)

This is secondary to bacterial overgrowth in the duodenal stump and may result in malabsorption. As a result, mild diarrhoea is not uncommon following gastrectomy (in 70% of patients) but it is rarely severe. Tests for malabsorption and bacterial overgrowth will be discussed under small bowel resection.

Vitamin B$_{12}$ deficiency

Vitamin B$_{12}$ deficiency secondary to loss of intrinsic factor secretion is invariable after a total gastrectomy but rare after partial resections. The patient will experience symptoms secondary to anaemia. A full blood count will reveal a macrocytic anaemia and B$_{12}$ deficiency can be confirmed using a Schilling test.

Iron deficiency anaemia

This can result from a decrease in iron absorption. The overall incidence following gastrectomy is approximately 30%. The patient will experience symptoms secondary to anaemia. A full blood count will reveal a microcytic anaemia and iron indices will be reduced.

Duodenum

The duodenum is primarily a fixed, retroperitoneal structure. It is likely to be damaged in blunt, crushing injuries to the upper abdomen. The diagnosis of duodenal trauma may be difficult and hence is often delayed. In only 5% of cases is the injury to the duodenum isolated (Snyder et al., 1980), with associated damage to the liver, colon, pancreas and inferior vena cava occurring most commonly.

If the duodenal injury results in intraperitoneal contamination the diagnosis is clinical, with signs of upper abdominal peritonitis. Retroperitoneal tears result in more subtle signs and contrast radiology with CT scanning or ultrasound examination may be required. Retroperitonal air is seen in only 50% of cases although non-specific abnormalities on the plain abdominal film such as scoliosis or obliteration of the right psoas shadow are seen more frequently.

At laparotomy, primary repairs are commonly performed when the diagnosis is made early. Delay in diagnosis usually requires a more complex procedure, sometimes including 'diverticulisation' of the duodenum, which results in its exclusion from the gastrointestinal tract. Such repairs are commonly associated with drainage of the duodenum, stomach and jejunum. Mortality from duodenal injury is directly proportional to the delay in diagnosis and can approach 50% (Corley et al., 1975; Lucas and Ledgerwood, 1975). Such deaths are most commonly due to the sequelae of the duodenal injury such as sepsis, respiratory failure and haemorrhagic pancreatitis.

Complications following duodenal trauma and available outcome measures

Duodenal fistula

Duodenal fistula may develop following the breakdown of a surgical repair resulting in fistulation of gastric contents through a drain site or laparotomy incision.

Treatment of this condition is essentially to prohibit oral intake and to maintain hydration and nutrition via the parenteral route in order to allow the fistula to close. The volume of the fistula output, the duration of days on total parenteral nutrition and the need for further surgery can be used as crude measures to assess outcome following this complication.

Obstruction at the site of repair

This is manifested by vomiting, or profuse nasogastric aspirate. This complication is treated conservatively with parenteral nutrition. A similar clinical picture may be seen secondary to haematoma of the duodenal wall without any mucosal disruption.

Sepsis

Sepsis from delayed diagnosis is associated with a high mortality rate (see above) and may need a further laparotomy or laparostomy.

Other complications

Complications from the duodenostomy and jejunostomy tubes can occur. Haemorrhage from insertion sites, displacement of the tubes and fistulae following their removal are all reported.

Pancreas

The pancreas may be injured by both penetrating and blunt abdominal trauma. Injury to the pancreas is associated with duodenal injury in approximately 40% of cases (Lucas and Ledgerwood, 1975; Snyder *et al.*, 1980). Preoperative assessment of pancreatic damage may include CT or ultrasound scanning but peritoneal lavage is of limited use. Clinical suspicion of pancreatic damage may require laparotomy to exclude it and operative intervention comprises drainage, pancreatic resection or pancreatic repair. In common with duodenal trauma, the mortality rate of missed pancreatic injuries approaches 50%. A severe injury may require pancreaticoduodenectomy (Whipple's procedure), with reported good outcome.

Assessment of outcome following such surgery is directed at measurement of pancreatic function, both endocrine and exocrine. The function may be impaired either as a result of tissue loss secondary to surgical ablation or as a result of tissue damage resulting in chronic pancreatitis.

Complications following surgery for pancreatic trauma and available outcome measures

Endocrine dysfunction

Endocrine dysfunction may result in diabetes. Simple assessment of a starving blood glucose will usually be sufficient to assess endocrine function and a glucose tolerance test will yield little in the way of further information.

Exocrine dysfunction

Exocrine dysfunction will only occur if approximately 90% of the gland has been resected or damaged. This may result in symptoms of malabsorption with diarrhoea, steatorrhoea and weight loss. The degree of pancreatic exocrine malfunction can be estimated by a 3-day faecal fat collection which must occur on a regulated diet containing 100 g of oral fat. During this period less than 6 g should be excreted per 24 hours. A further estimate of exocrine dysfunction may be gained by the *para*-amino benzoic acid (PABA) test. *N*-benzoyl-L-tyrosyl-*para*-amino benzoic acid is a synthetic peptide hydrolysed by pancreatic chymotrypsin to release free PABA, which is then absorbed, metabolised and excreted in the urine. After an oral load of the peptide, a reduction in the absorption of free PABA occurs in cases of pancreatic insufficiency.

Small bowel and colon

Blunt trauma associated with sheering forces to the abdomen may result in the tearing of the small bowel or colonic mesentery with consequent blood loss and the potential for bowel ischaemia. Penetrating trauma may also result in either division of the blood supply or isolated or multiple bowel perforations. The clinical picture will be dictated by the relative mix of hypovolaemia secondary to haemorrhage and peritonitis secondary to either ischaemia or peritoneal contamination. The diagnosis of bowel trauma is clinical or is noted at the time of a full laparotomy for multiple trauma. Surgical management of such injuries may either include primary closure of the defects or resection (small bowel) or resection with exteriorisation (for the colon). The assessment of outcome will be dictated by the length and the position of the resected bowel.

Complications following surgery for bowel trauma and available outcome measures

Short bowel syndrome

Extensive small bowel resection results in diarrhoea and malabsorption. In severe cases, water and electrolyte imbalance may occur, resulting in postural hypotension, oedema, weight loss and cramps. The passage of frequent liquid stools may cause excoriation of the perianal skin and a barrier cream may be necessary. Some degree of adaptation of the small bowel can be expected over a period of 1 or 2 years, the capacity of the ileum to hypertrophy is greater than that of the jejunum and is enhanced in the presence of an intact colon. Twenty-four-hour stool weights may be measured to monitor stool volume and malabsorption can be estimated by serum measurement of zinc, magnesium, calcium, vitamin D, vitamin B_{12}, folate and total iron binding capacity. If bacterial overgrowth is suspected duodenal aspiration with subsequent culture can be performed.

The aims of managing the patient with small bowel syndrome should be to avoid symptoms of dehydration and lethargy. These aims are likely to have been achieved if the gut losses are under 2 litres a day, urine output is over 1 litre per day, urinary sodium levels are $> 20 \, \text{mmol} \, l^{-1}$, serum magnesium $> 0.7 \, \text{mmol} \, l^{-1}$ and the patient's body weight is within 10% of the premorbid weight (Lennard-Jones and Wood, 1991).

Nutritional status

From studies of small bowel resection following surgery for volvulus or Crohn's disease, it has been demonstrated that approximately 150 cm of small bowel is compatible with normal enteral nutrition, as long as the colon is intact. If massive resection of the small bowel plus the colon have been necessary (with a resultant end stoma), a patient with less than 100 cm of jejunum is likely to need parenteral supplements. It behoves the surgeon to estimate the length of the remaining small bowel following a resection so that a realistic approach to nutrition can be established. Malnutrition is associated with muscular weakness, lack of stamina and a permanent feeling of coldness. Specific deficiencies commonly encountered are magnesium and iron. Vitamin B_{12} deficiency is inevitable after resections of more than 100 cm of distal ileum. Many patients may need to take more nutrients by mouth to compensate for the malabsorption secondary to a short gut and feeding via a fine bore nasogastric tube overnight may have advantages for the patient. Measurements of patients' weight, grip strength and skin fold thickness can be used to assess nutritional state with serial measurements of serum albumin.

Conclusions

When reviewed prospectively, missed injuries or diagnostic delay are often the cause of mortality or morbidity secondary to abdominal trauma. They may result either from the failure to perform appropriate investigations or from the performance of an incomplete laparotomy. If re-exploration is necessary for a missed injury the mean time to second-look laparotomy is significantly less in those patients who survive compared with those who die (Scalea et al., 1988). Similarly, those patients who need multiple laparotomies because of missed injuries do worse than those patients whose injuries were diagnosed at the initial laparotomy. Distinguishing between a missed injury and a consequence of a severe injury may be difficult or indeed impossible as organ failure may be indicative of occult sepsis which may or may not be secondary to a missed injury (Polk and Shields, 1977). A large percentage of such patients require intensive care facilities and of these, on-going sepsis and multi-organ failure will result in the death of approximately 50% of patients. Strict adherence to surgical protocols, such as those employed in dedicated units, should decrease this unnecessary morbidity and mortality.

References

Corley RD, Norcross WJ, Shoemaker WC (1975) Traumatic injuries to the duodenum. *Ann. Surg.*; **181**: 92–98

Franke EL, Neu HC (1981) Post splenectomy infection. *Surg. Clin. North Am.*; **61**: 135–155

Ghosh S, Symes JM, Walsh TH (1988) Splenic repair for trauma. *Br. J. Surg.*; **75**: 1139–1140

Kaku N (1987) Short-term and long-term changes in hepatic function in 60 patients with blunt liver injury. *J. Trauma*; **27**: 607–614

Le Quesne LP, Hobsley M, Hand BH (1960) The dumping syndrome. *Br. Med. J.*; **i**: 141–146

Lennard-Jones JE, Woods (1991) Coping with the short bowel. *Hosp. Update*; **17**: 797–807

Lucas CE, Ledgerwood AM (1975) Factors influencing outcome after blunt duodenal injury. *J. Trauma*; **15**: 839–846

Mackie CR, Wisbey ML, Cuschieri ML (1982) Milk $^{99}Tc^m$ – EHIDA test for enterogastric bile reflux. *Br. J. Surg.*; **69**: 101–104

Olsen WR (1982) Late complications of central liver injuries. *Surgery*; **92**: 733–743

Patel J, Williams JS, Shmigel B, Hinshaw JR (1981) Preservation of splenic function by autotransplantation of traumatized spleen in man. *Surgery*; **90**: 683–688

Polk HC, Shields CL (1977) Remote organ failure: a valid sign of occult intra-abdominal infection. *Surgery*; **81**: 310–313

Scalea TM, Phillips TF, Goldstein AS, Selafani SJ, Duncan AO, Atmeh NA, Shaftan GW (1988) Injuries missed at operation: nemesis of the trauma surgeon. *J. Trauma*; **28**: 962–967

Sherman R (1980) Perspectives in management of trauma to the spleen. *J. Trauma*; **20**: 1–13

Snyder WH, Weigelt JA, Watkins WL, Bietz DS (1980) The surgical management of duodenal trauma. *Arch. Surg.*; **115**: 422–429

The Splenic Injury Study Group (1987) Splenic injury: a prospective multicentre study on non-operative and operative treatment. *Br. J. Surg.*; **74**: 310–313

Chapter 6

The urogenital tract

J. M. T. Perkins and D. Cranston

Introduction

Trauma to the urogenital tract may occur in isolation from blunt or penetrating injuries, but more often the magnitude of the force causing injury to the genitourinary tract is sufficient to injure other intra-abdominal and extra-abdominal structures. The management and treatment of genitourinary injury depends on the nature of the injury and the priority with which the associated injuries need treatment.

Outcome measures following injury to the urogenital tract can be quantified in terms of death, disability or full recovery. Disability may be the result of stricture, retention, stone formation, urinary infections and rarely renal failure, incontinence with its associated problems, or impotence.

Renal trauma

The majority of deaths in males and females under 40 years of age are due to trauma; 10% of trauma cases have genitourinary tract involvement with the kidney being the organ most frequently injured. In children the kidneys are relatively larger and less well protected than in the adult, and renal injury is second only to head injury in frequency, occurring more frequently than splenic injury and four times more frequently than liver or intestinal injury (Morse, 1975). A pre-existing congenital malformation is found in 10% of children who sustain a renal injury (Feins, 1979).

Clinical features of renal injury include abdominal and flank tenderness with flank ecchymosis and clinical evidence of rib fracture alerting the clinician to the possibility of renal injury. The presence of haematuria and shock (systolic BP < 90 mmHg) in patients with blunt trauma identifies a higher risk group with a 25% likelihood of major renal injury (Hardeman *et al.*, 1987). The presence or absence of haematuria in blunt renal trauma should be assessed on the first voided or catheter specimen of urine (Mendez, 1977) as it may be fleeting and clear rapidly.

Outcome measures

Detection of haematuria may be by dipstick testing or microscopy, and whilst the quantity of haematuria detected by dipstick testing correlates poorly with microscopic findings (Chandke and McAninch, 1988), dipstick testing shows a 97.5% sensitivity and specificity for detection of haematuria. In a series of 339 patients in whom haematuria was assessed by dipstick testing, no significant renal injury was missed (Goldner et al., 1985). The degree of haematuria does not correlate with the severity of renal injury and is absent in 25% of cases of renal pedicle injury (Stables et al., 1976).

Intravenous urography remains the key investigation in the initial assessment of renal trauma. This should be carried out in all cases of penetrating trauma, blunt renal injury with gross haematuria, and blunt renal injury with microscopic haematuria and shock (systolic BP < 90 mmHg). Using these criteria in three separate studies a total of 1671 patients with blunt renal trauma, microscopic haematuria and no shock were evaluated to assess the safety of conservative management without intravenous urography (IVU). In these 1671 patients only one serious renal injury was missed (< 0.05%) (Cass et al., 1986; Hardemann et al., 1987; Mee et al., 1989).

Intravenous urography may not accurately stage all renal injuries. From 33% to 60% of IVU films are inadequate for reliable interpretation (Elkin et al., 1966; Lang et al., 1971; Maggio and Brosman, 1978) and when abnormal, the findings are often non-specific showing only decreased opacification, irregular cortical margins or renal displacement. Non-function and extravasation are seen as reliable radiological findings for pedicle injury or major laceration, but in a series of 53 patients with non-visualisation on IVU, only 40% had sustained a renal pedicle injury (Cass and Luxenberg, 1984). Furthermore, 20% of IVUs in patients with renal pedicle injury are reported as normal (Carroll and McAninch, 1985).

In extensive trauma or in patients with equivocal IVU findings, CT scanning is the investigation of choice. It is less invasive and time-consuming than arteriography and more sensitive and specific than IVU (Bretan et al., 1986). The appearances of renovascular injury are characterised by lack of enhancement or excretion, rim enhancement, central haematoma or the abrupt cut off of an enhanced renal artery (Steinberg et al., 1984; Sclafani et al., 1985).

Surgery may be required to stage those patients incompletely assessed by clinical and radiological techniques, or who are known to have a major renal injury. In penetrating trauma to the abdomen or flank the kidney is injured in 6–8% of cases, and of these patients 40–60% will have a major or renovascular injury (Carroll and McAninch, 1985). The site of injury – flank, abdomen or lumbar – fails to predict severity of the renal injury sustained. In penetrating trauma exploration is mandatory, unless staging indicates that the nature of the injury justifies expectant management (Carlton et al., 1968). In blunt trauma exploration is seldom required and most series report an exploration rate of < 10% (McAninch and Carroll, 1982). Indications for exploration in blunt trauma may be absolute – the presence of an expanding or pulsatile retroperitoneal haematuria consistent with major laceration – or relative – urinary extravasation, non-viable tissue, incomplete staging and arterial thrombosis.

Controversy still exists regarding the relative merits of aggressive and conservative management in renal trauma. Proponents of prompt surgical intervention are motivated by the belief that conservative treatment provides a conducive environment for the development of complications, including delayed haemorrhage and parenchymal loss, and that early intervention spares renal function.

Delayed exploration rates as high as 45% and nephrectomy rates as high as 21% in conservatively managed patients are quoted to support this view. However nephrectomy rates for patients undergoing immediate surgical intervention may be as high as 58% in comparison to figures from 0.7% (Krieger et al., 1984) to 20% (Rosenthall and Amman, 1983) for those managed conservatively and nephrectomy has been cited as occurring three times more frequently in patients explored acutely (Cass and Ireland, 1973). Conservative management has been associated with a lower complication rate (Nation and Massey, 1963; Cass and Ireland, 1973), the potential for spontaneous recovery and the advances in percutaneous techniques for treatment of stricture, stone and the drainage of abscesses/fluid. Non-operative management is non-injurious to the kidney and offers opportunities for clinical stabilisation and appraisal of renal status. Eighty to ninety per cent of all renal injuries respond to this management.

Renovascular lesions comprise pedicle avulsion, main renal artery thrombosis, segmental artery interruption, arteriovenous aneurysm and fistula formation. A series of 1698 renal injuries quotes a 2.6% incidence of renovascular injury (Cass and Luxenberg, 1987a). The results of revascularisation remain disappointing and functional compromise characterised by reduced renal function, total or segmented atrophy, hypertension and rethrombosis is frequently encountered despite technical operative success. Warm ischaemic tolerance by the kidney is poor and intervention greater than 12 hours after injury carries little chance of parenchymal salvage (Cass and Luxenberg, 1983). Peripheral renal vascular injuries are not uncommon but non-operative management is preferred (Cass and Luxenberg, 1984). Other forms of renovascular injury – arteriovenous fistula and aneurysm formation – are rare.

Hypertension is an acknowledged outcome of renal trauma. The definition of hypertension varies according to the series, but is usually defined as a blood pressure exceeding 150–160 mmHg systolic or 90–95 mmHg diastolic, or both (Grant et al., 1971; Cass et al., 1987b).

Reported incidences generally range from 0.7% to 33%, but incidences as high as 55% have been reported in patients with blunt renal trauma managed conservatively (Cass et al., 1987b). Others have observed hypertension rates of 50% (Stables et al., 1976) and 57% (Maggio and Brosman, 1978) in patients with renal artery thrombosis not undergoing early successful revascularisation or nephrectomy. The onset of hypertension is usually seen within the first few months following injury but late onset up to 14 years later is recorded (Carini et al., 1981). Post-traumatic hypertension may be transient, and spontaneous resolution is documented after hypertensive periods from 9 days to 12 months.

Renal function as an outcome measure in renal trauma has only been assessed in the acute phase following injury and with conflicting results. A decrease in renal filtration and function, assessed by measurement of creatinine clearance, inulin clearance and osmolar clearance, has been shown in one series of trauma patients who underwent nephrectomy (McGonigal *et al.*, 1987), but others have not demonstrated any increase in acute renal failure or mortality (Cass and Luxenberg, 1987b).

Death rates from renal trauma are difficult to interpret due to multifactorial influences such as the presence of associated injuries and the timing and quality of resuscitation.

Death from renal injury alone is rare. Overall mortality varies from 8% to 29%, but within these series, death specifically from renal injury ranges from 0.8% to 4% (McCague, 1950; Bertini *et al.*, 1986; Cass *et al.*, 1987a).

One series correlated mortality with 4% of 607 renal contusions, 6% of 355 parenchymal lacerations and 29% of renal ruptures and pedicle injuries (Del Villar *et al.*, 1972).

Ureteric injury

Ureteric injury occurs rarely in trauma. Injury to the ureter should be suspected in penetrating abdominal trauma and in children with hyperextension injuries of the spine, who may suffer an avulsion injury at the pelvi-ureteric junction. Ninety-six per cent are associated with gunshot wounds and in 92% of ureteric injuries there is damage to other intra-abdominal organs (Guerriero, 1989). In penetrating injury haematuria is present in 80–90% of cases but is usually microscopic.

Extravasation secondary to ureteric injury is demonstrated on IVU. All penetrating injuries should be explored. The nature of operative repair is dependent on the site of injury, the timing of intervention and the extent of associated injury. Rarely, in severe injury with avulsion of the collecting system, nephrectomy is performed.

Outcome measures

The major long-term complication is stricture formation, diagnosed on intravenous urography and/or retrograde ureterography. This may lead subjectively to loin pain, and objectively to deterioration in renal function on the affected side. It will not lead to renal failure if the contralateral side is present and functioning normally.

Bladder injury

Bladder rupture is classified as extraperitoneal or intraperitoneal (or both). Approximately 60% of injuries are extraperitoneal, 35% intraperitoneal and 5% a combination of the two (Carroll and McAninch, 1984).

Bladder rupture occurs in patients who experience excessive force to the lower abdomen. It should be suspected in patients who experience a sudden deceleration force and who complain of lower abdominal pain, haematuria and an inability to void. Intraperitoneal rupture may present as an acute abdomen and may present with a rising blood urea nitrogen in the well-hydrated patient with no pre-existing renal impairment (Shah *et al.*, 1979).

Pelvic fractures account for 81% of traumatic bladder injuries, most in association with fractures of the pubic ramus (55%) (Cass, 1989). There is no relationship between the type of pelvic fracture and the nature of the bladder injury (intra- or extraperitoneal). In a 10-year review of 1080 pelvic fractures, 8.6% of patients sustained bladder or urethral injuries. Bladder injuries alone accounted for 6.2%, posterior urethral injuries for 1.9%, and combined bladder and posterior urethral injury for 0.4% (Cass, 1989).

Diagnosis is confirmed by cystography. It is important to distend the bladder during these studies, using at least 400 ml water soluble contrast medium, as small bladder ruptures may be concealed in states of lesser bladder distension (Weyrauch and Peterfry, 1940; Carroll and McAninch, 1983; Mee *et al.*, 1987).

Isolated extraperitoneal rupture of the bladder is treated by Foley catheter drainage. Using this regimen 87% will have healed by the tenth day and almost all by 3 weeks (Corriere and Sandler 1986). If surgery is necessary for associated injuries the bladder can be opened, repaired and drained via a suprapubic catheter. Any bony spicules found penetrating the bladder should be removed. Intraperitoneal bladder ruptures must be explored and repaired. The nature of the force required to produce an intraperitoneal bladder rupture causes a high incidence of associated injuries, most often bowel lacerations and injury to major vessels. In a series of 213 patients with an intraperitoneal bladder rupture and a white cell count greater than 20000 per ml, all but two had a laceration of the liver or spleen (Peters, 1989).

Outcome measures

Complications and mortality in bladder rupture are most frequently the result of associated injuries with an average of 2.4 associated injuries for intraperitoneal rupture and 2.6 for extraperitoneal rupture (Cass, 1988). Overall mortality ranges from 12% to 15% (Cass, 1988; Corriere and Sandler, 1986) with considerable difference depending on the type of bladder injury, ranging from 11% with contusion to 26% for intraperitoneal and 36% for intra- and extraperitoneal rupture combined. Bladder function is not compromised by rupture.

Urethral injury

Posterior urethral injury

Management of posterior urethral injuries remains controversial and a difficult challenge. The diagnosis must be considered in all patients who have a fracture of the bony pelvis or wide separation of the symphysis pubis. Posterior urethral injury occurs in approximately 5% of pelvic fractures (Palmer *et al.*, 1983). A rupture of the bladder is found in 10–20% of patients with a posterior urethral injury (Sandler *et al.*, 1981).

Clinical signs of posterior urethral rupture include blood at the external urethral meatus, and inability to void and a palpable bladder. Supporting signs are a high riding prostate gland on rectal examination and the presence of a perineal haematoma. The inability to pass a urethral catheter into the bladder has been used to diagnose urethral injury, but this practice should be discouraged as it introduces infection and may convert a partial tear to a complete injury. Diagnosis is by retrograde urethrography. Initial management is by one of three methods:

1. Suprapubic cystostomy is performed, continuity of bladder and urethra re-established with interlocking sounds and urethral continuity maintained over an indwelling silastic urethral catheter. A suprapubic catheter also drains the bladder. Modifications to this method include putting traction on the urethral catheter (DeWeerd, 1977), or the use of perineal traction sutures placed through the prostatic capsule and a fenestrated urethral catheter to drain urethral secretions (Turner-Warwick, 1973, 1977a,b).
2. Primary reanastomosis of urethral ends over a stenting urethral catheter.
3. The Johansen technique: immediate suprapubic drainage only combined later with elective reconstruction of stricturing.

Outcome measures

Clinically the presence of a stricture is apparent on patient questioning of urinary flow and this can be objectively supported by flow rate urodynamics to evaluate the velocity of the urinary stream.

In evaluating the nature of any stricture, the key investigation is the synchronous cystogram and retrograde urethrogram – the so-called 'up and downogram' – which demonstrates the length of the prostate bulbar gap and the presence of any fistulae or false passages that influence the surgical approach.

Moorehouse compares the results of failed conventional realignment or primary anastomosis (1 and 2 above) with the Johansen technique using a two-stage scrotal flap urethroplasty. Impotence rates were 8% using the Johansen technique and 26% using other methods, and incontinence rates were 5% and 16% respectively (Morehouse, 1988). In a later series of 36 patients treated by immediate suprapubic drainage and later one-stage perineal reanastomosis, the impotence and incontinence rates were 11% and 0 respectively. Stricture cure rate was 86% with five recurrent strictures cured by internal urethrotomy.

Incontinence may be caused by damage to the bladder neck or to the distal urethral sphincter mechanism, which is almost always damaged in abstraction defects (Turner-Warwick, 1973). This can be assessed by voiding cystourethrography. If the distal sphincter is compromised and damage occurs to the bladder neck, then incontinence will result. The commonest cause of bladder neck incompetence is circumferential tethering by haematoma fibrosis in the retroperitoneal space. This is easily visualised endoscopically, as is any segmental injury to the bladder neck mechanism indicated at endoscopy by a notched scar in one sector of the circumference.

Impotence, defined as the inability to produce an erection adequate for sexual intercourse, is more commonly the result of neural rather than vascular compromise. The nervi errigentes run in close proximity to the subprostatic urethra and neural damage in pelvic fracture urethral distraction injury is sufficient to cause erection failure in 20–37% (Gibson, 1980; Turner-Warwick, 1989) – this may be complete erection failure (17%), or partial (20%) with weak, infrequent and inadequate erections (Gibson, 1980). Many patients experience failure of erection for days or weeks after injury but this usually recovers although recovery can take up to a year or more (Turner-Warwick, 1989; Gibson, 1988).

Anterior urethral injury

Injury to the anterior urethra occurs most frequently in straddle-type injury and damage occurs in the bulbar urethra. Injuries to the pendulous urethra from blunt trauma are rare as the tissues of the penis are elastic to the limit of their compliance; injuries may occur from penetrating trauma.

Clinically the diagnosis of anterior urethral injury is acute urethral bleeding. Diagnosis is by retrograde urethrography and the initial step in management should be suprapubic cystostomy drainage alone (Pontes and Pierce, 1978). Attempts at primary closure should be avoided as more damage is often done than good (Kiracofe *et al.*, 1975).

Outcome measures

By conservative management more than 70% will heal without stricture.

Flow rate urodynamics will reveal patterns typical of stricturing, with a flow rate of $< 10 \mathrm{\,ml\,s^{-1}}$ on a voided volume of 100 ml or greater also suggestive of stricture formation (Milroy *et al.*, 1988). However, most strictures that occur are short (< 0.5 cm) and easily visualised endoscopically and treated by optical urethroplasty but the timing of intervention is at the discretion of the individual surgeon.

Genital injury

Male

This is rare and occurs in 7% of cases of male trauma with testicular trauma accounting for 43%, penile injury 32% and scrotal injury 20% (Cass, 1983a). In testicular injury the incidence of rupture after blunt trauma is 48% (Cass, 1983b) and early exploration is called for if doubt exists in diagnosis.

Outcome measures

Conservative treatment predisposes to infection and testicular necrosis. In conservative management the rate of testicular loss is 22% compared to a

7% loss rate in those cases explored acutely. Fertility following testicular trauma has only been assessed experimentally in rats, but has not been evaluated in humans. Experimentally induced unitesticular trauma in rats showed decreased fertility as assessed by successful or unsuccessful impregnation of female rats, and microscopic evaluation of the viability of the spermatogenic epithelium and extent of spermatogenesis (Stairs *et al.*, 1990). Changes were observed in the contralateral (non-traumatised) testicle, presumably as a result of immunological mechanisms following disruption of the blood–testis barrier at trauma. Penetrating injuries to penis or scrotum should be treated according to accepted principles of debridement, lavage, repair, drainage and systemic antibiotics.

Female

Female genital injury is rare. Vaginal injury in penetrating trauma may involve injury to the bladder, lower urinary tract and rectum also.

Outcome measures

Outcomes include sexual dysfunction and infertility either due to direct tubal injury or peritubal adhesions from infection.

Conclusions

Specific and detailed outcome measures are not often applicable in urogenital tract trauma. Grading systems for the degree of injury or the severity of complications have not been formally outlined, nor have specific scoring systems related to urogenital tract trauma; broader categories of outcome such as death or survival, renal parenchymal loss or salvage, or the presence or absence of stricture formation are more applicable.

References

Bertini JR Jr, Fletchner SM, Miller P *et al.* (1986) The natural history of traumatic branch renal artery injury. *J. Urol.*; **135**: 228–230

Bretan PN, McAninch JW, Federle MP *et al.* (1986) Computerised tomographic staging of renal trauma: 85 consecutive cases. *J. Urol.*; **136**: 561–565

Carlton CE, Scott DR, Goldman M (1968) The management of penetrating injuries of the kidney. *J. Trauma*; **8**: 1071–1075

Carini M, Selli C, Trippitelli A *et al.* (1981) Surgical treatment of reno-vascular hypertension secondary to renal trauma. *J. Urol.*; **126**: 101–104

Carroll PR, McAninch JW (1983) Major bladder trauma: the accuracy of cystography. *J. Urol.*; **130**: 887–888

Carroll PR, McAninch JW (1984) Major bladder trauma: a mechanism of injury and a modified method of diagnosis and repair. *J. Urol.*; **132**: 254–257

Carroll P, McAninch JW (1985) Operative indications in penetrating renal trauma. *J. Trauma*; **25**: 587–589

Cass AS (1983a) Male genital injury from external trauma. In *Genitourinary Trauma*. Boston: Blackwell Scientific Publications

Cass AS (1983b) Testicular Trauma. *J. Urol.*; **129**: 299–300

Cass AS (1988) External Bladder Trauma. In *Genitourinary Trauma*. Boston: Blackwell Scientific Publications

Cass AS (1989) Diagnostic studies in bladder rupture. *Urol. Clin. North Am.*; **16**: 267–273

Cass AS, Ireland GW (1973) Comparison of the conservative and surgical management of the more severe degrees of renal trauma in multiple injured patients. *J. Urol.*; **109**: 8–10

Cass AS, Luxenberg M (1983) Conservative or immediate surgical management of blunt renal trauma. *J. Urol.*; **130**: 11–16

Cass AS, Luxenberg M (1984) Unilateral non-visualisation on excretory urography after external trauma. *J. Urol.*; **132**: 225–227

Cass AS, Luxenberg M (1987a) Management of renal artery injuries from external trauma. *J. Urol.*; **138**: 266–268

Cass AS, Luxenberg M (1987b) Renal failure and mortality after nephrectomy for severe trauma in multiple injured patient. *Urology*; **30**: 213–215

Cass AS, Luxenberg M, Gleich P *et al.* (1986) Clinical indications for radiological evaluation of blunt renal trauma. *J. Urol.*; **136**: 370–371

Cass AS, Luxenberg M, Gleich P *et al.* (1987a) Death from urologic injury due to external trauma. *J. Trauma*; **27**: 319–321

Cass AS, Luxenberg M, Gleich P *et al.* (1987b) Long term results of conservative and surgical management of blunt renal lacerations. *Br. J. Urol.*; **59**: 17–20

Chandke P, McAninch JW (1988) Detection and significance of microscopic haematuria in patients with blunt renal trauma. *J. Urol.*; **140**: 16–18

Corriere JN Jr, Sandler CM (1986) Management of the ruptured bladder: seven years of experience with 111 cases. *J. Trauma*; **26**: 830–833

Del Villar RG, Ireland GW, Cass AS (1972) Management of renal injury in conjunction with the immediate surgical treatment of the acute severe trauma patient. *J. Urol.*; **107**: 208–211

DeWeerd JH (1977) Immediate realignment of posterior urethral injury. *Urol. Clin. North Am.*; **4**: 75–80

Elkin M, Meng C-H, de Paredes RG (1966) Correlation of intravenous urography and renal angiography in kidney injury. *Radiology*; **86**: 496–498

Feins NR (1979) Multiple trauma. *Paediatric Clin. North Am.*; **26**: 759–771

Gibson GR (1980) Impotence following fractured pelvis and ruptured urethra. *Br. J. Urol.*; **42**: 86–88

Goldner MP, Mayron R, Ruiz E (1985) Are urine dipsticks reliable indicators of haematuria in blunt renal trauma patients? *Ann. Emerg. Med.*; **14**: 580–582

Grant RP, Gifford RW, Pudvan WR *et al.* (1971) Renal trauma and hypertension. *Am. J. Cardiol.*; **27**: 173–176

Guerriero WG (1989) Ureteral injury. *Urol. Clin. North Am.*; **16**: 237–248

Hardemann S, Husman DA, Chin HKW *et al.* (1987) Blunt urinary trauma: identifying those patients who require radiological studies. *J. Urol.*; **138**: 99–101

Kiracofe HL, Pfister RR, Peterson NE (1975) Management of non-penetrating distal urethral trauma. *J. Urol.*; **114**: 57–62

Krieger JN, Algood CB, Mason JT *et al.* (1984) Urological trauma in the Pacific Northwest. *J. Urol.*; **132**: 70–73

Lang EK, Tridnel BE, Turner RW *et al.* (1971) Arteriographic assessment of injury resulting from renal trauma: An analysis of 74 patients. *J. Urol.*; **106**: 1–8

Maggio AJ, Brosman S (1978) Renal artery trauma. *Urology*; **11**: 125–130

McAninch JW, Carroll PR (1982) Renal trauma: kidney preservation through improved vascular control – a refined approach: *J. Trauma*; **22**: 285–290

McCague EJ (1950) Renal trauma: conservative management. *J. Urol.*; **65**: 773–776

McGonigal MD, Lucas CE, Ledgerwood AM (1987) The effects of treatment of renal trauma on renal function. *J. Trauma*; **27**: 471–476

Mee SH, McAninch JW, Federle MP (1987) Computerised tomography in bladder rupture: diagnostic limitations. *J. Urol.*; **137**: 207–209

Mee SL, McAninch JW, Robinson AL *et al.* (1989) Radiographic assessment of renal trauma: a 10 year prospective study of patient selection. *J. Urol.*; **142**: 1095–1098

Mendez R (1977) Renal trauma. *J. Urol.*; **118**: 698–703

Milroy EG, Charple CR, Cooper JE (1988) A new treatment for urethral strictures. *Lancet*; **i**: 1424–1427

Morehouse DD (1988) Management of posterior urethral rupture. A personal view. *Br. J. Urol.*; **61**: 375–381

Morse TS (1975) Renal injuries. *Paediatric Clin. North Am.*; **22**: 379–391

Nation EF, Massey BD (1963) Renal trauma. *J. Urol.*; **89**: 775–778

Palmer JK, Benson GS, Corriere JN Jr (1983) Diagnosis and initial management of urological injuries associated with 200 consecutive pelvic fractures. *J. Urol.*; **130**: 712–714

Peters PC (1989) Intraperitoneal rupture of the bladder. *Urol. Clin. North Am.*; **16**: 279–282

Pontes JE, Pierce JM, Jr (1978) Anterior urethral injuries: four years of experience at the Detroit General Hospital. *J. Urol.*; **120**: 563–564

Rosenthall L, Amman W (1983) Renal trauma. *Semin. Nucl. Med.*; **13**: 238–241

Sandler CM, Phillips JM, Harris JD *et al.* (1981) Radiology of the bladder and urethra in blunt pelvic trauma. *Radiol. Clin. North Am.*; **19**: 195–208

Sclafani SJA, Goldstein AS, Panetta T *et al.* (1985) CT diagnosis of renal pedicle injury. *Urol. Radiol.*; **7**: 63–65

Shah PM, Kim K, Samirez-Schon G *et al.* (1979) Elevated blood urea nitrogen: an aid to diagnosis of intraperitoneal rupture of the bladder. *J. Urol.*; **122**: 741–743

Stables DP, Fouche RF, de Villiers VN (1976) Traumatic renal artery occlusion: 21 cases. *J. Urol.*; **115**: 229–233

Stairs SA, Schulz JN, Hewitt CW *et al.* (1990) The effects of testicular trauma on fertility in the Lewis rat and comparisons to iso-immunised recipients of syngeneic sperm. *J. Urol.*; **143**: 638–641

Steinberg DL, Jeffrey RB, Federle MP *et al.* (1984) The computerised tomographic appearances of renal pedicle injury. *J. Urol.*; **132**: 1163–1164

Turner-Warwick R (1973) Observations on the treatment of traumatic urethral injuries and the value of the fenestrated urethral catheter. *Br. J. Surg.*; **60**: 775–781

Turner-Warwick R (1977a) A personal view of the immediate management of pelvic fracture urethral injuries. *Urol. Clin. North Am.*; **4**: 81–93

Turner-Warwick R (1977b) A personal view of the management of traumatic posterior urethral strictures. *Urol. Clin. North Am.*; **4**: 111–124

Turner-Warwick R (1989) Prevention of complications of urethral injuries. *Urol. Clin. North Am.*; **16**: 335–358

Weyrauch HM Jr, Peterfy RA (1940) Tests for leakage in early diagnosis of ruptured bladder. *J. Urol.*; **44**: 264–266

Chapter 7

Burns

A. Phipps

It is estimated that well over 100 000 burn victims are treated in accident and emergency departments in the UK every year. The injuries occupy a spectrum of severity from the trivial to the devastating; whilst the majority of patients may be treated outside hospital, about 14 000 per year are admitted, of whom about 6% die.

Some of those who survive burn injuries are temporarily inconvenienced by the experience; for others, the course of their lives is irreversibly altered by disability or disfigurement, which may inflict major changes on their personal, social or professional capabilities.

In the face of this immense diversity of injury and consequences, the measurement of treatment outcomes is beset with difficulties. In the first half of this century, the very survival of even moderately severe burns was highly unlikely (Colebrook, 1950; Jackson, 1981). The prevention of burn shock by early intravenous fluid resuscitation and the establishment of the first dedicated burns units in the 1940s had a major impact on the fatality of burn injuries, and it is on quantifying and predicting this easily identified outcome of survival according to the characteristics of the injury and the patient that most analytical effort has been expended.

Minor burns

The huge majority of burns are small in scale and do not threaten life. In the main the patients who have suffered them do not require or receive inpatient treatment, and outcomes are usually only formally documented when patients are being treated as part of a clinical trial, for instance of a new dressing material (e.g. Lawrence, 1977; Phipps and Lawrence, 1988). In such cases, the morbidity parameters which may be measured are healing times, bacteriological efficacy and pain control. The cost of a treatment method and factors reflecting patient convenience (e.g. the frequency of dressing changes, or the ability to continue work and everyday activities whilst treatment is in progress) may also be included in its overall evaluation. An attempt may also be made to rate the healed wound by scoring qualities of the resultant scar such as hypertrophy, texture, colour, etc.

The assessment of healing times is made more difficult by the fact that most dressings obscure the wound, and their removal at frequent intervals, purely for the purpose of viewing to check whether healing has occurred, is unacceptable to patients and may itself delay healing. Many dressings may and should be left in place undisturbed for periods of up to a week; measurements of healing times for minor burns, which are likely to fall in the range of 1–3 weeks, may thus contain a significant degree of imprecision.

Delays in burn wound healing and the risk of sepsis depend upon the ability of a treatment schedule to control colonisation of the wound with bacteria. This may be evaluated by monitoring bacterial acquisition times on serial wound swabs, and recording the prevalence of locally invasive infection in the form of cellulitis or lymphangitis. Pain in the wound during and between dressing changes may be scored by the patient using one of the established methods, such as verbal scoring or visual analogue scales (c.f. Chapter 2).

Mortality probability

Outcome measures and severity indicators which can accurately describe the mortality probability of a burn injury have several potential uses (Roi et al., 1983): to act as a guide to management policy for individual patients; to assist in counselling patients and their relatives; to characterise a patient population in terms of severity; to identify for clinical audit purposes those patients whose outcome differs significantly from that expected; and to provide benchmarks for the evaluation of institutions or therapeutic policies.

Rough appraisals of a patient's survival after a major burn are regularly made, particularly in cases where an injury appears to be so severe that survival would be unprecedented, and 'comfort care' may be more appropriate than attempts at resuscitation. For example, survival is generally considered unlikely if the numerical sum of the total percentage body surface area burned and the patient's age exceeds 100. Similar rules of thumb have been formalised in American papers as the 'Baux rule' (sum of age plus percentage burn greater than 75 predicts poor outcome) or the 'modified Baux rule' (for patients over 20 years old, sum of age plus percentage burn greater than 95 predicts less than 50% survival) (Stern and Waisbren, 1978).

More complex systems to predict the likelihood of death from burn injuries were pioneered by the work of Bull and Squire in the burns unit of the Birmingham Accident Hospital (Bull and Squire, 1949). They used probit analysis of retrospective case fatality rates to calculate the mortality probability for burns of different extent (total percentage body surface area burned) in patients falling into banded age groups. Subsequent revisions of this work have been published for later series of patients (Bull and Fisher, 1954; Bull, 1971). Mortality probability according to Bull's tables continues to be used widely, both in the UK and elsewhere, to ascribe a measure of severity to burns in individual patients for everyday audit, and to describe the severity profile of patient populations in comparative studies.

Numerous scoring systems have been reported which use probit analysis, discriminant analysis or multiple logistic regression analysis to model fatality rates to prognostic variables in series of burned patients, and many articles have been published proposing and comparing mortality indices in patient populations from one or more institutions. All of these models incorporate age and the total burn extent and/or the area of full-thickness burning as the most heavily weighted factors. Systems such as Bull's, which ignore full-thickness burning as an explicit variable, reflect in their mortality predictions the consideration that larger total area burns are on average more inclined to be associated with significant areas of full-thickness skin loss. Thus the risk for unusual individuals who, by the nature of their injury, have sustained significantly smaller or larger areas of deep burning than average for their total burn extent may differ from that forecast by these systems.

Other predictors of mortality which have been proposed include: indications of an inhalation injury (Clark et al., 1986; Thompson et al., 1986; Shirani et al., 1987; Zöch et al., 1992); inhalation injury and the presence of prior bronchopulmonary disease (Zawacki et al., 1979); the sex of the patient, perineal involvement by the burn wound and delay in admission (Roi et al., 1983); patient sex and inhalation injury (Tobiasen et al., 1982); and haematological and biochemical measurements and maximum daily body temperature during initial treatment (Peterson et al., 1988).

In general these indices have all been found to forecast fatality rates in the institutions by which they have been developed with an overall prediction accuracy in the region of 90%. Significant variations in treatment protocols between different units may, however, limit the validity of models developed by one unit when applied to patient populations in another (Bowser et al., 1983).

It might be expected that severity indices specifically oriented to burns would correlate more closely with burn mortality than scoring systems designed for trauma in general. This has been confirmed in a retrospective study (Krob et al., 1991), in which various general trauma indices (Trauma Score, Injury Severity Score and Glasgow Coma Scale) were compared with a range of burn scoring systems (Baux Rule, Edlich Burn Score (Tobiasen et al., 1982) and Zawacki Score (Zawacki et al., 1979)), all based principally on the age of the patient and the extent of the cutaneous burn. The burn-specific systems predicted both mortality and length of hospital stay more accurately than the non-burn scores.

Over the years in which mortality has been scrutinised, burn victims have benefited from many developments (Monafo, 1992), including progress in intensive care techniques, the advent of effective antimicrobials (in part offset by the emergence of resistant organisms) (Lawrence, 1992), advances in wound care and methods of achieving skin cover, changes in surgical techniques and philosophy, and the increasing concentration of the treatment of serious burns into specialised burns units. Stratification of the burn population by age and some measure of burn wound severity has defined injuries of comparable gravity sufficiently to allow some historical comparisons to be made. It appears that, overall, developments in burn care over the last four decades have resulted in a general shift in the direction of reduced mortality over much of the severity spectrum. For a given age cohort, this may alternatively be expressed as an increase in the size of burn which carries a 50% mortality (LA_{50}) (Curreri *et al.*, 1980).

Dominant amongst trends in burn management over the past two decades has been the adoption by many burns units of more aggressive surgical policies, stimulated by, but not confined to, the introduction in the early 1970s of early tangential excision (ETE) and grafting of the burn wound as an alternative to more conservative treatment (Janzekovic, 1970; Jackson and Stone, 1972). This shift towards earlier surgery has been widely credited with reducing mortality (Feller *et al.*, 1980; Wolfe *et al.*, 1983; Heimbach, 1987; Tompkins *et al.*, 1988; and others). Studies have been published which compare directly the results of early excision methods with those of conventional management, using mortality as the principal outcome measure, but with varying conclusions.

Of recently reported series, one (Cryer *et al.*, 1991) demonstrated increases in LA_{50} values in patients treated by ETE in comparison with other published studies, but only for patients aged between 41 and 60 years. Mortality was significantly lower in this age group for victims of burns of between 20% and 65% total body surface area. Duration of hospital stay also appeared to be shorter than in the compared series.

Another study (McManus *et al.*, 1989) appeared to show a survival advantage of early tangential excision of large area burns (greater than 30% total body surface area). However, in this series the basis for comparison had been age- and area-stratified mortality statistics from the same unit at least 20 years previously. The authors cautioned that not only had patients from the 1980s undergoing ETE been selected for the absence of physiological contraindications (most commonly pulmonary problems as a result of inhalation injury, itself a significant contributor to burn mortality (Clark *et al.*, 1986)), but they had also had the benefit of other advances, particularly in the control of burn wound infection, the effect of which could not be excluded from the comparison. Similarly, a large retrospective study reported a significant historical fall in mortality amongst paediatric burn patients (Tompkins *et al.*, 1988). The adoption of aggressive early excision was the most dramatic change identifiable over the study period, but the advent of this surgical modality had been accompanied by, and to some extent may have required, other improvements in the total care of these patients.

An earlier, randomised controlled trial of very early excision versus exposure treatment in Denmark (Sorensen *et al.*, 1984) showed no mortality advantage in any of the stratified patient groups, but shorter periods of hospitalisation and fewer infective episodes in patients with small burns of less than 15% BSA.

In another controlled trial, decreased mortality has been reported in young adults between 17 and 30 years old undergoing early total excision of burns over 30% BSA in the absence of inhalation injuries (Herndon *et al.*, 1989). These patients did not, however, appear to differ significantly from controls treated more conservatively on morbidity measures such as length of stay, number of septic episodes and total number of operative procedures.

Morbidity measures

The important parameters of overall morbidity such as the length of hospital stay, the number of operations required, time from first to last grafting procedure, total anaesthesia time and transfusion requirements have already been mentioned. The principal correlates of these criteria again appear to be the total percentage burn area and the extent of full-thickness burns, but the analysis may be influenced on the one hand by the surgical policy adopted (Heimbach, 1987), and on the other by the discharge criteria applied in a burns unit (Bowser *et al.*, 1983).

The nature and prevalence of infective episodes is often specifically cited in comparative reviews (Sorensen *et al.*, 1984; Herndon *et al.*, 1989), and is clearly relevant in a condition in which infection remains the single largest cause of death (Sevitt, 1966; Peck and Heimbach, 1989), and frequently underlies prolonged wound healing. Criteria for measurement of infection vary from study to study; Herndon *et al.* (1989) defines days of systemic infection on the basis of any of four of the following criteria being met:

- Temperature greater than 38.5 °C or less than 36.5 °C.
- Respiratory rate over 30/min.
- Blood glucose over 150 mg/dl (8.3 mmol).
- Platelet count less than $100 \times 10^3/l$.
- White-cell count greater than 15 or less than $5 \times 10^9/l$.
- Gastric aspirates greater than 200 ml/h.
- Wound containing more than 10^5 organisms/g on on quantitative bacteriology.

These are essentially correlates of a clinical diagnosis of septicaemia. Blood cultures in burns are notoriously unreliable, with only 15–20% positive cultures from clinically septicaemic patients (J. A. Clarke, personal communication). The use of biopsies to diagnose invasive wound infections is accepted (Pruitt and Foley, 1973) but not widely used because of its expense and inconvenience.

The rate at which burn wounds heal is a complex reflection of the depth of the original injury and the effectiveness of the measures employed for managing the burn wound, including surgical intervention and non-surgical treatment such as dressings and nutritional support. A wound closure index (WCI) has been proposed which defines an objective measurement of the rate of healing by the use of serial planimetry mapping, followed by the fitting of a graphical plot of unhealed burn area versus time with a regression line, the negative gradient of which is the wound closure index (Scott-Conner *et al.*, 1986). The authors applied logistic regression analysis of the WCI together with age and initial burn area to produce a rule to predict mortality probability, which reflected the observed tendency in most patients for mortality to decrease with more rapid wound closure. It could be recalculated at intervals during treatment to provide feedback on individual patient progress (Scott-Conner *et al.*, 1988).

In the context of modern burn management, survival of the burn victim should no longer be the sole indicator of successful outcome (Blades *et al.*, 1979; Petro and Salisbury, 1986; Patterson *et al.*, 1987). In burns as in major trauma in general (Yates, 1990), measures are needed which reflect long-term functional recovery of the patient both physically and psychologically.

The length of time before return to work or school following a major burn depends upon many factors, including time spent in treatment of the acute episode, in physical and psychological rehabilitation and in the early stages of reconstruction. As such it may serve as a broad measure of recovery (Chang and Herzog, 1976). It appears that time off work may be predicted mainly from the total extent of the burn wound, or by a regression analysis which also includes the extent of partial- and full-thickness burn and the time under active treatment (Helm and Walker, 1992). Ability to maintain preburn socioeconomic status has also been used qualitatively as an indicator of functional rehabilitation (Bartlett *et al.*, 1978).

In the elderly, the equivalent measure may be the degree of independence preserved after a burn injury. Whilst even small burns carry a higher mortality risk in the elderly, it appears that those who survive to be discharged do not show an accelerated death rate when compared with life tables for a similar, unburned population. However, a shift in lifestyle towards higher dependency is apparent for some patients both in the short and long term (Manktelow *et al.*, 1989).

The number and complexity of reconstructive operations required by survivors of burns are highly pertinent from a patient's own viewpoint; such measures reflect the amount of postburn deformity and disability, particularly from contracted scars, and the extent to which the overall therapeutic strategy has been able to limit such adverse outcomes. Reconstructive surgery is more likely to be required after large-area burns or burns with a large deep component, and the nature of this surgery has been studied (Prasad *et al.*, 1991). It appears that, in one unit at least, the trend over a 15-year period has been for survivors of all but the very largest burns to require fewer reconstructive operations. This decrease was attributed to improved burn wound management, and to the more liberal use of physiotherapy and splintage. Similarly, other authors (Huang *et al.*, 1978) had found a marked reduction in the frequency with which scar contracture release was required after the introduction of rigorous splintage and pressure garment therapy.

The disability which may result from burns of the hand affects the long-term functional outcome of a burn quite independently of the overall severity of the whole injury. Hand function may be represented by meticulous measurements of ranges of motion and sensation, with the addition of a functional assessment related to everyday tasks, to which may be added an aesthetic evaluation (Frist *et al.*, 1985). One report (Luster *et al.*, 1990) has suggested that finger joint stiffness or reactive torque could also be measured, and has introduced a method for making this measurement electronically.

A burn scar assessment scale has been devised (Sullivan *et al.*, 1990) which scores various physical parameters of a scar (pigmentation changes, vascularity, pliability and height above the normal skin surface). Interobserver agreement was acceptably reliable, and it was suggested that this type of rating could be used to evaluate the influence of treatment on scar maturation. There is, however, no agreed measure of the cosmetic acceptability of scars.

Much has been written on the psychological effects of a burn injury and the deformity and disability which may result (Malt, 1980). Patients react to the consequences of their burn in many different ways (Bernstein *et al.*, 1992), and their individual subjective responses may not correlate quantitatively with the apparent severity of their disfigurement. Many of the factors involved in psychosocial adjustment are not easily measured or quantified, although it is possible to describe aesthetic disfigurement in a reasonably consistent fashion.

Among recent surveys, adult burn victims discharged from the burns unit in Birmingham were studied using pre-existing psychological questionnaire-based scoring methods (Hospital Anxiety Depression Scale – HADS; Psychosocial Adjustment to Illness Scale – PAIS) (Wallace and Lees, 1988). Strong correlations were found between psychological morbidity at discharge and at 6 months and 2 years later, with little diminution in morbidity over time. Although other studies had found a relationship between psychological morbidity and burn severity (White, 1982), the main physical correlate in this series was the visibility of the disfigurement. This was also found in a recent survey of burn patients in Edinburgh (Williams and Griffiths, 1991), which used one of the same assessment methods (HADS) together with a questionnaire (Impact of Event Scale) designed to measure post-traumatic stress.

Australian burn patients were studied (Tucker, 1987), also using questionnaires (PAIS and Diagnostic Interview Schedule for Post-Traumatic Stress Disorder (DIS-PTSD)) as well as six self-report inventories of psychological well-being. Here also, a poor association was found between indicators of physical severity and psychological outcome measures. In addition, this study identified a group of patients with late-onset post-traumatic stress disorder (PTSD). PTSD has been reported as a sporadic outcome of both major and minor burns. It may arise in patients injured in particularly stressful circumstances, or in some cases in those with a vulnerable personality (Courtemanche and Robinow, 1989).

Thus conventional severity scores and measures of physical morbidity or mortality probability may not on their own be appropriate tools to predict the psychological outcome of an individual burn injury. However, a separate, early psychological evaluation using established measures appears to be able to anticipate some longer-term problems.

Children and adolescent burn victims have been studied using specific psychological profiles. Patients between 8 and 16 years of age (Sawyer *et al.*, 1983) were examined by a technique which examines several potential psychological problem areas and evaluates school, home and social functioning. This study found different levels of adjustment in adolescent and pre-adolescent children, and suggested that apparently well-adjusted children might develop adverse psychological outcomes in adolescence. Other authors (Stoddard *et al.*, 1989) have found anxiety and depressive disorders existing in patients assessed several years after a childhood burn. Thus psychosocial outcomes may only be assessed fully in these patients in the long term.

Overall quality of life after burns has been examined using existing measures such as the Sickness Impact Profile (SIP), which measures recovery in a range of areas including physical well-being and independence (Patterson *et al.*, 1987). A Burn-Specific Health Scale (Blades *et al.*, 1982) has also been constructed by extracting items considered to be most relevant to burn patients from existing American inventories designed to assess general health (SIP), physical functioning (Index of Activities of Daily Living) and psychological well-being (General Well-Being Schedule), to which were added items suggested by burn patients and staff. It was suggested that the resulting 114-item scale might be valuable in identifying areas of rehabilitation requiring additional support, both in individual cases and in patient populations.

Multicentre databases

It has increasingly been recognised that many aspects of burn care cannot be studied adequately using the numbers of patients treated in individual burns units.

A voluntary registry of burn care and outcome was established in the USA in 1970 as the National Burn Information Exchange (NBIE) (Feller and Crane, 1970). A central database is maintained which contains a record of the nature of patients' burn wounds and their extent, together with epidemiological information regarding predisposing factors, burning agent and location, and details of concurrent injuries. Resuscitation requirements and details of wound closure surgery are recorded, as well as a checklist of complications and a broad evaluation of the condition at discharge. Further information is gathered about subsequent reconstructive procedures. Participating units receive an annual report on their own cases and on combined, summarised data for the entire database, and have access to specific analyses of similar data on request.

This large database, reported to contain information on 99 000 patients by 1985 and increasing by about 6000 records per year, has been used to investigate prognostic factors (Roi *et al.*, 1983; Feller and Jones, 1987), whilst indicating a steady improvement in survival rates and hospitalisation times over a 20-year period (Feller *et al.*, 1976, 1980; Feller and Jones, 1987). A comparison of contemporary survival rates between different hospitals within the NBIE showed positive correlations with speed of achieving wound closure, and with organisational factors which could together be described broadly as 'quality of care'.

A National Burn Injury Database (NBID) is currently being established as a collaborative venture between the British Burn Association (BBA) and the UK Major Trauma Outcome Study (MTOS) (K. Dunn, 1992, personal communication). Information is being collected from accident departments and burns units.

The MTOS incorporates information collected about patients at all stages from the scene of the accident and at all subsequent stages of their management; these data are accumulated anonymously on a central computer. The joint initiative which forms the NBID is part of a widening of the area of interest of the MTOS to include all forms of trauma nation-wide. Like the NBIE, the NBID aims to provide a regular overview of mortality and morbidity trends, as well as comparative performance figures for individual participating units, and details of specific patients whose outcome falls outside the expected range.

Data are at present being collected for patients who meet one or more of the following three criteria:

- Those admitted to hospital for formal resuscitation. This will therefore include adults with burns of 15% body surface area and greater and children with 10% or more BSA burns.
- All patients dying in hospital with a burn, scald or inhalation injury.
- All patients who are admitted for a proven or suspected inhalation injury.

Information gathered by the burn centre includes basic demographic and epidemiological data, an evaluation of the burn and associated injuries, and a record of the general status of the patient on arrival (Glasgow Coma Scale parameters; physiological variables such as core temperature, pulse, blood pressure and capillary refilling; plus clinical signs such as pallor, sweating, restlessness or cyanosis). Signs of smoke inhalation and the results of any confirming investigations are noted, and the presence of any pre-existing disease. All resuscitation measures are recorded.

Subsequent care is represented by the timing of the first grafting procedure and the grade of personnel involved, and the date of achieve-ment of complete skin cover. Details of nutritional support are recorded.

Morbidity and outcome measures requested include survival; lengths of stay in an ITU, in the burns unit and in hospital; time to complete healing; maintenance of body weight; and the presence of listed complica-tions. A semiquantitative estimate and description of physical disability at discharge is made.

The stated aims of the NBID are to provide a large, match-controlled database for outcome and other studies which may be beyond the numer-ical limitations of individual units, and to establish norms for participating units to use for comparative audit. In addition the database will be used by the MTOS to improve the Abbreviated Injury Scale, which at present characterises burn injuries poorly. This will allow greater comparability between Injury Severity Scores for injuries with a significant burns com-ponent and non-burn trauma. It is also the intention that epidemiological and outcome data together will allow effective planning of burn care in the UK for the future.

Acknowledgements

The author gratefully acknowledges the assistance of Mr K. Dunn FRCS, Co-ordinator, National Burn Injury Database. Enquiries about the NBID should be addressed to Mr Dunn care of the Department of Plastic Surgery, Withington Hospital, Manchester M20 8DR, UK.

References

Bartlett RH, Wingerson E, Simonton S, Allyn PA, Martinez S, Feinberg SD (1978) Rehabilitation following burn injury. *Surg. Clin. North Am.*; **58**: 1249

Bernstein NR, O'Connell K, Chedekel D (1992) Patterns of burn adjustment. *J. Burn Care Rehabil.*; **13**: 4–12

Blades BC, Jones C, Munster AM (1979) Quality of life after major burns. *J. Trauma*; **19**: 556–558

Blades BC, Mellis N, Munster AM (1982) A burn specific health scale. *J. Trauma*; **22**: 872–875

Bowser BH, Caldwell FT, Baker JA, Walls RC (1983) Statistical methods to predict morbidity and mortality: self assessment techniques for burn units. *Burns*; **9**: 318–326

Bull JP (1971) Revised analysis of mortality due to burns. *Lancet*; **ii**: 1133

Bull JP, Fisher AJ (1954) A study of mortality in a burns unit; a revised estimate. *Ann. Surg.*; **139**: 269–274

Bull JP, Squire JR (1949) A study of mortality in a burns unit. *Ann. Surg.*; **130**: 160–173

Chang FC, Herzog B (1976) Burn morbidity: a follow up study of physical and psychological disability. *Ann. Surg.*; **183**: 34–37

Clark CJ, Reid WH, Gilmour WH, Campbell D (1986) Mortality probability in victims of fire trauma: revised equation to include inhalation injury. *Br. Med. J.*; **292**: 1303–1305

Colebrook L (1950) *A New Approach to the Treatment of Burns and Scalds.* London: Fine Technical Publications

Courtemanche DJ, Robinow O (1989) Recognition and treatment of the post-traumatic stress disorder in the burn victim. *J. Burn Care Rehabil.*; **10**: 247–250

Cryer HG, Anigian GM, Miller FB, Malangoni MA, Weiner L, Polk HC (1991) Effects of early tangential excision and grafting on survival after burn injury. *Surg. Gynecol. Obstet.*; **173**: 449–453

Curreri PW, Luterman A, Braun DW, Shires GT (1980) Burn injury. Analysis of survival and hospitalization time for 937 patients. *Ann. Surg.*; **192**: 472–477

Feller I, Crane KH (1970) National burn information exchange. *Surg. Clin. North Am.*; **50**: 1425–1436

Feller I, Jones CA (1987) The National Burn Information Exchange. *Surg. Clin. North Am.*; **67**: 167–189

Feller I, Flora JD, Bawol R (1976) Baseline results of therapy for burned patients. *JAMA*; **236**: 1943–1947

Feller I, Tholen D, Cornell RG (1980) Improvements in burn care, 1965 to 1976. *JAMA*; **244**: 2074–2078

Frist W, Ackroyd F, Burke J, Bondoc C (1985) Long-term functional results of selective treatment of hand burns. *Am. J. Surg.*; **149**: 516–521

Heimbach DM (1987) Early burn excision and grafting. *Surg. Clin. North Am.*; **67**: 93–107

Helm PA, Walker SC (1992) Return to work after burn injury. *J. Burn Care Rehabil.*; **13**: 53–57

Herndon DN, Barrow RE, Rutan RL, Rutan TC, Desai MH, Abston S (1989) A comparison of conservative versus early excision therapies in severely burned patients. *Ann. Surg.*; **209**: 547–552

Huang TT, Blackwell SJ, Lewis SR (1978) Ten years experience in managing patients with burn contractures of axilla, elbow, wrist and knee joints. *Plast. Reconstr. Surg.*; **61**: 70–76

Jackson DM (1981) Foreword. In Cason JS (ed) *The Treatment of Burns.* London: Chapman and Hall

Jackson DM, Stone PA (1972) Tangential excision and grafting of burns: the method and a review of fifty consecutive cases. *Br. J. Plast. Surg.*; **25**: 416–426

Janzekowic A (1970) A new concept in the early excision and immediate grafting of burns. *J. Trauma*; **10**: 1103–1108

Krob MJ, D'Amico FJ, Ross DL (1991) Do trauma scores accurately predict outcomes for patients with burns? *J. Burn Care Rehabil.*; **12**: 560–563

Lawrence JC (1977) The treatment of small burns with a chlorhexidine-medicated tulle-gras. *Burns*; 3: 239-244

Lawrence JC (1992) Burn bacteriology during the last 50 years. *Burns*; 18: (suppl) S23-29

Luster SH, Patterson PE, Cioffi WG, Mason AD, McManus WF, Pruitt BA (1990) An evaluation device for quantifying joint stiffness in the burned hand. *J. Burn Care Rehabil.*; 11: 312-317

Malt U (1980) Long-term psychosocial follow-up studies of burned adults: review of the literature. *Burns*; 6: 190

Manktelow A, Meyer AA, Herzog SR, Peterson HD (1989) Analysis of life expectancy and living status of elderly patients surviving a burn injury. *J. Trauma*; 29: 203-207

McManus WF, Mason AD, Pruitt BA (1989) Excision of the burn wound in patients with large burns. *Arch. Surg.*; 124: 718-720

Monafo WW (1992) Then and now: 50 years of burn treatment. *Burns*; 18: (suppl) S7-10

Patterson DR, Questad KA, Boltwood MD, Covey MH, de Lateur BJ, Dutcher KA, Heimbach DM, Marvin JA (1987) Patient self-reports three months after sustaining a major burn. *J. Burn Care Rehabil.*; 8: 274-279

Peck MD, Heimbach DM (1989) Does early excision of burn wounds change the pattern of mortality? *J. Burn Care Rehabil.*; 10: 7-10

Petro JA, Salisbury RE (1986) Rehabilitation of the burn patient. *Clin. Plast. Surg.*; 13: 145-149

Peterson VA, Murphy JR, Haddix T, Ford P, Anderson SJ, Bartle EJ (1988) Identification of novel prognostic indicators in burned patients. *J. Trauma*; 28: 632-637

Phipps AR, Lawrence JC (1988) Comparison of hydrocolloid dressings and medicated tulle-gras in the treatment of outpatient burns. In Ryan TJ (ed) *Beyond Occlusion – an environment for recovery*, London: Royal Society of Medicine Congress and Symposium series, no 136

Prasad JK, Bowden ML, Thomson PD (1991) A review of the reconstructive needs of 3167 survivors of burn injury. *Burns*; 17: 302-305

Pruitt BA Jr, Foley FD. (1973) The use of biopsies in burn patient care. *Surgery*; 73: 887-897

Roi LD, Flora JD, Davis TM, Wolfe RA (1983) Two new burn severity indices. *J. Trauma*; 23: 1023-1029

Sawyer MG, Minde K, Zuker R (1983) The burned child – scarred for life? *Burns*; 9: 205-213

Scott-Conner CEH, Coil JA, Conner HF, Mack ME (1986) Wound closure index: a guide to prognosis in burned patients. *J. Trauma*; 26: 123-127

Scott-Conner CEH, Meydrech E, Wheeler WE, Coil JA (1988) Quantitation of rate of wound closure and the prediction of death following major burns. *Burns*; 14: 373-378

Sevitt S (1966) Death after burning. *Med. Sci. Law.*; 1: 36-44

Shirani KZ, Pruitt BA, Mason AD (1987) The influence of inhalation injury and pneumonia on burn mortality. *Ann. Surg.*; 205: 82

Sorensen B, Fisker NP, Steensen JP, Kalaja E (1984) Acute excision or exposure treatment? Final results of a three-year randomised controlled clinical trial. *Scand. J. Plast. Reconstr. Surg.*; 18: 87-93

Stern M, Waisbren BA (1978) Comparison of methods of predicting burn mortality. *Burns*; 6: 119

Stoddard FJ, Norman DK, Murphy M (1989) A diagnostic outcome survey of children and adolescents with severe burns. *J. Trauma*; 29: 471-477

Sullivan T, Smith J, Kermode J, McIver E, Courtemanche DJ (1990) Rating the burn scar. *J. Burn Care Rehabil.*; 11: 256-260

Thompson PB, Herndon DN, Traber DL, Abton S (1986) Effect on mortality of inhalational injury. *J. Trauma*; 26: 163-165

Tobiasen J, Hiebert JM, Edlich RF (1982) The abbreviated burn severity index. *Ann. Emerg. Med.*; 11: 260-262

Tompkins RG, Remensnyder JP, Burke JF, Tompkins DM, Hilton JF, Schoenfeld DA,

Behringer GE, Bondoc CC, Briggs SE, Quinby WC (1988) Significant reductions in mortality for children with burn injuries through the use of prompt eschar excision. *Ann. Surg.*; **208**: 577–585

Tucker P (1987) Psychological problems among adult burn victims. *Burns*; **13**: 7–14

Wallace LM, Lees J (1988) A psychological follow-up study of adult patients discharged from a British burn unit. *Burns*; **14**: 39–42

White AC (1982) Psychiatric study of patients with severe burn injuries. *Br. Med. J.*; **ii**: 465–467

Williams EE, Griffiths TA (1991) Psychological consequences of burn injury. *Burns*; **17**: 478–480

Wolfe RA, Roi LD, Flora JD, Feller I, Cornell RG (1983) Mortality differences and speed of wound closure among specialised burn care facilities. *JAMA*; **250**: 763–766

Yates DW (1990) Scoring systems for trauma. *Br. Med. J.*; **xi**: 1090–1094

Zawacki BE, Azen SP, Imbus SH, Chang YC (1979) Multifactorial probit analysis of mortality in burned patients. *Ann. Surg.*; **189**: 1–5

Zöch G, Schemper M, Kyral E, Meissl G (1992) Comparison of prognostic indices for burns and assessment of their accuracy. *Burns*; **18**: 109–112

Chapter 8

Missile and gunshot wounds

S. J. E. Matthews

Introduction

Surgery for the victims of war is different from the type of surgery practised for civilian injuries. War wounds are associated with massive destruction of tissues and are always grossly contaminated.

Missiles not only include bullets and shrapnel but any other object from the path or shockwave of an explosion. These fragments may then become secondary missiles. Secondary missiles, depending on their ballistics, would present with different injury profiles.

There is a trend in modern warfare to cause maiming rather than death, so as to overload logistic support routes. The introduction, in 1985, by Haywood of Battlefield Trauma Life-Support (BATLS) Scheme (Advanced Trauma Life Support in a battlefield setting) resulted in individuals trained in BATLS and ATLS in forward areas of the battlefield, for the first time, in the Gulf war. This philosophy has resulted in the survival of casualties with unprecedented injury severity (Ryan, 1992).

The battlefield casualties would have a diverse range of injuries, not only of an orthopaedic nature, but multisystem, such as burns, chemical or otherwise. Chemical agents may be mixed with high explosive and permanent respiratory damage may be inflicted. Isolated injuries to one system are unusual. The psychological and neurological impact to these patients are major outcome factors and, these may be compounded by auditory and ocular deficit.

Recognised systems

There is no single unifying outcome measure for use in battlefield casualties. The nearest recognized system which fits this description is the Army Fitness Score, known by the acronym of PULHHEEMS, which is in regular use (Ministry of Defence, 1987).

Another system currently in use is the Army Personnel Fitness Assessment (APFA) which gives a combined overall fitness score. Both the PULHHEEMS and APFA have been used as outcome measures before (Bowyer and Matthews, 1991; Hoad and Clay, 1992).

APFA

The usual purpose of the test is to measure the basic physical structure of a military unit and random samples such as 20% may be taken. It is also used to indicate the physical level of a recruit and to monitor the effectiveness of his training as it proceeds. The APFA consists of a strength test and an endurance test. The strength test is in two sections. First, the maximum number of repetitions of press-ups, trunk curls, heaves and dips are all added together. There is no time limit set for any of these exercises but any particular set must be performed continuously without rests. The second part consists of measuring the maximum height reached by the outstretched hand which is corrected for height. This is called the vertical jump test (VJT).

The score of both parts is added to the endurance score. Endurance is tested by the time taken on a 1.5-mile best-effort run with a score being read from a table (Figure 8.1). The combined scores give the overall APFA score.

Heaves

The subject hangs on a beam by the hands with the feet clear of the floor. The arms are bent until the bottom of the chin is level with the top of the beam. A score of 1 is awarded for each heave.

Trunk curls

This is performed on an inclined balancing bench, one end fixed into no. 10 wall bar up from the ground. From the supine position, feet secured,

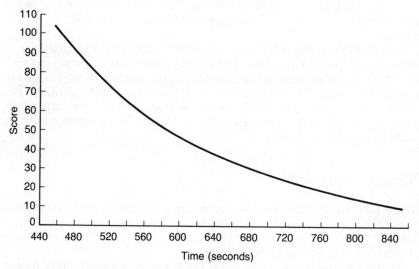

Figure 8.1 Scoring for the APFA endurance test. The test is scored depending on how quickly one-and-a-half miles can be run. The score is read from a table, here it has been presented graphically for convenience and to illustrate the non-linear relationship between the score and the time taken

hands clasped behind the neck, the trunk is curled forwards until the vertical position is reached. A slight knee bend is permitted. Score 1 point for each curl.

Dips

With the body supported with straight arms on parallel bars with feet clear of the ground, the body is lowered to achieve at least a right angle at the elbow and then up again to full extension at the elbow.

The vertical jump test

The subject is stood by a wall. The arm nearest the wall is raised and the fullest extent of reach with fingers outstretched is marked. The arm is lowered, the knees are bent and a standing jump is performed to touch the wall as high as possible. The difference in the two marks is measured. One point is scored for every inch, or part-inch, jumped above 10 inches.

In the heave, dip and trunk curl tests, a half point is awarded when over 50% of movement is achieved in each case. The total score is rounded down to a complete number.

A grade is awarded according to performance (Table 8.1) of either an individual or the mean value of a group or military unit.

Grade A is for individuals or units requiring a high standard of physical fitness and grade B represents a good all-round standard of fitness. Grade C is associated with reduced arm, shoulder and trunk strength and grade D as with C but with reduced stamina too. Grade E is considered a minimum standard of fitness and individuals who fail to meet it should be referred to a medical officer before training is commenced.

PULHHEEMS

The PULHHEEMS is a system of medical classification and is designed to:

A. Provide a functional assessment of the individual's capacity for work.
B. Assist in expressing the physical and mental attributes appropriate to individual employments with the army.
C. Assist in posting people to the employment for which they are most suited in the light of their physical, intellectual and emotional make-up.
D. Provide a system which is administratively simple to apply.

Table 8.1 The APFA performance grading

Grades	Stamina	Heaves	Dips	Curls	VJT	Total
A	55	11	11	22	11	110
B	50	10	10	20	10	100
C	50	8	7	15	10	90
D	40	8	7	15	10	80
E	33	5	5	10	7	60

A 'P' value of 0 to 8 is awarded to an individual. The P value awarded depends on the scores allocated in the PULHHEEMS categories known as qualities (see below). In the quality category, a score of 1–8 in declining function is awarded for each category, the score is referred to as a degree. (Appendix 8.1). The degree of the P quality will determine the individual's PULHHEEMS employment standard or PES. The PES categories available are:

1. Forwards everywhere (FE): this means employable on full combatant duties in any area and in any part of the world.
2. Forward temperate (FT): this means employable on combatant duties in any area in temperate climates only.
3. Lines of communication everywhere (LE): this means normally employed in communication zones or bases in any part of the world, but may be employed in a combatant zone in any role that is not primarily a fighting one.
4. Lines of communication temperate (LT): as for LE, but in temperate climates only.
5. Bases everywhere (BE): employable in the base area only in any part of the world.
6. Bases temperate (BT): as for BE but in temperate climates only.
7. Home only (HO): employable in countries close to home provided adequate and suitable medical facilities are available to treat the condition for which the individual has been so graded. This may be designated as HO (UK), i.e. employable in the UK only.
8. None: unfit for duty either indefinitely or temporarily.

The qualities assessed under the PULHHEEMS system are as follows:

Physical capacity (P)

Indicates an individual's general physical characteristics and his potential capacity to develop physical stamina with training.

Upper limbs (U)

Indicates the functional use of the hands, arms, shoulder girdle and upper spine, and in general the individual's ability to handle weapons. Pathological conditions of the upper limbs, having a constitutional basis, may also affect the assessment under P.

Locomotion (L)

This indicates the individual's ability to march. Pathological conditions affecting marching ability which have a constitutional basis, will also affect the assessment under P.

Hearing (HH)

This simply records the ability to hear. Diseases of the ear are assessed under the quality of P.

Eyesight (EE)

This records the ability to see with the right and left eye. Diseases of the eyes are assessed under the quality of P.

Mental capacity (M)

This indicates the individual's ability to learn army duties. Assessment is the psychologist's problem and is based on:

1. Impression given on personal interview with particular regard to alertness and the ability to apply intelligence possessed.
2. Record of school and occupational progress.
3. Selection test results with particular reference to those tests most closely concerned with the measurement of intelligence itself and acquired ability.

Stability (S)

Indicates emotional stability and is the psychiatrist's province.

Appendix 8.1 demonstrates the measure of degrees under different qualities.

Discussion

Although both the APFA and PULHHEEMS systems are flawed, there are advantages to be found in both systems. The advantage of the APFA is that a direct measurement can be made and therefore comparison and statistical handling is facilitated. Measurement is accurate and fairly reproducible and can be assessed by unskilled personnel without special equipment. The disadvantages are that the APFA score is really a measure of fitness and does not reflect the generalised level of function. Furthermore certain injuries will not be reflected by a change in APFA score. Another disadvantage to the APFA system is that the score depends on the tester's motivation. This effect has been eliminated in the past by using this score to assess highly motivated individuals as in those who are undergoing recruit training (Hoad and Clay, 1992).

The PULHHEEMS system is certainly a better overall assessment than the APFA score of the total functional capacity of an individual. It is, in a sense, modular, and each quality can be used as an outcome measure in isolation of the others. It is in routine use in the army and every serviceman has a PULHHEEMS rating on recruitment and is periodically assessed at set ages throughout his career. Furthermore medical boards are held regularly when specialist opinions are sought at military hospitals. Current PULHHEEMS grade are recorded in the patient's own personal medical documents which are readily available. The PULHHEEMS system has also previously been used as an outcome measure for the purposes of research (Bowyer and Matthews, 1991). It is long established in the Services and as recognized implications for employment according to functional capacity.

The PULHHEEMS system, however, is complex and unwieldy. It is inaccurate due to the relatively subjective nature of some of the 'quality' definitions and is open to misinterpretation. The scoring system itself is relatively illogical as it does not progress in simple numerical steps. Furthermore the definitions of the different quality will vary according to sex and rank. Another disadvantage is that it is not directly comparable with the Royal Navy or Royal Air Force scoring systems. Nevertheless it can be, and has been, utilised as an outcome measure of function. It is applicable to multisystem disorders, such as those encountered with missile and gunshot wounds and, in a military setting, can be used to compare the outcome with a previous score, taking into account pre-injury functional level. This, of course, assumes a meaningful pre-injury score which, not uncommonly, has been awarded with bias and according to individuals' socioeconomic circumstance and usefulness to his service.

References

Bowyer GW, Matthews SJE (1991) Anterior cruciate ligament reconstruction using the Gore-tex ligament. *J.R. Army Med. Corps.*; **137**: 69–75

Hoad NA, Clay DN (1992) Smoking impairs the response to a physical training programme. *J.R. Army Med. Corps.*; **138**: 115–117

Ministry of Defence (1987) *PULHHEEMS Administrative Pamphlet 1987.* Ministry of Defence D-DM (A)-1-77-9E.

Ryan JM (1992) Editorial. *J.R. Army Med. Corps.*; **138**: 6–7

Appendix 8.1 Guide to PULHHEEMS – factors to be considered in functional interpretation of degrees of each quality – men

	P	U	L	HH	EE	M	S
Degrees	*Age, build, strength and stamina*	*Strength, range of movement and general efficiency of upper arm, shoulder, girdle and upper back*	*Strength, range of movement and efficiency of feet, legs, pelvic girdle and lower back*	*Acuity of hearing*	*Visual acuity. The degrees entered under EE are simple records of visual acuity, and bear no relationship to the degrees under the remaining qualities. Eye disease may, however, affect the degree entered under P*	*Mental capacity*	*Emotional stability*
1	Fit after training for full strain and fatigue on combatant duty. Fit to withstand exposure to all kinds of weather. A front line fighter in any part of the world	Muscle power above average. Must be able to handle a rifle and do heavy manual work including digging, pushing, dragging, heaving, lifting and climbing. All tasks carried out with rapidity and efficiency	Capable of very severe locomotor strain for 5 or 6 days. Can undertake forced marches and fight at the end of such marches. Can run, climb, jump, crawl, dig and perform all kinds of labour quickly	Good hearing	Normal vision		

Appendix 8.1 *Cont*

	P	U	L	HH	EE	M	S
2	Fit after training for normal work or strain but unable to endure 'extreme' degrees for long periods. A front line fighter in any part of the world	Muscle power average. Able to do all a U1 man can do but at a slower pace	Same as L1 but pace may be slower	Acceptable practical hearing for Service purposes	Minor defect of vision	Ability under Army conditions to learn to perform successfully full combatant duties. Includes those who can be trained as tradesmen and specialists	Emotionally fit to perform Army duties adequately under full combatant conditions in any part of the world
3	Fit for ordinary work. Has not the stamina even after training to endure the strain and fatigue of full combatant duty. Fit for restricted service in any part of the world	Must be able to use a weapon for defensive purposes and be capable of less severe forms of manual work than U2	Capable of marching 5 miles or further in an emergency. Able to stand for periods of at least 2 hours. Fit for guard duties	Impaired hearing. At this level most personnel are unfit for entry into the Services. Serving personnel are fit for duty consonant with their impairment	Moderate defect of vision but able to shoot with reasonable accuracy	Ability under Army conditions to learn to perform simple labouring duties, including fitness to bear arms in self-defence	Although having a history of emotional instability, are at present well adjusted and fit to serve in any part of the world in a role which is not primarily a fighting one
4	Fit in temperate climates, after training, for full strain and fatigue on combatant duty. A front-line fighter in temperate climates			Very poor hearing. This grading will be awarded only exceptionally	Able to read only half-way down the chart. Unfit to drive if both eyes are 4		

5	Fit in temperate climates, after training, for normal work or strain, but unable to endure extreme degrees for long periods. A front-line fighter in temperate climates			All detail blurred but able to shoot in self-defence		
6	Fit for ordinary work. Has not the stamina even after training to endure the strain and fatigue of full combatant duties. Fit for restricted service in temperate climates			All detail severely blurred		While having a history of emotional instability are sufficiently well adjusted to serve in temperate climates in a role which is not primarily a fighting one
7	Capable of performing useful Army duties within limits of his disabilities. Not likely to break down if suitably employed which includes time for regular meals and rest. Service in the UK only	Capable of sedentary and routine work of a higher type. Includes personnel unable to bear arms on account of physical disability (ankylosis of elbow, etc.). Service in the base area at home or overseas	Able to walk 2 miles a day at own pace. Can stand for moderate but not prolonged periods. Service in the base area at home or overseas	Able to read only top letter of the chart	Because of low mental capacity are unfit to bear arms, but are capable of simple labouring duties under supervision including a minimum of responsibilities. Service in the UK only	Emotionally fit to perform Army duties adequately under living conditions favourable to the individual in the UK

Appendix 8.1 *Cont*

	P	U	L	HH	EE	M	S
8	Medically unfit for any form of service	Medically unfit for any form of service	Medically unfit for any form of service	Medically unfit for any form of service	Unable to read the top letter of the chart but able to move across country and engage targets at close range	Medically unfit for any form of service	Medically unfit for any form of service

Chapter 9

Union and non-union of fractures

J. G. Andrew and P. R. Kay

Fracture healing is a complex biological process which ultimately can restore complete functional integrity to a bone. Unlike most tissues, which repair by scarring, this tissue can restore itself to bone which is indistinguishable from the original (McKibbin, 1978). In children, and occasionally in adults, the remodelling may be so complete that, eventually, there is no radiographic trace of the fracture having occurred.

The desired outcome from a fracture is sound union within a reasonably short time frame. Usually, if a fracture is not united at 4 months it is considered to have delayed union, and if not united at 6 months to be a non-union. However, in clinical terms fracture union cannot be viewed in isolation, various associated problems must be assessed before the outcome for a particular patient can be assessed as satisfactory. At a minimum, these include freedom from pain (from algodystrophy or other causes), satisfactory fracture alignment, good soft tissue healing, freedom from infection and normal or near normal function of the associated joints. Thus a patient with a soundly united os calcis fracture who still has pain and severe limitation of subtalar movement at 1 year can only be regarded as a poor result, even though the fracture may have been soundly united within the first 2 months. Therefore, measures of union and non-union of fractures generally only give a small part of the overall outcome measure of a particular fracture; they are more important in those fractures which are at a relatively high risk of slow healing or non-union. It will become clear that there are no entirely satisfactory measures available for this process. However, further investigation would be worthwhile as:

- Early detection of abnormal responses may indicate changes in management to avoid morbidity and disability.
- Detection of union would reduce overtreatment of fractures.
- Precise detection of non or delayed union may reduce the problem of re-fracture.

The fractures which are at high risk of delayed union or non-union fall into two groups. First, fractures within or associated with joints and second, high energy fractures with associated soft tissue stripping. Fractures of the first type include subcapital fractures of the femoral and humeral necks, scaphoid fractures and odontoid peg fractures. The prime example of the second type of high risk fracture is the tibial shaft fracture. This bone has a relatively incomplete muscular envelope, so that soft tissue stripping may jeopardise the blood supply of this bone more than in other fractures. Further, the fractured tibia is at a high risk of being open because of its subcutaneous surface. The measures of union and non-union appropriate to these two types of fracture are often different.

The overall size of the problem of delayed union of fractures is not clear. Estimates of the incidence of delayed union in tibial fractures have varied from 2% to 17%. Similarly, there are varying estimates of delayed union of scaphoid fractures (reviewed in Gelberman *et al.*, 1989). Non-union frequently affects the victims of high energy injuries. Patients with non-unions are often young men who are wage earners, so that the social costs of the resulting morbidity are high.

Measurement of the problems of fracture healing may be divided into three phases. First, various predictive measures may be employed. These are used at an early stage after the fracture and include clinical and radiological assessment of the injury for poor prognostic indicators. Second, the process of fracture healing may be measured in various ways. This is the phase which has attracted most interest, and a wide variety of tools have been tried. The plethora of available techniques reflects the value which would be placed upon a reliable test to discriminate between fractures which will heal without assistance and those which will require intervention to obtain healing within a reasonable period of time. This requirement for a predictor of fracture healing is particularly felt with tibial fractures; such fractures are often treated conservatively for many months before it is acknowledged that a problem of fracture healing exists. For fractures which have not united after this period of expectant management, it is perceived that this time has been wasted.

The final phase which may be measured is outcome of fracture healing, essentially when the processes of fracture healing are complete. It is very difficult to state when the process has run its course, and to say when a delayed union becomes a non-union. Measurement of this phase of fracture healing has attracted much less interest than measurement of the process of healing; a chapter devoted to final outcome measures of fracture healing would be extremely short!

Tools to measure the various stages

Predictive tools

The tools available to measure fracture healing may be used in various ways. These include individual clinical assessment, scientific examination of process and surgical techniques and audit of clinical performance. In all of these except the first, patients are considered as groups. Under these circumstances, valid conclusions can only be drawn from results if some assessment and grading is made of the presenting patients and their injuries. Accordingly, when considering outcomes it is important to consider factors which are known to have prognostic significance for fracture union, so that groups of patients are not compared inappropriately.

Factors predictive of fracture union or non-union fall into two groups, those about the patient's overall condition and those specific to the particular fracture. In the first category, systemic factors known to adversely affect fracture healing include diabetes mellitus (Loder, 1988), osteogenesis imperfecta (Gamble *et al.*, 1988), scurvy and rickets and other abnormalities of vitamin D metabolism. There is some anecdotal evidence that advanced HIV infection may cause problems with fracture healing. This might be expected given the important role that inflammatory cells are thought to play in wound and fracture healing, and may become a more important consideration in the future. Rheumatoid arthritis may adversely affect fracture healing (Bogoch *et al.*, 1991): this is probably due to the diffuse osteopenia associated with rheumatoid arthritis (Hartel *et al.*, 1976).

There are at least two factors which are known to enhance fracture healing. The first is youth: fractures in children are common but delayed union is extremely rare, and times to union are short. Results of severe tibial fractures are worse in the elderly than in young adults, with amputation being more frequently required (Court Brown *et al.*, 1990). The second factor is head injury. The link between severe head injury and enhanced callus formation is now well established, and may be related to a circulating factor (Bidner *et al.*, 1990).

A wide variety of fracture-specific factors have been noted to be associated with a poor prognosis for fracture union; assessment of this risk is one reason for the many fracture grading systems which have been developed. Some of these are listed in Table 9.1. Grading systems exist for fractures of most other bones, but in the context of union and non-union they are of less relevance. One severe problem with radiological grading systems is interobserver variability (Frandsen *et al.*, 1988). This must be specifically considered as a source of error in studies of outcomes. The grading systems listed are mostly based on radiological appearances. Exceptions include the Gustilo and Edwards grading systems. The Gustilo grading describes the severity of soft tissue damage in open fractures. The value of this method is that it reflects both the risk of infection and the degree of soft tissue and vascular damage. Bone infection after fracture is little short of disastrous (Kelly, 1984; Cattaneo *et al.*,

Table 9.1 Fracture grading systems

Grading system	Bone/injury	Reference	Reference on relevance to fracture union
Neer	Neck of humerus	Neer, 1970	
Garden	Intracapsular fracture neck of femur	Garden, 1961	Nieminen and Satokari, 1975; Frandsen and Andersen, 1981
Pauwels	Intracapsular fracture neck of femur	Pauwels, 1935	Nieminen and Satokari, 1975
Herbert	Scaphoid fracture	Herbert and Fisher, 1984	Herbert and Fisher, 1984
Edwards	Tibia	Edwards, 1965	Edwards, 1965
Gustilo	Tibia	Gustilo *et al.*, 1984	Court Brown *et al.*, 1990

1992). The original system used grades 1, 2 and 3. It quickly became clear that the major problems of union and infection arose within the grade 3 group, so that this has now been divided into three subcategories (Gustilo *et al.*, 1984). This system has proven to be a good predictor of union (Court Brown *et al.*, 1990). The system allows a simple assessment of the soft tissue damage sustained by the bone, which is likely to reflect the degree of vascular damage incurred, which has a profound effect on fracture healing (Brueton *et al.*, 1990).

The Edwards system for tibial fractures includes elements of both soft tissue and radiological assessment; however, it is complex and has not been widely adopted. Despite this, it is clear that fracture position is crucial in assessment of the probability of normal healing. Displacement of the fracture reflects both the degree of soft tissue damage which has occurred at the time of injury and the distance which the reparative process has to bridge. The healing process is capable of spanning a moderate distance, but overdistraction of fractures leads to non-union (Nicol, 1964). This is confirmed experimentally in many animal models of non-union which use a fracture gap of greater than a critical size to cause non-union (Nilsson *et al.*, 1986). Grading systems for other fractures generally include elements reflecting the amount of displacement.

Radionuclide bone scanning offers a method of assessing response by the bone ends in a fracture. If it is performed in the early postfracture stage (in the first week) it may indicate the likelihood of problems with fracture healing due to impaired vascularity. This has proved useful with displaced femoral neck fractures (Stromqvist *et al.*, 1984; Alberts *et al.*, 1987; Alberts, 1990). Its value at this stage after tibial shaft fractures is less clear (Oni *et al.*, 1989c). Bone scanning has been extensively employed at an early stage after scaphoid fractures (e.g. Ganel *et al.*, 1979), but appears to have been used exclusively to determine whether an occult fracture is present, rather than whether it will unite. Most bone scan studies of fractures have not examined blood phase images, so their indication of vascularity of a fracture is indirect. Magnetic resonance imaging (MRI) is a powerful method of investigating the vascularity of bones. MR spectroscopy has been employed experimentally to investigate fracture site pH – it was found that abnormally healing fractures have a lower pH than normal fractures (Newman *et al.*, 1985, 1987) – however this technique remains experimental. MRI has been use to investigate tibial fractures (Laasonen *et al.*, 1989), but no useful conclusions were reached about whether it was of value in predicting non-union. Further investigations of this modality of imaging will be required to determine whether it has a prognostic value for fracture union. A final prognostic tool for assessing risk of non-union is measurement of fracture site stability. Most mechanical tests have been employed later in the course of fracture repair. However, Rehnberg and Olerud (1989) measured stability of intracapsular femoral neck fractures using a strain gauge during the course of operation to fix the fractures. Instability at this stage was strongly correlated with failure of union later.

Finally, the influence of modality of treatment on the prospects for healing must be appreciated. At one extreme, it is possible to abolish the callus response in diaphyseal fractures by rigid fixation (Terjesen and

Apalset, 1988; O'Sullivan *et al.*, 1989). Conversely, excessive movement of a fracture may be associated with hypertrophic non-union. Ideally a mechanical prescription could be made for each fracture to optimise the prospects for healing, however, at present insufficient knowledge of the healing process is available to permit this. Axial fracture fixation may empirically be associated with improved results and several groups have reported good results with intramedullary nailing of tibial fractures (Collins *et al.*, 1990; Folleras *et al.*, 1990). Additional risks occur with internal fixation, where surgical approaches may increase the amount of soft tissue damage and permit ingress of bacterial contaminants to areas of damaged tissue. Under some circumstances, these risks are worth taking to obtain a good fracture position and stability but the potential for later problems is undeniable. The depressing sight of a patient with an infected non-union after plating is less common today than in the past but does still occur.

Process tools

As indicated above, the largest group of tools for measurement of fracture union and non-union are related to assessing the process of fracture healing. The most commonly employed method is a combination of clinical history, clinical stiffness testing and examination of plain X-rays. There is evidence that none of these is sufficient alone, although the combined power of the three methods does not appear to have been formally tested against a more objective method. There are no recent reports of the value (or otherwise) of the patient's assessment of fracture union. This may reflect a hopeless degree of subjectivity and interobserver error which would arise in such a study, none the less, the results might be of interest. Clinical history is frequently used as the ultimate arbiter of satisfactory union; few clinicians would discount a complaint of persistent pain on weight bearing in the early postfracture period. This form of assessment may be formalised by measuring the amount of weight born by the patient via the injured limb.

The reliability of clinical (manual) stiffness testing was examined by Matthews *et al.* (1974) and Hammer and Norrbom (1984). Both devised experimental models simulating fractured bones. Hammer and Norrbom's model permitted the stiffness of the model to be varied. It was found that the minimum angulation which could be detected was about 4°; this remained roughly constant with varying stiffness of the model. Relatively large forces will have to be applied to fractures to achieve angulations of this magnitude (especially with distal tibial fractures, where the lever arm between the heel, where the angulatory force is usually applied, and the fracture, is short). Accordingly, it is unlikely that this angulation is often achieved in practice in fractures which are clinically healed. Clinical testing may determine whether grossly low stiffness is present, or whether there is severe pain on stressing. Neither of these is objective and both will depend on the force exerted by the examiner. The value of manual evaluation of fracture union remains uncertain.

Plain X-rays are probably the most widely used way of examining the process of fracture union. Methods which have been used in examination of plain radiographs include assessment of callus size, haziness and obliteration of the fracture gap and whether bony trabeculae can be seen to cross the fracture gap. Several authors have examined the reliability of orthopaedic surgeons in determining union from plain X-rays. Nicholls *et al.* (1979) examined interobserver agreement for union of X-rays of rabbit experimental fractures, which were subsequently tested for strength of union. They concluded that orthopaedic surgeons were not very reliable at determining early bone union. Given the standardised nature of the fractures, this is discouraging to say the least!

Hammer *et al.* (1985) examined the reliability of X-ray assessment of fracture healing in human tibial fractures. They measured fracture stiffness using a radiographic method of determining angulation to an applied load and compared these results with clinical evaluation of the X-rays for union. Fifty-five per cent of fractures judged to be unstable on stiffness measurement were assessed as united by clinicians examining the standard X-rays. Conversely, in those fractures thought to be stable on stiffness testing 44% were judged not to be united by clinical evaluation of X-rays. Similar results were found for scaphoid fractures by Dias *et al.*, (1988). It appears that clinician evaluation of plain X-rays is not a satisfactory method of assessing fracture union, with significant interobserver variation and a risk of both under- and overestimating the degree of union. In Hammer's study, the chance of a clinician predicting whether or not a fracture was mechanically sound was only 50%.

Attempts have been made to quantify the interpretation of plain radiographs of healing fractures. At the simplest level, X-ray scoring methods have been proposed. Lane and Sandhu (1987) gave scores to evidence of bone formation, evidence of union at the fracture gap and evidence of remodelling. Panjabi *et al.* (1985) found that, in experimental fractures, the best predictors of fracture stiffness were cortical continuity, callus area and overlap of the bony fragments. Both of these were suggested in papers describing animal models. Many of the suggested parameters remain subjective, and the methods do not appear to have been tested on clinical fractures against any more objective measure of fracture healing. Oni *et al.* (1991) examined the relationship of clinical factors pertinent to fracture healing (trauma severity, fracture morphology, displacement and fracture gap) and callus size and volume. No relationship was found between the clinical factors examined and the amount of callus produced. These results are thus at a degree of variance with those in animal models. This indicates that measurement of callus area and other elements of X-ray scoring require specific validation in clinical fractures before being recommended for widespread use.

Tiedeman *et al.* (1990) produced experimental fractures in dogs and measured the intensity of light transmitted through standard X-rays. They termed this roentgenographic densitometry. They found a high degree of correlation between the density of the callus (as measured by the lowest measurable density in the osteotomy gap using a 0.5 × 14 mm window) and the stiffness of the bones. They suggested that this method might be clinically useful. One of the more obvious problems with this is achieving standard X-ray projections in a clinical setting. It is possible to both record and repeat tube to bone distances and exposures, to monitor fracture healing. However most orthopaedic and X-ray departments have not so far managed to overcome the logistic difficulties involved. An alternative method of approaching this problem is to use computerised analysis of brightness levels on plain X-rays (De Palma et al., 1991). This may prove useful in the future, but so far has neither been widely used or validated in either animal or human fractures against fracture stiffness or strength.

Radionuclide bone scanning has been widely investigated for the measurement of the process of fracture healing. The fractures which have been best investigated with this method are tibial shaft fractures (Matin, 1979; O'Reilly et al., 1981; Smith et al., 1987; Oni et al., 1989c) and subcapital fractures of the femoral neck (Stromqvist et al., 1984; Alberts et al., 1987; Sonne Holm et al., 1987). The value of this investigation in tibial shaft fractures remains controversial, although the more recent studies have generally concluded that scintigraphy is a useful aid to prediction of delayed fracture union. Smith et al. (1987) used a ^{99}Tc-MDP scan in 73 patients after tibial fracture. A surprisingly high number (32) of these failed to unite normally (defined as union by 4 months). They employed a regimen of three postfracture scans, which were supposed to be at 2, 6 and 12 weeks postfracture. In the event, the first scan was obtained at a variable time postfracture, between 2 and 4 weeks. Scans were obtained at an early and late period after injection and compared, in addition, measurements from the fracture site, the bone adjacent to the fracture site and the contralateral limb examined. Despite the variation in times of the scan, they found that the ratio of uptake at the fracture site and in normal bone in the same limb adjacent to the fracture was a good predictor of delayed union. Using a value of 1.3 for this ratio gave a sensitivity of about 70% and a specificity of 90% in predicting delayed union. These varied slightly depending on the gamma camera operator, as the precise area chosen as normal bone within the tibia varied. Similar results were found by Oni et al. (1989c), although these authors employed a value of two for the ratio described above.

Bone scanning as a predictor of union in femoral neck fractures was investigated by Sonne Holm et al. (1987). These authors employed bone scans at 6 weeks, and 3, 6 and 12 months postfracture in 35 patients. Non-union occurred in six patients (and avascular necrosis of the femoral head in a further five). They employed a ratio of uptake at the injured and normal hips (head:head ratio, HHR), and found that this was not predictive of the non-unions which occurred. Alberts et al. (1987) and Stromqvist et al. (1984) performed similar studies. Both groups found that the HHR was predictive of non-union when measured in the first month after operation, giving a prognostic accuracy of 0.87. The first group also found it predictive at 6 weeks and 3 months, but the second group did not. The HHR was > 1 in the normally healing hips, but < 1 in the patients with non-union. Both groups also measured neck:neck ratios, but their results differed. It may be seen that there are a variety of conflicting results for this method of assessing the outcome of femoral neck fracture. The situation might be improved by avoiding ratios between normal and injured sides, which has been shown to be unsatisfactory in tibial fractures (discussed by Smith et al., 1987). The test might prove more valuable if a ratio of uptake at the fracture site and a normal part of the same bone was employed. Stromqvist et al. (1984) examined the use of such a ratio and found that there was a high degree of correlation with HHR; they did not specifically address its correlation with delayed union.

It may be seen that bone scintigraphy is of value in prediction of delayed union of the tibia. Its role in femoral neck fractures is not completely clear, but it is likely that, with appropriate technical refinements, it will prove reasonably accurate. Bone scanning has not, however, gained wide acceptance as a screening tool for delayed union of fractures. This may be for cost or logistical reasons; it may well merit more widespread use. A definite use for this method of investigation already exists in infected fractures. As mentioned above, the presence of active infection dramatically worsens the prognosis for fracture union. Initially, gallium-labelled scans were employed for this purpose, more recently indium-labelled white cell scans (where the patient's own leucocytes are labelled with radioactive indium and then retransfused) have proved more sensitive in demonstrating both the presence and extent of infection (Seabold et al., 1989). Because of the serious import of fracture infection, the use of these methods should be considered at an early stage (i.e. before further surgery).

Many types of imaging have been investigated in bone as an adjunct to investigation of osteoporosis. Markel et al. (1990) investigated the healing of tibial osteotomies in dogs, using quantitative CT (QCT), single photon absorptiometry (SPA), dual energy X-ray absorptiometry (DEXA) and MRI. They compared the results for the imaging techniques with torsional testing, indentation hardness testing, microradiography and histology. They found that the results for SPA, QCT and DEXA all correlated with the ultimate torque and torsional stiffness of the osteotomies, but not with energy to failure. Reassuringly, the best correlations were with measurements of the gap area of the osteotomy. MRI performed relatively poorly. These results are not surprising, as all three satisfactory methods have been used for bone mineral determination previously, return of bone mineral content is known to be well correlated with return of mechanical stiffness and strength (Powell et al., 1989). Similar results with SPA were found in a sheep model (Watkins et al., 1987). All three of these methods offer a hope for future non-invasive monitoring of the fracture process.

Various other imaging modalities have been employed in investigation of the process of fracture healing. These include thermography (Hartel et al., 1976) and impedance osteography (Kulkarni et al., 1990; Ritchie and Kulkarni, 1990). The former was described but does not appear to have been used again in this context. The latter uses an array of electrodes; two pass current through the limb, while the others are employed to measure the voltage at different points around the circumference of the limb. Using output from these voltage sensors, a computerised map of the impedance of the tissues of the limb at the level of the device is produced. The group investigated a small number of fractures but further results are awaited before the method can be properly evaluated.

Serum measurements

There has been considerable interest in development of a serum measure of fracture union. The best validated serum measure of bone turnover is serum osteocalcin measurements, which can be measured in many diagnostic biochemistry laboratories. The relationship of serum osteocalcin to the rate of metabolic bone turnover as measured by histomorphometry of iliac crest trephine biopsies is now well established (Vanderschueren *et al.*, 1990; Coen *et al.*, 1991; Iwasaki, 1991; Parviainen *et al.*, 1991; Power and Fottrell, 1991). Consequently, it is not surprising that it has been investigated by several groups as a possible marker of failure of fracture union (Oni *et al.*, 1989d; Obrant *et al.*, 1990; Nyman *et al.*, 1991). All have found that osteocalcin is elevated after fracture. Oni *et al.* (1989d) and Nyman *et al.* (1991) both found that osteocalcin levels were lower after fracture in slowly healing fractures and, in the first study, this reached statistical significance despite only 14 patients being included. The measurements at 8 and 16 weeks were both significant. They did not comment on the predictive value of osteocalcin for delayed fracture union. Osteocalcin synthesis is vitamin K dependent, and vitamin K levels after fracture have been measured (Bitensky *et al.*, 1988). Levels were depressed, after fracture, but it is not known whether the level of vitamin K reflects the degree of trauma or the risk of non-union. Both Oni *et al.* (1989d) and Nyman *et al.* (1991) also examined total serum alkaline phosphatase. Although the levels were elevated after fracture, neither groups' results reached statistical significance. Other, less bone specific, serum markers have been measured after fracture. These include somatomedin C (IGF I) (Oni *et al.*, 1989a), endothelial cell stimulating angiogenesis factor (ESAF) (Wallace *et al.*, 1991), creatine kinase (CPK) (Oni *et al.*, 1989b) and C reactive protein (CRP) (Kallio *et al.*, 1990). All of these were elevated after fracture, but none has been well enough investigated to be recommended as a serum indicator for delayed union. CPK and CRP are the most likely to be of value at present. CPK is a marker of muscle damage; unusually high levels after fracture may indicate severe soft tissue damage and hence a high risk of delayed union. Oni *et al.* (1989b) found CPK to be elevated after fracture but to be higher in high energy slow healing injuries. CRP may be a useful measure of prolonged inflammation at the fracture site and hence of occult osteomyelitis, rather than a direct measure of fracture healing. Since bone infection is known to have deleterious effects on fracture union, this test may be useful.

Histology

Histology is a method which has been used to stage many processes of surgical and medical importance. There are very few reports of histological examination of human fracture delayed and non-unions. The most comprehensive reports are probably by Urist *et al.* (1954) and Sevitt (1981). Both were descriptive and neither offered a satisfactory grading system with histological predictors of failure to heal. One of the problems in developing adequate predictive measures of delayed union is that, although a good deal is known about the biology of normal fracture healing, especially in animal models, very little is known of the genesis of clinical non-union. Because of this, it is difficult to apply data from normal healing (e.g. Markel *et al.*, 1990) to the main clinical problem of delayed union. Further work in this field is required.

End point measures

Diagnosis of an established non-union is sometimes fairly easy. Non-unions of intra-articular fractures (scaphoid, neck of femur) are often painfully obvious on plain X-ray by 6 months postfracture, as they are generally associated with some degree of dying back and sclerosis of the bone ends. Long bone non-unions will similarly become obvious with time but, in general, a much greater duration is required for these changes to occur. Consequently, diagnosis of non-union in these bones can cause problems for a considerable period. In the case of markedly 'atrophic' non-unions, fracture site mobility may be obvious, or stiffness testing may be helpful. The main problem arises with hypertrophic non-unions, where X-ray visualisation of the fracture line may be very difficult. These fractures will frequently appear to be soundly healed on stiffness testing. Few studies have specifically addressed this problem; perhaps the most useful was by Kuhlman *et al.* (1988). These authors used CT scanning and multiplanar reconstruction to visualise the persisting fracture gap. This allowed a definite diagnosis of non-union to be made and appropriate reconstructive surgery planned.

Mechanical methods of assessing fracture healing and union

Mechanical methods of assessing union and non-union can provide measures of both process and end point. Bones subserve mechanical functions: they support, act as levers and protect softer structures. The stiffness and strength of a bone are the qualities that govern its success in mechanical functions. A bone must be sufficiently stiff to resist gross deformation (Perren, 1979, Black *et al.*, 1984). It must also have strength so that it does not irreversibly fail by fracture during function (Currey, 1970). Following fracture, stiffness and strength are markedly altered. Thus, measuring the return of these prime mechanical properties should theoretically offer both a functional and fundamental measure of fracture healing.

Superficially, strength would appear to be the most fundamental property. This is particularly true as we spend much of our time treating fractures in which an injury has overcome the bone's strength. In reality, whilst strength is one of an intact bone's prime qualities, it is a poor and inappropriate measure of fracture healing. Analysis of normal skeletal loading (Nordin and Frankel, 1980) and the quantification of peak strains *in vivo* suggest that bones have between a three and ten times excess of strength above that required to withstand normal loads (Rubin and Lanyon, 1982). This design margin only comes into play during trauma or violent activity. Thus the return of normal strength may occur months after everyday function has returned.

Tests of strength, by definition, demand destruction of the material tested. Such tests obviously cannot be employed clinically as they would involve refracture ('The good news is that your fracture had healed perfectly – the bad news is that we had to break it again to find out'). Early animal studies tended to look at strength alone (Lindsay and Howes, 1931; McKeown et al., 1932; Wray and Goodman, 1963). From these studies it was noted that there were marked variations in the gross strength of healing fractures measured at the same time postfracture, in the same bone and species. Even when the cross-sectional area of bones was taken into account (Falkenberg, 1961), variations between similar specimens still existed.

Fracture site stiffness presents a property that can be measured without destruction of the specimen. By definition, tests for stiffness should not exceed the elastic limit of the material tested. Support was given to stiffness as a useful parameter of fracture healing by Lettin (1965), who noted it to be more consistent for similar fractures after similar periods of healing.

The theoretical basis for using stiffness measurement is worthy of comment. The increase in stiffness that is apparent at the fracture site represents far more than just a transition from gross mechanical disruption to bony union; it is in fact an intrinsic measurement of both the mechanics and biology of fracture healing. Without an increase in stiffness at the fracture site the developing sequence of tissues in fracture repair cannot occur.

Granulation tissue has a strain tolerance of about 100% (the tissue can tolerate being stretched to twice its original length), and thus can survive at the early fracture site despite its lack of stiffness and high strain. Because of the remarkable cellular proliferation which occurs in early fracture callus, the radius of the callus mass increases. The stiffness of the callus increases by a factor proportional to the fourth power of the radius of this mass. Cartilage can then develop with a stiffness of about 1000 times that of granulation tissue. Cartilage can only tolerate a strain level of about 10%. Thus whilst it provides increasing stiffness because of its moduli of elasticity, it needs to ensure that the strain level is reduced by the corresponding increase in fracture site stiffness to survive. Finally bone develops. As a tissue, bone's stiffness is some 400000 times that of granulation tissue but its strain tolerance is only about 2%, thus it also can only survive if the structural stiffness is again increased to maintain low strain levels.

Many authors have proposed that fracture site deflections, controlled by fracture site stiffness, govern the healing response (Henry et al., 1968; Lightowler and Swanson, 1972). Animal and human studies have demonstrated the great effect that altering fracture site movement has on fracture healing (Goodship and Kenwright, 1985). At the end of the healing process normal strength has been achieved.

In practical terms, the return of stiffness indicates when normal activity can resume, whilst the return of ultimate strength is a mechanical measure of the end of the fracture healing and bone remodelling processes (Black *et al.*, 1984). Many studies point to a very late return to normal strength long after clinical healing has occurred. Stiffness itself returns much more rapidly (Henry *et al.*, 1968; Lightowler and Swanson, 1972) and its rate of change is much greater during early healing, the period up to clinical union which occurs long before complete remodelling and normal strength.

There are five basic ways to attempt to assess the return of stiffness:

1. Direct stiffness measurement by bending the healing bone.
2. Load sharing tests where an instrumented implant or external fixator measures the pattern of load sharing between itself and the fracture as the bone heals.
3. Velocity of sound across a fracture.
4. Transfer functions measuring the mechanical effect the fracture has on energy transmission along a fractured bone.
5. Vibration analysis.

Direct stiffness measurements

The displacement of fractures during normal activities has been measured by means of X-ray photogrammetry (Lippert *et al.*, 1974) and by placing load sensors beneath plaster casts (Rymaszewski, 1984). The recorded displacements decreased during healing, but the values are not numerically comparable between cases. The displacement of fractures under quantified loading can be measured by X-rays taken before and after loading (Hammer and Norrbom, 1984), providing a measure of fracture stiffness. It is possible to routinely measure fracture stiffness by performing a quantifiable bending test on conservatively treated tibial fractures (Kay *et al.*, 1992) and by measuring angulation between external fixator bone pins (Richardson *et al.*, 1992).

The introduction of temporary bone screws into healing tibial fractures in patients attending outpatients has allowed the measurement of fracture stiffness using a strain gauged beam (Jernberger, 1970). This approach is obviously repeatedly invasive. In the presence of bone pins from external fixation, the stiffness of healing bones can be measured by detecting movement of the pins following application of a load to the healing bone with the fixator body removed or adapted to measure movement (Jorgensen, 1972; Richardson *et al.*, 1992; Kay *et al.*, 1989).

Load sharing tests

In the presence of any form of fracture fixation, it is possible to apply a known force and measure the amount of force being carried by the fixation. The force carried by the healing fracture, and hence its stiffness, may then be calculated. This has been most commonly performed with external fixation but has also been used with intramedullary nails and plates (Burny *et al.*, 1984; Evans *et al.*, 1988; Richards, 1987). There are, however, significant technical problems with estimating stiffness by load sharing techniques. As the fracture becomes stiffer, it becomes more and more difficult to calculate the stiffness, particularly if there is any loosening of the fixation to bone.

Velocity of sound

The measurement of the velocity of ultrasound through bones and across fractures has been studied in animals and human subjects (Anast *et al.*, 1958; Abendschein *et al.*, 1972; Gerlanc *et al.*, 1975; Brown and Mayer, 1976; Gill *et al.*, 1989; Mawhinney, 1989; Cunningham *et al.*, 1990). The velocity of longitudinal waves is described by the simple formula:

$$c = \frac{E}{\sigma}$$

where E is Young's modulus and σ the material density.

The velocity is dependent on the mass as well as the stiffness of the bone. As the mechanical properties return to normal at the fracture site, so the velocity of sound increases. The problem is that most fracture lines or gaps are only a small fraction of the length of a fractured bone. Thus, a delay at the fracture site tends to be masked by the large amount of normal bone. Second, the normal bone on either side of the fracture tends to become porotic, thus altering the velocity. Third, comparisons with the opposite side provide only relative and not absolute measurements of fracture healing. The technique is best used with long lengths of healing bone, with occasional extended fractures or following bone transport producing relatively long lengths of normal bone (Lowet *et al.*, 1992).

The velocity of sonic waves has also been measured for both longitudinal and bending waves. Longitudinal sonic waves have the same limitations as ultrasonic waves, but bending waves have been considered in more detail (Sonstegard and Matthews, 1976; Wong *et al.*, 1976, 1983). Phase velocity has also been studied, where one specific wavelength is measured out of the spectrum present (St Üssi and Fäh, 1988).

Transfer functions

A variety of transfer functions have been calculated in which the dissipation of energy from an impulse is measured across a fracture site, or the change in frequencies crossing a fracture site is measured. There is an overlap of these methods with various forms of vibrational resonance testing. None of these methods have really proved to be successful, as they are grossly affected by soft tissues swelling rather that fracture site stiffness.

Vibration analysis

The stiffness of a structure can be estimated by observing the frequency at which it vibrates when stimulated. In its simplest form the natural frequency of a simple beam is given by:

$$f_n = x \cdot \frac{EI}{ml^4}$$

In this case EI is the bending stiffness (E is Young's modulus and I is the second moment of cross-section of the beam), m is the mass of the beam and l its length. x is a coefficient dependent on the mode of vibration. Thus the stiffness is proportional to the square root of the resonant frequency. Because of this relationship, resonance studies have been performed on bones. Two basic approaches have been used: continuous stimulation of the bone and observation of the steady state vibration (Christensen *et al.*, 1982, 1986), and stimulation of the bone with a single impact and analysis of the response (Van der Perre and Cornelissen, 1983).

The results of clinical trials using vibration have not met the expectations based on clinical research (Van der Perre, 1992). This is due to variations in reproducibility and the absence of trends during healing in some patients. The main reason for this is that a variety of factors affect the resonance of a bone besides the stiffness of the fracture site (Steele *et al.*, 1988).

Mechanical testing has limitations. Most importantly, it is rendered difficult or impossible by internal fixation. Further, stiffness cannot be measured directly. Either the bone has to be bent or vibrated. As discussed, vibration depends on many other changing variables that obscure fracture site stiffness, we are left with bending. Applying a load and measuring displacement allows calculation of stiffness, but the relationship is a reciprocal – twice as stiff, half the displacement. When the fracture site is very mobile there is a lot of displacement for an applied force, thus the calculation of stiffness is accurate and precise. When the bone at the fracture site is approaching normal stiffness, there is very little displacement despite large forces, so the measurement becomes inaccurate and is not precise (Figure 9.1). Thus, stiffness measurement can provide a good measurement of the process of healing early on but is less reliable towards the end of healing. The relationship between displacement and strength is fundamental and cannot be altered. The bone at the fracture site becomes like the normal bone surrounding it as it heals, so an absolute end point is impossible to measure. However, the

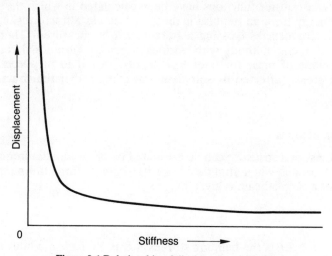

Figure 9.1 Relationship of displacement and stiffness

point at which clinical union occurs is at stiffness of the order of 25% of normal stiffness (Jernberger, 1970; Hammer and Norrbom, 1984; Richardson *et al.*, 1992) and this is just within the reach of such techniques (An *et al.*, 1988). Stiffness measurement can also provide a rate of healing, thus it can be used to compare groups of patients with healing fractures.

Conclusions

Fracture healing, along with all complex biological processes, is accompanied by a multitude of ever-changing parameters. The parameters are diverse and include chemical, mechanical, electrical, thermal, cellular, humoral, neural, vascular, muscular and psychological factors. Whilst it is possible to quantify almost all of these with varying degrees of accuracy in their own right, not all of these parameters necessarily parallel mechanical restitution of the healing bone itself. However, scintigraphy does appear to be a relatively non-invasive method of following some of these processes. Its value in routine (as opposed to experimental) clinical practice remains to be determined. Measurement of serum osteocalcin may be valuable in prediction of fracture healing but the wide variation in normal ranges described in the literature will hinder routine use of this test (B. Mawer, personal communication, 1993).

Mechanical methods offer a direct measurement of recovery of functional properties. Stiffness measurement has proved to be the most popular and promising but the use of vibration in the form of resonance has been disappointing. Stiffness calculation by bending long bones (measured via external fixation pins, imaged by X-ray or by quantifiable bending tests) is the most useful but can only be used in long bones, and usually only in the tibia. However, tibial fractures are probably the major clinical problem with respect to fracture healing.

In conclusion, a useful and widely applicable measure of fracture healing eludes us at present.

References

Abendschein WF, Hyatt GW (1972) Ultrasonic and physical properties of healing bone. *J. Trauma*; **12**: 297–301

Alberts K (1990) Prognostic accuracy of pre-operative and post-operative scintimetry after femoral neck fracture. *Clin. Orthop. Rel. Res.*; **250**: 221–5

Alberts KA, DahlBorn M, Ringertz H (1987) Sequential scintigraphy after femoral neck fracture. Methodological aspects and prediction of healing complications. *Acta Orthop. Scand.*; **58**: 217–222

An KN, Kasman RA, Chao EY (1988) Theoretical analysis of fracture healing monitoring with external fixators. *Eng. Med.*; **17**: (1) 11–15

Anast GT, Fields T, Siegel IM (1958) Ultrasonic techniques for the evaluation of bone fractures. *Am. J. Phys. Med.*; **37**: 157–159

Bidner SM, Rubins IM, Desjardins JV, Zukor DJ, Goltzman D (1990) Evidence for a humoral mechanism for enhanced osteogenesis after head injury. *J. Bone Joint Surg.*; **72A**: 1144–1149

Bitensky L, Hart JP, Catterall A, Hodges SJ, Pilkington MJ, Chayen J (1988) Circulating vitamin K levels in patients with fractures. *J. Bone Joint Surg.*; **70B**: 663–664

Black J, Perdigon P, Brown N, Pollack SR (1984) Stiffness and strength of fracture callus. *Clin. Orthop.*; **182**: 278–288

Bogoch E, Ouellette G, Hastings D (1991) Failure of internal fixation of displaced femoral neck fractures in rheumatoid patients. *J. Bone Joint Surg.*; **73B**: 7–10

Brown SA, Mayor MB (1976) Ultrasonic assessment of early callus formation. *Biomed. Eng.*; **11**: 124–127

Brueton RN, Brookes M, Heatley FW (1990) The vascular repair of an experimental osteotomy held in an external fixator. *Clin. Orthop. Rel. Res.*; **257**: 286–304

Burny F, Dankerwolke M, Bourgois R, Domb M, Saric O (1984) Twenty years experience in fracture healing measurement with strain gauges. *Orthopaedic*; **7**: 1823

Cattaneo, R Cattagni AB, Johnson EE (1992) The treatment of non-unions and segmental defects of the tibia by the method of Ilizarov. *Clin. Orthop. Rel. Res.*; **280**: 143–152

Christensen AB, Tougaard L, Dyrbye C (1982) Resonance of the human tibia. *Acta Orthop. Scand.*; **53**: 867–874

Christensen AB, Ammitzboll F, Dyrbye C, Cornelissen M, Cornelissen P, Van der Perre G (1986) Assessment of tibial stiffness by vibration testing *in situ* I. Identification of mode shapes in different supporting conditions. *J. Biomech.*; **19**: 53–60

Coen G, Mazzaferro S, Ballanti P, Bonucci E, Bondatti F, Pasquali M, Perruzza I, Manni M, Sardella D (1991) Plasma insulin-like growth factor-1 and bone formation parameters in predialysis chronic renal failure. *Miner Electrolyte Metab.*; **17**: 153–159

Collins DN, Pearce CE, McAndrew MP (1990) Successful use of reaming and intramedullary nailing of the tibia. *J. Orthop. Trauma*; **4**: 315–322

Court Brown CM, Wheelwright EF, Christie J, McQueen MM (1990) External fixation for type III open tibial fractures. *J. Bone Joint Surg.*; **72B**: 801–804

Cunningham JL, Kenwright J, Kershaw CJ (1990) Biomedical measurement of fracture healing. *J. Biomech. Eng. Technol.*; **14**(3): 92–101

Currey JD (1970) The mechanical properties of bone. *Clin. Orthop.*; **73**: 210–231

De Palma L, Greco F, Specchia N, Rizzi L (1991) [Evaluation of fracture healing with the computerized analysis of radiographic images.] Valutazione dell'evoluzione del callo di frattura mediante analisi computerizzata di immagini radiografiche. *Radiol. Med. (Torino)*; **82**: 44–47

Dias JJ, Taylor M, Thompson J, Brenkel IJ, Gregg PJ (1988) Radiographic signs of union of scaphoid fractures. An analysis of inter-observer agreement and reproducibility. *J. Bone Joint Surg.*; **70B**: 299–301

Edwards P (1965) Fracture of the tibial shaft: 492 consecutive cases in adults. *Acta Orthop. Scand.*; Suppl 76, 1–82

Evans M, Kenwright J, Cunningham JL (1988) Design and performance of a fracture monitoring transducer. *J. Biomed. Eng.*; **10**(1): 64–69

Folleras G, Ahlo A, Stromsoe K, Ekeland E, Thoresen BO (1990) Locked intramedullary nailing of fractures of femur and tibia. *Injury*; **21**: 385–388

Frandsen PA, Andersen PE (1981) Treatment of displaced fractures of the femoral neck. *Acta Orthop. Scand.*; **52**: 547–552

Frandsen PA, Andersen E, Madsen F, Skjodt T (1988) Gardens classification of femoral neck fractures. An assessment of interobserver variation. *J. Bone Joint Surg.*; **70B**: 588–590

Gamble JG, Rinsky LA, Strudwick J, Bleck EE (1988) Non-union of fractures in children who have osteogenesis imperfecta. *J. Bone Joint Surg.*; **70A**: 439–443

Ganel A, Engel J, Oster Z, Farine I (1979) Bone scanning in assessment of fractures of fractures of the scaphoid. *J. Hand Surg.*; **4**: 540–543

Garden RS (1961) Low angle fixation in fractures of the femoral neck. *J. Bone Joint Surg.*; **43B**: 647–663

Gelberman RH, Wolock B, Siegel DB (1989) Fractures and non-unions of the carpal scaphoid. *J. Bone Joint Surg.*; **71A**: 1560–1565

Gerlanc M, Haddad D, Hyatt GW, Langloh JT, St. Hilaire P (1975) Ultrasonic study of normal and fractured bone. *Clin. Orthop.*; **111**: 175–180

Gill PJ, Kernohan G, Mawhinney IN, Mollan RA, McIlhagger R (1989) Investigation of the mechanical properties of bone using ultrasound. *Proc. Instn Mech. Engrs.*; **203**: 61–63

Goodship AE, Kenwright J (1985) The influence of induced micro-movement upon the healing of experimental tibial fractures. *J. Bone Joint Surg.*; **67B**: 650–655

Gustilo RB, Mendoza RM, Williams DN (1984) Problems in the management of type III (severe) open fractures; a new classification of type III open fractures. *J. Trauma*; **24**: 742–746

Hammer R, Norrbom H (1984) Evaluation of fracture stability. A mechanical simulator for assessment of clinical judgement. *Acta Orthop. Scand.*; **55**: 330–333

Hammer RR, Hammerby S, Lindholm B (1985) Accuracy of radiological assessment of tibial shaft fracture union in humans. *Clin. Orthop. Rel. Res.*; **199**: 233–238

Hartel J, Sonnenburg M, Birr H (1976) Thermometrische Unersuchungen des Fraktur-heilungsverlaufs am Unterkiefer. *Beitr. Orthop. Traumatol.*; **23**: 280–284

Henry AN, Freeman MAR, Swanson SAV (1968) Studies on the mechanical properties of healing experimental fractures. *Proc. R. Soc. Med.*; **61**: 902–906

Herbert TJ, Fisher W (1984) Management of the fractured scaphoid using a new bone screw. *J. Bone Joint Surg.*; **66B**: 114–123

Iwasaki T (1991) Effect of glucocorticoids on bone Gla protein values – BGP as a good marker of osteoporosis. *Acta Paediatr. Jpn.*; **33**: 310–316

Jorgensen A (1972) Measurement of stability of crural fractures of the tibia treated with Hoffman osteotaxis. *Acta Orthop. Scand.*; **43**: 207–218 and 264–291

Kallio P, Michelsson JE, Lalla M, Holm T (1990) C reactive protein in tibial fractures. *J. Bone Joint Surg.*; **72B**: 615–617

Kay P, Freemont A, Edwards J, Taktak A, Laycock D (1992) Quantification of fracture repair by direct stiffness measurement and vibration analysis. *J. Bone Joint Surg.*; **74B**: Suppl II, 134

Kay P, Ross ERS, Powell ES (1989) Development and clinical application of an external fixator monitoring system. *J. Biomed. Eng.*; **11**: 240–244

Kelly PJ (1984) Infected non-union of the femur and tibia. *Orthop. Clin. North Am.*; **15**: 481–490

Kuhlman JE, Fishman EK, Magid D, Scott WW, Brooker AF, Siegelman SS (1988) Fracture non-union: CT assessment with multiplanar reconstruction. *Radiology*; **167**: 483–488

Kulkarni V, Hutchison JMS, Ritchie IK, Mallard JR (1990) Impedance imaging in upper limb fractures. *J. Biomed. Eng.*; **2**: 219–227

Laasonen EM, Kyro A, Korhola O, Bostman O (1989) Magnetic resonance imaging of tibial shaft fracture repair. *Arch. Orthop. Trauma Surg.*; **108**: 40–43

Lane JM, Sandhu HS (1987) Current approaches to experimental bone grafting. *Orthop. Clin. North Am.*; **18**: 213–225

Lippert F, Hirsch C (1974) The three-dimensional measurement of tibial fracture motion by photogrammetry. *Clin. Orthop. Rel. Res.*; **105**: 130–143

Loder RT (1988) The influence of diabetes mellitus on the healing of closed fractures. *Clin. Orthop. Rel. Res.*; 210–216

Lowet G, Buelens W, Goossens S, Lammens J, Ven der Perre G (1992) *In vivo* assessement of callus consolidation after bone lengthening with the Illizarov technique. *VII Meeting Eur. Soc. Biomech., Rome*; 136

McKeown RM, Lindsay MK, Harvey SC, Howes EL (1932) The bending strength of healing fractured fibulae of rats: Part 2: – observations on a standard diet. *Arch. Surg.*; **24**: 458–488

McKibbin B (1978) The biology of fracture healing in long bones. *J. Bone Joint Surg.*; **60B**: 150–162

Markel MD, Wikenheiser MA, Morin RL, Lewallan DG, Chao E (1990) Quantification of bone healing. Comparison of QCT, SPA, MRI and DEXA in dog osteotomies. *Acta Orthop. Scand.*; **61**: 487–498

Matin P (1979) The appearance of bone scans following fractures, including immediate and long term studies. *J. Nucl. Med.*; **20**: 1227–1231

Matthews LS, Kaufer H, Sonstegard DA (1974) Manual sensing of fracture stability: a biomechanical study. *Acta Orthop. Scand.*; **45**: 373–381

Mawhinney IN (1989) Bone and Ultrasound. MD Thesis, Queen's University of Belfast

Neer CS (1970) Displaced proximal humeral fractures. Part I: classification and evaluation. *J. Bone Joint Surg.*; **52A**: 1077–1089

Newman RJ, Duthie RB, Francis MJ (1985) Nuclear magnetic resonance studies of fracture repair. *Clin. Orthop. Rel. Res.*; 297–303

Newman RJ, Francis MJ, Duthie RB (1987) Nuclear magnetic resonance studies of experimentally induced delayed fracture union. *Clin. Orthop. Rel. Res.*; 253–261

Nicol EA (1964) Fractures of the tibial shaft. *J. Bone Joint Surg.*; **46B**: 373–387

Nieminen S, Satokari K (1975) Classification of medial fractures of the femoral neck. *Acta Orthop. Scand.*; **46**: 775–781

Nilsson OS, Urist MR, Dawson EG, Schmalzried TP, Finerman GA (1986) Bone repair induced by bone morphogenetic protein in ulnar defects in dogs. *J. Bone Joint Surg.*; **68B**: 635–642

Nyman MT, Paavolainen P, Forsius S, Lamberg-Allardt C (1991) Clinical evaluation of fracture healing by serum osteocalcin and alkaline phosphatase. *Ann. Chir. Gynaecol.*; **80**: 289–293

Obrant KJ, Blandine MS, Bejui J, Delmas P (1990) Serum bone-GLA protein after fracture. *Clin. Orthop. Rel. Res.*; **258**: 300–303

Oni OO, Brenkel I, Valance D, Iqbal SJ, Gregg PJ (1989a) Serum somatomedin activity following adult tibial shaft fractures. *Injury*; **20**: 269–270

Oni OO, Fenton A, Iqbal SJ, Gregg PJ (1989b) Prognostic indicators in tibial shaft fractures: serum creatinine kinase activity. *J. Orthop. Trauma*; **3**: 345–347

Oni OO, Graebe A, Pearse M, Gregg PJ (1989c) Prediction of the healing potential of closed adult tibial shaft fractures by bone scintigraphy. *Clin. Orthop. Rel. Res.*; **245**: 239–245

Oni OO, Mahabir JP, Iqbal SJ, Gregg PJ (1989d) Serum osteocalcin and total alkaline phosphatase levels as prognostic indicators in tibial shaft fractures. *Injury*; **20**: 37–38

Oni OO, Dunning J, Mobbs R, Gregg P (1991) Clinical factors and the size of the external callus in tibial shaft fractures. *Clin. Orthop. Rel. Res.*; **273**: 278–283

O'Reilly RJ, Cook DJ, Gaffney RD, Angel KR, Patterson DC (1981) Can serial scintigraphic studies predict delayed fracture union in man? *Clin. Orthop. Rel. Res.*; **175**: 139–146

O'Sullivan ME, Chao EY, Kelly PJ (1989) The effects of fixation on fracture healing. *J. Bone Joint Surg.*; **71A**: 306–310

Panjabi MM, Walter SD, Karuda M, White AA, Lawson JP (1985) Correlations of radiographic analysis of healing fractures with strength: a statistical analysis of experimental osteotomies. *J. Orthop. Res.*; **3**: 212

Parviainen MT, Pirskanen A, Mahonen A, Alhava EM, Maenpaa PH (1991) Use of non-collagen markers in osteoporosis studies. *Calcif. Tissue Int.*; **49**: suppl, S26–30

Pauwels F. (1935) *Der Schenkelhalsbruch. Ein mechanisches Problem: Grundlagen des Heilingvorganges Prognose und kausale Therapie.* Stuttgart: Ferdinand Enke Verlag

Perren SM (1979) Physical and biological aspects of fracture healing with special reference to internal fixation. *Clin. Orthop. Rel. Res.*; **138**: 175–196

Powell ES, Lawford PV, Duckworth T, Black MM (1989) Is callus calcium content an indicator of the mechanical strength of healing fractures? An experimental study in rat metatarsals. *J. Biomed. Eng.*; **11**: 277–281

Power MJ, Fottrell PF (1991) Osteocalcin: diagnostic methods and clinical applications. *Crit. Rev. Clin. Lab. Sci.*; **28**: 287–335

Rehnberg L, Olerud C (1989) The stability of femoral neck fractures and its influence on healing. *J. Bone Joint Surg.*; **71B**: 173–177

Richardson JB, Kenwright J, Cunningham JL (1992) Fracture stiffness measurement in the assessment and management of tibial fractures. *Clin. Biomech.*; **7**: 75–79

Ritchie IK, Kulkarni V (1990) Impedance osteography: clinical applications of a new method of imaging fractures. *J. Biomed. Eng.*; **12**: 369–373

Rubin CT, Lanyon LE (1982) The functional strain and fatigue life in bone. *Trans. Orthop. Res. Soc.*; **7**: 83

Rymaszewski LA (1984) A Preliminary Clinical Investigation into the Use of 'Flexigage' as a Sensor to Monitor Tibial Fracture Healing. MSc Thesis, University of Strathclyde, Glasgow

Seabold JE, Nepola JV, Conrad GR, Marsh JL, Montgomery WJ, Bricker JA, Kirchner PT (1989) Detection of osteomyelitis at fracture non-union sites: comparison of two scintigraphic methods. *AJR*; **152**: 1021–1027

Sevitt S (1981) *Bone Repair and Fracture Healing in Man*. Edinburgh: Churchill Livingstone

Smith MA, Jones EA, Strachan RK, Nicholl JJ, Best JJK, Tothill P, Hughes SPF (1987) Prediction of fracture healing in the tibia by quantitative radionuclide imaging. *J. Bone Joint Surg.*; **69B**: 441–447

Sonne Holm S, Nordkild P, Dyrbye M, Jensen J (1987) The predictive value of bone scintigraphy after internal fixation of femoral neck fractures. *Injury*; **18**: 33–35

Sonstegard DA, Matthews LS (1976) Sonic diagnosis of bone fracture healing – a preliminary study. *J. Biomech.*; **9**: 689–694

Steele CR, Zhou LJ, Guido L, Marcu R, Heinrichs WL, Cheema C (1988) Non-invasive determination of ulnar stiffness and bone mineral contents in humans. *J. Biomech. Eng.*; **110**: 86–96

Stromqvist B, Brismar J, Hansson L, Palmer J (1984) Technetium 99 methylene diphosphonate scintimetry after femoral neck fracture. A three year follow-up study. *Clin. Orthop. Rel. Res.*; **182**: 177–189

St Üssi E, Fäh D (1988) Assessment of bone mineral content by *in vivo* measurment of flexural wave velocities. *Med. Biol. Eng.*; 349–354

Terjesen T, Apalset K (1988) The influence of different degrees of stiffness of fixation plates on experimental bone healing. *J. Orthop. Res.*; **6**: 293–299

Tiedeman JJ, Lippiello L, Connolly JF, Strates BS (1990) Quantitative roentgenographic densitometry for assessing fracture healing. *Clin. Orthop. Rel. Res.*; **253**: 279–286

Urist MA, Mazet R, McLean FC (1954) The pathogenesis and treatment of delayed union and non-union. *J. Bone Joint Surg.*; **36A**: 931–968

Vanderschueren D, Gevers G, Raymaekers G, Devos P, Dequeker J (1990) Sex and age-related changes in bone and serum osteocalcin. *Calcif. Tissue Int.*; **46**: 179–182

Van der Perre G (1992) Non-invasive monitoring of fracture healing. *Int. Soc. Fract. Repair Belgium*; 85–117

Van der Perre G, Cornelissen P (1983) On the mechanical resonances of a human tibia *in vitro*. *J. Biomech.*; **16**: 549–552

Wallace AL, McLaughlin B, Wiess JB, Hughes SPF (1991) Increased endothelial cell stimulating angiogenesis factor in patients with tibial fractures. *Injury*; **22**: 375–376

Watkins PE, Kelly DJ, Leendertz JA, Rigby HS, Walker PC, Kenwright J, Goodship AE (1987) The application of photon absorption densitometry to the assessment of fracture healing. *J. Bone Joint Surg.*; **69B**: 495

Wong ATC, Goldsmith W, Sackman JL (1976) Flexural wave propagation in discontinuous model and *in vitro* tibiae. *J. Biomech.*; **9**: 812–825

Wong FY, Pal S, Saha S (1983) The assessment of *in vivo* bone condition in humans by impact response measurment. *J. Biomech.*; **16**: 849–856

Chapter 10

Osteoarthritic risks of intra-articular fractures

S. J. Gregg-Smith and S. H. White

Introduction

The aims of management of intra-articular fractures are relief of pain, promotion of healing and prevention of complications. Of the many complications the most feared is probably post-traumatic osteoarthritis (PTOA). The incidence of PTOA varies with the joint involved and the specific nature of the fracture, but has been quoted as ranging from 10% to 100% (Wright, 1990). The diagnosis of osteoarthritis has most often been based on radiographic appearance, rather than on clinical symptoms and signs. Radiographic criteria were proposed by Kellgren and Lawrence in 1957 and adopted by the World Health Organisation in 1961 (Altman *et al.*, 1986).

The clinician faced with a fracture is usually obliged to make a rapid decision about treatment and it is very difficult to study the natural history of intra-articular fractures. Thus, in considering the outcome for any particular patient, not only must account be taken of the original injury, but also of the nature of the treatment given. All forms of treatment may themselves impose additional insults to the patient. It is well recognised that a measure as simple as wearing a sling or taking to a wheelchair may result in permanent stiffness of the joints. More invasive forms of treatment may so interfere with the pathophysiology of fracture healing as to produce complete non-union.

An important consideration of the long-term outcome of intra-articular fractures is the distinction between permanent sequelae and osteoarthritis. From a medicolegal standpoint lawyers and patients often seem more concerned about the risk of developing osteoarthritis than the overall disability resulting from the injury. This problem was highlighted by Wright (1990), when a judge had asked him to provide guidelines on the incidence of arthritis after fracture and how reliable the medical profession could be at predicting its occurrence given a specific fracture in a specific patient. The lawyers in assessing damages for personal injury are particularly concerned that the state of the individual will not deteriorate after financial settlement and leave that person with less money than would be a reasonable recompense for their total degree of disability. Thus, PTOA which develops over a variable period of time following the initial insult has become a particular focus of interest. In many cases the risk of osteoarthritis is irrelevant since the permanent sequelae of the injury may be worse than the effects of osteoarthritis. For example, a patient with an intra-articular fracture of the head of the proximal phalanx of the little finger is highly likely to develop permanent stiffness of that joint. A significant part of grip strength is dependent upon power flexion of the little finger and the debilitating effect of loss of grip strength vastly overshadows the mild pain that may ensue should osteoarthritis occur.

Lawyers and their clients have a specific interest in the outcome of an intra-articular fracture. Three possible courses of symptoms are shown conceptually in Figure 10.1, where the ill effects of injury are shown against time. Popular opinion is that, following initial recovery, disability increases with time as shown by line 1. However, the reality more often resembles lines 2 or 3 in Figure 10.1, where patients tend to divide into different groups. Line 3 represents those patients whose disability decreases as they recover from their injury and have only a small risk of developing osteoarthritis. Line 2 represents those patients who never really recover from the ill effects of their injury. These ill effects frequently consist of stiffness, instability or chronic pain in the region of a joint and may occur in the absence of radiologically apparent osteoarthritis. In the earlier literature on the results of fractures emphasis was placed on the overall functional outcome for the patient (Apley, 1956). More recently much greater attention has been focused on the development of osteoarthritis, measured both by symptoms and radiographic changes (Knirk and Jupiter, 1986).

Most papers reviewing the long-term outcome of fractures rely on scoring systems based on such factors as range of movement, grip strength, degree of malalignment and radiological evidence of arthritis.

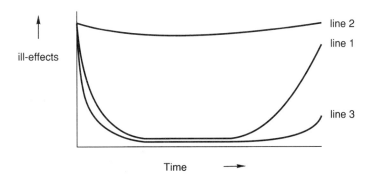

Possible outcomes of intra-articular injury:
Line 1 indicates early recovery but late arthritis.
Line 2 indicates permanent sequelae, very nearly as bad as late arthritis.
Line 3 indicates good recovery with only a small late risk of arthritis.

Figure 10.1 Probability of ill-effects after intra-articular fracture

There is enormous variation in the weighting given to the different factors. Each author promotes the system that he has used and the reader obtains a spurious idea of the true objectivity of the result. This was elegantly demonstrated by Bradway *et al.* (1989) who applied several different scoring systems to the same group of intra-articular fractures of the distal radius and found a wide variation in the apparent result.

Clinical post-traumatic osteoarthritis

Not all osteoarthritis is symptomatic and there are three criteria which need satisfying for post-traumatic arthritis to be defined adequately:

1. There must be objective evidence of permanent damage to the joint such as radiological changes, deformity or limitation of range of movement.
2. The individual must have some symptoms from the affected joint.
3. The individual must have an appreciation of the limitations imposed upon him by the objective findings or the symptoms.

These concepts match the World Health Organisation's definitions of impairment, disability and handicap. *Objective deficit, or impairment,* such as the loss of range of movement of a joint may be compensated for by movement of other joints. *Symptoms, or disability,* which are subjective, will not manifest themselves in a person well motivated to carry on a favoured activity despite pain (for economic or social reasons). *Functional limitation, or handicap,* may be exaggerated by an individual's reaction. For example, someone not enjoying their work may find minor damage to the patellofemoral joint produces sufficiently severe pain to prevent him working, whereas an enthusiastic footballer with major damage to the knee may continue to play as often as possible.

Symptoms and functional limitation are by their very nature subjective and it is difficult to objectively define outcome. Nevertheless, it is also most desirable to be able to predict these criteria from the viewpoint of the patient, the doctor and the lawyer.

Pathomechanics of osteoarthritis after trauma

If osteoarthritis may arise from an intra-articular fracture, what is the mechanism of joint deterioration? There are a number of distinct mechanisms by which osteoarthritis can be theoretically predicted after an intra-articular fracture:

1. A gap in the joint surface.
2. A step in the joint surface.
3. Abnormal soft tissues around the joint.
4. Malalignment of the bone in the diaphysis or metaphysis.
5. Any combination of these factors.

A gap in the joint surface

The effect of a chondral or osteochondral gap will be similar in that higher concentrations of stress will be borne at the margins of the defect. Figure 10.2 illustrates various ways in which a gap may be produced. The near-perfect congruity of a normal joint (Figure 10.2(a)) will be affected by the loss of a fragment or its impaction into underlying bone (Figure 10.2(b)). However, an osteochondral defect may also be due to imperfect reduction of the fracture even if bone and cartilage are not lost (Figure 10.2(c)). It has been shown that a small gap in the articular surface may lead to osteoarthritis. Ovadia and Beals (1986) studied 145 fractures of the tibial plafond of the ankle with a mean follow-up of 57 months and a minimum of 24 months. A gap of 1–4 mm on the post-reduction X-ray was identified in 35 of 83 patients who were otherwise judged to have a good reduction. Of these, 80% had good clinical results, whereas those with no articular gap achieved good results in 98% of patients. This difference was statistically significant ($P < 0.05$) but the analysis did not distinguish between poor results due to osteoarthritis and poor results due to other sequelae. If a gap of 1–4 mm is unacceptable what is the critical size of gap that can be tolerated? There are no studies in which there is a satisfactory multivariant analysis when the problem of the gap has been isolated as an independent variable from the other confounding influences, such as the fracture pattern, age, method of treatment and associated soft tissue injuries.

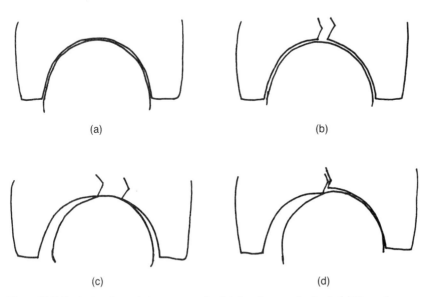

(a)

(b)

(c)

(d)

Figure 10.2 Contact patterns between opposing joint surfaces under load. (a) Normal, congruent joint. (b) A gap due to loss of a fragment or impaction into underlying bone. (c) Incomplete reduction, or over reduction have far more serious consequences on cartilage stresses. (d) A step in the articular surface similarly increases local contact stresses

Steps in the articular surface

A step in the articular surface has long been regarded as a poor prognostic feature influencing the development of osteoarthritis (Figure 10.2(d)). Articular surfaces of dissimilar shape can touch only over small areas, either at a point or along a line in the unloaded state. The contact pressure under load is equal to the value of the compressive contact force divided by the area of contact. If the contact area is small, the contact pressure is large, and the classical theory of wear of sliding surface predicts a high wear rate (Bowden and Tabor, 1964). Where point contact occurs then the stresses are theoretically infinite. Hyaline cartilage is designed to resist compression and to permit sliding. It follows therefore that point or line contact resulting from an articular step may result in unacceptable levels of stress and this in turn will cause hyaline cartilage failure. Theoretically any surface irregularity will produce the phenomenon and in practice there must be a step in nearly all intra-articular fractures how ever well treated they may appear to be.

Most studies to date have concentrated on the very large steps seen radiographically on postfixation films. For instance, Porter (1970) in a study of 137 lateral tibial plateau fractures found a direct correlation between the depth of depression of the tibial plateau and the prognosis. The results in cases with mild depression were good, whereas almost half the patients with over 14 mm of depression had a poor result. Porter also found that the prognosis was related to the area of the plateau which had been depressed if the step exceeded 10 mm.

Hohl and Luck (1956) also found that the depth of radiographic depression was related to functional results: patients with under 10 mm of depression had 77% acceptable results (excellent or good by their standards) whereas those with over 10 mm had only 61% acceptable results. These findings have been confirmed by a number of other studies (Schatzker et al., 1979; Jensen et al., 1988; Volpin et al., 1990). However, the striking finding, common to all these studies, is the lack of correlation between radiological appearance and functional result.

Fractures of the femoral condyles are likely to go on to develop arthritis within 1–5 years if any step is left in the articular surface (Egund and Kolmert, 1982; Smith et al., 1989). This occurrs both in the patellofemoral and tibiofemoral compartments, although the patellofemoral joint seemed to be at higher risk.

In the wrist joint symptomatic arthritis is even more prevalent with minor degrees of surface irregularity. Knirk and Jupiter (1986) studied a group of 43 patents with distal radial intra-articular fractures that were managed in a variety of ways. There was a mean follow-up of 6.7 years. Of those patients with a step of 2 mm or greater 100% had radiological arthritis and if the step was between 1 mm and 2 mm this incidence only fell to 91%. Ninety-three per cent of those with X-ray changes were symptomatic. This has been confirmed by other series of similar injuries (Bradway et al., 1989; Verhaven et al., 1991). Fractures of the scaphoid seem to be equally unforgiving, where rates of symptomatic arthritis approaching 100% have been reported (Ruby and Leslie, 1987; Vender et al., 1987).

Recently the validity of a policy of restoration of articular congruity at the expense of devascularisation has been questioned. Extensive open exposure to achieve anatomical perfection may inhibit fracture union. The AO/ASIF group has discussed the adverse effects of slavish adherence to the goal of perfect reduction at the expense of bone viability (Gautier *et al.*, 1992). Although this 'new concept of internal fixation' is most applicable to diaphyseal fractures, the increasing use of ligamentotaxis in the management of comminuted intra-articular fractures demonstrates the general applicability of this concept. Like many of the ideas currently fashionable in medicine this is not really new. Apley (1956) in a classical study of 60 patients with tibial plateau fractures evaluated at 1–10 years by his functional method showed no correlation between radiographic appearance and function. This was such a striking feature that Apley stated '. . . radiographs are irrelevant to treatment'. In all, 83% had excellent or good knees. The same group was studied 8 years later and there was no deterioration in function. The patients had all been treated by skeletal traction and early joint movement.

The marked differences in outcome of joints left with an articular step are not easy to explain. Some joints seem less tolerant than others. Intra-articular fractures of the wrist and the hip lead to rapid and symptomatic arthritis, while similar injuries to the ankle and elbow are much better tolerated. In the knee the picture is more confusing as the tibial and femoral sides of the articulation behave in a completely different manner.

Abnormal soft tissues around the joint

The soft tissues around the joint also have an important rôle in determining the forces applied to the articular surface. Ramsey and Hamilton (1976) have shown that widening of the medial part of the ankle mortice following trauma alters the contact area of the tibiotalar joint. As little as 1 mm of lateral talar shift results in a 42% decrease in the tibiotalar contact area. It follows that a proportional increase in stress will be borne in the remaining areas of contact. Clinical evidence shows that osteoarthritic changes after such injuries do indeed start at these sites, with thinning of the cartilage at the lateral border of the tibial plafond, and sclerosis of the subchondral bone.

There is increasing evidence that post-traumatic joint instability may lead to arthritis. This is not to say that the instability alone is the culprit; acquired instability, in which specific ligaments fail and the joint becomes unstable, seems to present a special risk.

Harrington (1979) showed that ankle osteoarthritis commonly follows lateral ligament rupture. The study group consisted of 36 patients with at least 10 years of recurrent symptomatic lateral ligament instability. Weight-bearing radiographs showed narrowing of the joint space over the medial half of the talar and tibial surfaces. In all cases where arthroscopy was utilised the extent of the degeneration was found to exceed that which had been anticipated on the X-rays.

The carpus is particularly prone to developing arthritis following disruption of the scapholunate ligaments, even in the absence of apparent bone injury (Harrington *et al.*, 1987). The scaphoid, which normally sits in the elliptical scaphoid fossa of the distal radius, rotates when its normal constraints are disrupted so that it rests on the edge of the fossa, like an egg balanced across a teaspoon. Not only does this lead to high forces on the articular surface of this joint, leading to early degenerative change, but also causes a change in the normal relationship of the other carpal bones and widespread arthritis throughout the wrist joint.

Similarly, anterior cruciate ligament (ACL) rupture is known to predispose the knee joint to osteoarthritis. Joint instability occasioned by anterior cruciate rupture increases the risk of meniscal damage to 50% within 5 years. Meniscectomy results in a high incidence of osteoarthritis (Fairbank, 1948; Dandy and Jackson, 1975). Tapper and Hoover (1969) found the incidence to be as high as 85% after 10 years. Lynch and Henning (1988) in a study of 1081 patients with chronic ACL deficiency concluded that osteoarthritis was directly related to the inability of the ACL deficient knee to protect the meniscus and that the only real variable was the rate at which degeneration will occur.

If such ligament damage can result in a chain of events leading to arthritis, consider the added effect of ligamentous injury on fracture of a joint. Disruption of a joint by fracture is always associated with some degree of soft tissue damage. In the assessment of the prognosis of joint fractures it is often difficult to ascertain the extent of damage to the soft tissue constraints. Ideally this information should be recorded and its impact prospectively assessed.

Malalignment of the bone in the diaphysis or metaphysis

Although this is not strictly related to intra-articular injury, many fractures have components extending into the metaphysis or the diaphysis and malalignment may then result from malunion. Malalignment of long bones is often said to produce premature arthritis in joints, especially in the lower limb. This is thought to be true both after trauma and in other disease processes leading to deformity. Koostra (1973) observed varus or valgus deformities exceeding 10° in 14 of 63 patients after femoral fracture, none of whom were symptomatic.

Kettlekamp et al. (1988) used a biomechanical model to demonstrate a correlation between varus or valgus deformity and arthritis in a group of 14 patients presenting with unicompartmental arthritis of the knee at an average of 31 years after femoral or tibial shaft fracture. There was a strong correlation with the angle and degree of malunion. There are major difficulties using a static biomechanical model in a self-selecting group of patients in a retrospective study. It was conceded that this did not provide evidence that malalignment always leads to degenerative arthritis.

Egund and Kolmert (1982), in a review of 62 supracondylar fractures of the knee, concluded that there was little connection between residual angular deformity and the developement of gonarthritis. Only 12 of these patients had no intra-articular component to the fracture and only five had a deformity greater than 5°. Two were reviewed at more than 4 years after injury of whom one had arthritis. In conclusion, there is little objective evidence to confirm that angular deformity per se causes arthritis and the verdict remains open.

Aggravating factors for osteoarthritis after intra-articular fractures

There are other factors apart from those caused by mechanical derangement of the joint secondary to injury that may operate to alter the risk of deterioration. These may pre-exist in the patient or be caused by the mode of treatment selected.

The influence of age

The final common pathway leading to arthritis is the same regardless of the mechanism leading to abnormal loading of the articular surface. This concept was neatly encapsulated by Harrington *et al.* (1987) when discussing wrist arthritis who pointed out that 'disruption of ligamentous or osseous support alters the normal carpal kinematics and degenerative arthrosis then follows, regardless of the inciting pathologic event'. Abnormal loading leads to cartilage failure and surface damage. The surface damage results in further abnormalities of load bearing and the cycle becomes self-sustaining. Aborting this process requires regeneration of hyaline cartilage but such a capacity has never been convincingly demonstrated in humans, although some fibrocartilage may be produced. It seems reasonable to suppose that surface hyaline cartilage damage is a permanent insult. As a consequence less cartilage is available to resist the natural processes of wear and degeneration and early osteoarthritis is likely to occur.

It has been estimated that the thickness of hyaline cartilage of the human hip is sufficient to resist 200 years of normal wear before the development of clinical osteoarthritis (Sokoloff, 1980). Any reduction in hyaline cartilage thickness will risk accelerating the onset. Irregularity of the articular surface following fracture healing will not only interfere with normal cartilage function but also produce elevations of stress which may be unacceptably high. These factors will be even more important in the third of the population who would normally develop osteoarthritis.

The body of evidence supports the theoretical deduction that older patients are more susceptible to osteoarthritis after injury than the young. The stress/strain properties of a material depend, in part, on the thickness of that material; thinner cartilage generates greater tensile forces in its basal layers for a given load. These observations may explain the different risks of osteoarthritis following trauma in young and old joints. It has been demonstrated experimentally that an impulsive force, when applied repetitively, can cause mechanical failure of cartilage. Simon *et al.* (1972) and Weightman (1976) concluded that cartilage exhibited typical fatigue behaviour, since the number of stress cycles required to produce failure increases as the applied stress is decreased. Kempson (1990) looked at the tensile properties of cartilage from the femoral condyles of human knees in the range 8–91 years of age. The stress required to produce fracture of the cartilage decreased with increasing age. In effect repetitive strain of a joint occasioned by normal use will cause more rapid failure of older, and thus thinner and weaker cartilage, than in younger, thicker and stronger cartilage.

Iatrogenic factors

Stiffness alone may be a risk factor for joint deterioration. Immobilisation is a common way of producing atrophic changes in the experimental animal (Palmostei *et al.*, 1979; Woo *et al.*, 1987). There is also clinical evidence that the longer and more profound the stiffness, the greater the likelihood of cartilage integrity being impaired (Enneking and Horowitz, 1972; Mayall *et al.*, 1963). Salter *et al.* (1980) have demonstrated that articular cartilage relies for its nutrition on the passage of healthy synovial fluid over its surface. This provides a rationale for the treatment of fractures by functional casts allowing early joint movement (Sarmiento *et al.*, 1977, 1989), the use of continual passive motion, and the use of internal fixation. Joint movement spreads cartilage loading and enhances chondrocyte nutrition. Stiffness of the joint, in contrast, will reduce the lubrication of the joint and reduce the load distribution across the joint. For instance, a knee which is unable to flex beyond 70° will experience stress protection of the cartilage at both the posterior aspects of the femoral and tibial condylar surfaces, since the sliding and rolling movements of the knee will be confined to the anterior portion. The confinement of stress to one part of the joint may have deleterious effects on the overloaded and underloaded areas, not to mention the remodelling of the underlying subchondral bone plate. Indeed late surgery to release contractures followed by intense physiotherapy may have a theoretical risk of accelerating arthritis in areas of atrophy. Stiffness therefore, per se, may have far-reaching effects and may be a direct consequence of the joint injury, but will in most cases be difficult to distinguish from the iatrogenic effects of restrictive or overinvasive management regimens.

Measurements of outcome

Assessment of initial joint damage

Plain radiography is not a satisfactory instrument for the measurement of the osteoarthritic risk following fracture repair. In trauma, undue emphasis has been placed on the interpretation of radiographs which do not show the articular surface. They are the tool of the surgeon interested in fractures of the metaphyses and diaphyses of bone. The joint consists of radiolucent hyaline cartilage which separates the radio dense subchondral bone plates. To provide a prognosis of a distal femoral fracture solely on the basis of plain radiographs is as risky as a structural surveyor pronouncing on a building by looking at a house without considering the foundations. Despite this knowledge it is astonishing how few surgeons when reporting the outcome of fracture management by internal fixation make use of their opportunity to directly observe the joint surfaces. For example, in one very detailed outcome study of severe ankle fractures, no mention was made of the chondral surface as seen at 23 internal fixations, the authors preterring to deduce postoperative joint anatomy by radiographic interpretations of the bone contours (Philips et al., 1985). Surgeons who practise internal fixation will be familiar with the scratches, deep clefts and areas where articular cartilage has been gouged out. In such fractures the damage on one side of the joint is meted out by the 'hammer effect' of one side on the other.

Arthroscopy after acute dislocation of the patella often reveals major damage to the cartilage of the lateral facet of the trochlea and the undersurface of the patella in patients whose radiographs show no evidence of injury. The mearest flake of radiodense material after patella dislocation signifies a major complete thickness chondral detachment. Since the degree of chondral damage can only be assessed by direct inspection, it follows that the outcome of openly reduced and internally fixed fractures deserves special consideration in studies of outcome.

Since plain radiographs are ineffective at showing surface damage is there a satisfactory alternative? The answer is no.

Tomography still has a rôle in the assessment of some fractures but does not help in the demonstration of the articular cartilage.

Ultrasound has been tried in the assessment of femoral cartilage ulceration but it is generally poor at determining surface damage. Its theoretical relevance is only for cartilage surfaces over which a probe can be placed and this would have little relevance in the ankle, hip or wrist.

Computerised tomography is also ineffective at showing surface cartilage, but is at its most helpful in demonstrating gaps or steps in the subchondral bone plate. It has gained wide acceptance as a tool in the delineation of intra-articular fractures in areas difficult to visualise with conventional radiographs, such as the subtalar joint (Giachino and Uhthoff, 1989). Unfortunately it cannot give much valuable information after internal fixation due to the artefact caused by the metal implants. However there are new developments in software processing of the image to compensate for these metal shadows which may soon find their way into clinical practice.

It had been hoped that *magnetic resonance imaging (MRI)* would be a useful instrument for measuring both hyaline cartilage loss as a result of injury and hyaline cartilage ulceration as a result of late osteoarthritis. However, this hope has not yet been realised. Spiers and colleagues have shown in a study of patients with knee pain, all of whom underwent arthroscopy and MRI, that the sensitivity of MRI in showing full thickness cartilage defects is only 18% (Spiers et al., 1993). MRI does show subchondral bruising and microfractures after injury that cannot be easily discerned by plain radiography. MRI images are also corrupted by metallic implants, but this may be minimised by the use of titanium implants.

Contrast arthrography is possible, but is not generally applied to this problem, being invasive and of no obvious practical therapeutic benefit. Full thickness defects in the articular cartilage are likely to be recognised, but small surface abrasions will be invisible using this technique.

Arthroscopy is a most effective means of inspecting the articular surface, but is only applicable in certain joints. Arthroscopy in a fluid-filled joint space also explains why MRI is poor at delineating cartilage damage. Whilst at an open arthrotomy cartilage damage may appear as a crevice or scratch and osteoarthritis appear as a ulcer, under arthroscopic conditions, when these types of lesion are not seen, the cartilage is frequently seen to be fibrillated, with fronds of cartilage remnants rising perpendicular to the subchondral bone plate. This appearance strongly suggests degrees of abnormality which are not perceivable by any imaging modality yet available.

Assessment of the soft tissue damage is difficult and has been neglected. The classification of open fractures by Gustilo *et al.* (1984) has been an important contribution but is not directed at injuries involving the joint. *Stress radiography* has been widely used in the management of knee and ankle injuries but, in common with *examination under anaesthesia*, is observer dependant and difficult to quantify. Attempts to make these sort of observations less variable by the use of mechanical arthrometers are still under evaluation.

Assessment of established joint damage

Osteoarthritis remains the most important outcome determined after intra-articular fractures, although, as we have already discussed, it is not the only endpoint relevant to the patient or to the clinician. Superficially the presence of osteoarthritis seems a hard endpoint, allowing comparisons to be made between groups of patients. Radiological criteria for the assessment of osteoarthritis remain the standard available method for the classification of the changes.

The grading system described by Kellgren and Lawrence (1957) remains the one in most widespread use. They identified five radiographic features of osteoarthritis (osteophytes, periarticular ossicles, joint space narrowing and subchondral sclerosis, subchondral cysts and alteration in shape of the bone ends) and synthesised these into a 5-point grading system.

None	0	absence of X-ray changes
Doubtful	1	minute osteophytes
Minimal	2	definite osteophyte, minimal joint space narrowing
Moderate	3	moderate loss of joint space, small or moderate osteophyte
Severe	4	severe loss of joint space, subchondral sclerosis, large osteophytes

Standardised, single views of the joints are used. They examined whether this system resulted in low levels of inter- and intra-observer error and concluded that one observer was reliable in repeatedly grading at the same score. The variation between observers was much greater and, in the hip joint, would result in up to four times as much definite arthritis being diagnosed. Combining and averaging the score of two observers gave the most accurate results, with an error of ±3%. This method is rarely described in clinical papers using their classification.

The question of standardisation of readings has also been addressed by a group of American rheumatologists interested in the definition of osteoarthritis (Altman *et al.*, 1987). They used series of radiographs of the hand, hip and knee, taken at different times in the same patients, and demonstrated that using three trained people to score the radiographs resulted in the most accurate identification of disease grading and disease progression. In addition it appeared that different features were required to correctly identify the time sequence in the different joints. This suggests that osteoarthritis may differ between joints and that one all-encompassing grading system may not be appropriate.

There are a number of problems in applying this system. Ahlback (1968), in a detailed analysis of the radiological features of osteoarthritis of the knee, drew attention to a number of important confounding factors. Radiographs have to be taken parallel to joint surface. In the knee, nine out of ten patients have greater joint space narrowing when the joint is loaded by weight bearing. Evaluation of osteophytes in a complex shaped joint is not possible with a simple anteroposterior X-ray projection; this is readily confirmed by considering the appearance and distribution of osteophytes seen during total knee replacement. Although rarely considered, these difficulties must apply to many other sites of arthritis.

The heavy reliance of this grading system on osteophytes has also been criticised (Bagge *et al.*, 1991; Hart *et al.*, 1991). The view that osteophyte formation is part of physiological ageing and that joint space narrowing is a more relevant finding has not been discounted. Direct measurement of the joint space has been proposed as a more accurate measure of cartilage loss, but has not always been found to give more reliable results (Altman *et al.*, 1987).

The most major criticism is based on the lack of correlation between clinical symptoms and signs and the radiological demonstration of joint changes. Lawrence, as early as 1966, noted that there was no correlation between joint pain and the presence of arthritis using his own scale. More recent studies (Bagge *et al.*, 1991; Hart *et al.*, 1991) have confirmed this, showing that the relationship between clinical features and X-ray findings is poor, with patients with marked clinical features and normal X-rays as well as patients with marked X-ray changes but no symptoms.

Recently the American College of Rheumatology has attempted to address the difficulties of defining the diagnosis of osteoarthritis (Altman *et al.*, 1986, 1990, 1991). In a series of papers they have drawn up algorithms using clinical, laboratory and radiological data to give sensitive and specific means of identifying the disease. The joints so far subjected to this process are the small joints of the hand, the hip and the knee. A number of different options are presented. Using more criteria results in greater sensitivity, but at the expense of specificity. Again, they draw attention to the differences between joints and emphasise the need to select appropriate combinations of features for the joint under consideration. They propose methods suitable for different purposes, such as prevalence surveys, reporting series of patients and individual diagnosis of patients in the clinic. They recommend caution in the use of these systems as they have not yet been subjected to independent verification. If this method can be validated the prospect of producing series of consistent data should improve considerably.

References

Ahlback S (1968) Osteoarthrosis of the knee: a radiographic investigation. *Acta Radiol. Suppl.*; **277**: 1–71

Altman R, Asch E, Bloch D, Bole G, Borenstein D *et al.* (1988) Development of criteria for the classification and reporting of osteoarthritis. *Arthr. Rheum.*; **29**: 1039–1050

Altman R, Fries J, Boch D, Carstens J, Cooke TD *et al.* (1987) Radiographic assessment of progression in osteoarthritis. *Arthr. Rheum.*; **30**: 1214–1225

Altman R, Alarcon G, Appelrouth D, Bloch D, Borenstein D *et al.* (1990) The American College of Rheumatology criteria for the classification and reporting of osteoarthritis of the hand. *Arthr. Rheum.*; **33**: 1601–1610

Altman R, Alarcon G, Appelrouth D, Bloch D, Borenstein D *et al.* (1991) The American College of Rheumatology criteria for the classification and reporting of osteoarthritis of the hip. *Arthr. Rheum.*; **34**: 505–514

Apley AG (1956) Fractures of the lateral tibial condyle treated by skeletal traction and early mobilisation. *J. Bone Joint Surg.*; **38B**: 699–708

Bagge E, Bjelle A, Eden S, Svanborg A (1991) Osteoarthritis in the elderly: clinical and radiological findings in 79 and 85 year olds. *Ann. Rheum. Dis.*; **50**: 535–539

Bowden FP, Tabor D (1964) *Friction and Lubrication of Solids*, Part II. London: Oxford University Press.

Bradway JK, Amadio PC, Cooney WP (1989) Open reduction and internal fixation of displaced, comminuted intra-articular fractures of the distal end of the radius. *J. Bone Joint Surg.*; **71A**: 839–847

Dandy DJ, Jackson RW (1975) The diagnosis of problems after meniscectomy. *J. Bone Joint Surg.*; **57B**: 349–352

Egund N, Kolmert L (1982) Deformities, gonarthrosis and function after distal femoral fractures. *Acta Orthop. Scand.*; **53**: 963–974

Enneking WF, Horrowitz M (1972) The intra-articular effects of immobilisation on the human knee. *J. Bone Joint Surg.*; **54A**: 973–978

Fairbank TJ (1948) Knee joint changes after meniscectomy. *J. Bone Joint Surg.*; **30B**: 664–670

Gautier E, Perren SM, Ganz R (1992) Principles of internal fixation. *Curr. Orthop.*; **6**: 220–232

Giachino AA, Uhthoff HK (1989) Current concepts review – intra-articular fractures of the calcaneus. *J. Bone Joint Surg.*; **71A**: 784–787

Gustilo RB, Mendoza RM, Williams DN (1984) Problems in the management of type III (severe) open fractures: a new classification of type III open Fractures. *J. Trauma*; **24**: 742–746

Harrington KD (1979) Degenerative arthritis of the ankle secondary to long-standing lateral ligament instability. *J. Bone Joint Surg.*; **61A**: 354–361

Harrington RH, Lichtman DM, Brockmole DM (1987) Common pathways of degenerative arthritis of the wrist. *Hand Clin.*; **3**: 507–525

Hart DJ, Spector TD, Brown P, Doyle DV, Silman AJ (1991) Clinical signs of early osteoarthritis: reproducibility and relation to X-ray changes in 541 women in the general population. *Ann. Rheum. Dis.*; **50**: 467–470

Hohl M, Luck JV (1956) Fractures of the tibial condyle. *J. Bone Joint Surg.*; **38A**: 1001–1018

Jensen DB, Bjerg-Nielsen A, Laursen N (1988) Conventional radiographic examination in the evaluation of sequelae after tibial plateau fracture. *Skeletal Radiol.*; **17**: 330–332

Kellgren JH, Lawrence JS (1957) Radiological assessment of osteoarthrosis. *Ann. Rheum. Dis*; **16**: 494–501

Kempson G (1980) The mechanical properties of articular cartilage and bone. In Owen R, Goodfellow J, Bullough P (eds) *Foundations in Orthopaedics and Traumatology*. London: Heinemann Medical, chap. 8, pp. 49–57

Kettlekamp DB, Hillberry BM, Murrish DE, Heck DA (1988) Degenerative arthritis of the knee secondary to fracture malunion. *Clin. Orthop. Rel. Res.*; **234**: 159–169

Knirk, JL, Jupiter JB (1986) Intra-articular fractures of the distal end of the radius in young adults. *J. Bone Joint Surg. (Am.)*; **68A**: 647–659

Koostra G (1973) *Femoral Shaft Fractures in Adults: a study of 329 consecutive cases with statistical analysis of different methods of treatment.* Assen, The Netherlands: Van Gorcum.

Lawrence JS, Bremner JM, Bier F (1966) Osteoarthrits. Prevalence in population and relationship between symptoms and X-ray changes. *Ann. Rheum. Dis.*; **25**: 1–24

Lynch MA, Henning CE (1988) Osteoarthritis in the ACL-deficient knee. In Feagin JA Jr, (ed) *The Crucial Ligaments.* Edinburgh: Churchill Livingstone, pp. 385–391

Mayall G, Douglas RR, Templeton JS, Merry PH (1963) Long term effects of fractures of the lower leg; a review of 34 cases. *Ann. Phys. Med.*; **9**: 223–238

Ovadia DN, Beals RK (1986) Fractures of the tibial plafond. *J. Bone Joint Surg.*; **68A**: 543–551

Palmostei M, Perricone E, Brandt KD (1979) Development and reversal of a proteoglycan aggregation defect in normal canine knee cartilage after immobilisation. *Arthritis Rheum.*; **22**: 508–512

Phillips WA, Schwartz HS, Keller CS, Woodward HR, Rudd WS, Spiegel PG, Laros GS (1985) A prospective, randomized study of the management of severe ankle fractures. *J. Bone Joint Surg.*; **67A**: 67–78

Porter BB (1970) Crush fractures of the lateral tibial table. *J. Bone Joint Surg.*; **52B**: 676–687

Ramsey PL, Hamilton W (1976) Changes in the tibiotalar area of contact caused by lateral talar shift. *J. Bone Joint Surg.*; **58A**: 356

Ruby LK, Leslie BM (1987) Wrist arthritis associated with scaphoid nonunion. *Hand Clin.*; **3**: 529–537

Salter RB, Simmonds DF, Malcolm BW (1980) The biological effect of continuous passive motion on the healing of full-thickness defects in articular cartilage. *J. Bone Joint Surg.*; **62A**: 1232–1251

Sarmiento A, Schaeffer JF, Beckerman L, Latta LL, Enis JE (1977) Fracture healing in rat femora as affected by functional weight bearing. *J. Bone Joint Surg.*; **59A**: 369–375

Sarmiento A, Gersten LM, Sobol PA, Shankwiler JA, Vangsness CT (1989) Tibial shaft fractures treated with functional braces: experience with 780 fractures. *J. Bone Joint Surg.*; **71B**: 602–609

Schatzker J, McBroom R, Bruce D (1979) The tibial plateau fracture. The Toronto Experience 1968–1975. *Clin. Orthop.*; **138**: 94–104

Simon SR, Radin EL, Paul IL, Rose RM (1972) The response of joints to impact loading. *J. Biomech.*; **5**: 267–272

Smith SJ, Crichlow TPKR, Roberts PH (1989) Monocondylar fractures of the femur: a review of 13 patients. *Injury*; **20**: 371–374

Sokoloff L (1980) The pathology of osteoarthritis and the role of ageing. In Nuki G (ed) *The Aetiopathogenesis of Osteoarthrosis.* London: Pitman Medical, pp. 1–15

Spiers ASD, Meagher T, Ostlere SJ, Wilson DJ, Dodd CAF (1993) Can MRI of the knee affect arthroscopic practice? *J. Bone Joint Surg.*; **75B**: 49–52

Tapper WM, Hoover NW (1969) Late results after meniscectomy. *J. Bone Joint Surg.*; **51A**: 517

Vender MI, Watson KH, Wiener BD, Black DM (1987) Degenerative change in symptomatic scaphoid nonunion. *J. Hand Surg.*; **12A**: 514–519

Verhaven E, Boeck H, Haentjens P, Opdecam P (1991) External fixation for comminuted intra-articular wrist fractures. *Acta Orthop. Belg.*; **57**: 362–373

Volpin G, Dowd GSE, Stein H, Bentley G (1990) Degenerative arthritis after intra-articular fractures of the knee. *J. Bone Joint Surg.*; **77B**: 634–638

Weightman BO (1976) Tensile fatigue of human articular cartilage. *J. Biomech.*; **9**: 193–200

Wright V (1990) Post-traumatic osteoarthritis – a medico-legal minefield. *Br. J. Rheumatol.*; **29**: 474–478

Woo SL-Y, Gomez MA, Sites TJ, Newton PO, Orlando CA, Akeson WH (1987) The biomechanical and morphological changes in the medial collateral ligament of the rabbit after immobilization and remobilization. *J. Bone Joint Surg.*; **69A**: 1200–1211

Chapter 11

Growth plate injuries

D. M. Eastwood

Fractures in childhood are common. It is surprising that although the physis is the weakest link in the immature skeleton, only some 18% of bony injuries actually involve the growth plate (Mizuta *et al.*, 1987). Physeal injuries are generally considered to have a favourable outcome 'healing quickly' and 'remodelling with time'; nevertheless, any surgeon who has been involved in the management of these cases is haunted by the prospect of residual deformity or premature growth arrest. It has been said that the dread complication of serious growth disturbance is usually predictable and, in certain circumstances, preventable (Salter and Harris, 1963). However, before outcome can be so confidently assured, a sound understanding of the pathological anatomy is required to ensure that similar injury patterns have been compared.

Applied anatomy of the growth plate

The anatomical structure of the physis and its surrounding tissues differs considerably between children and adults, so the effects of trauma to this region vary with age. The immature skeleton consists of two types of growth plate or physis:

1. *The traction epiphysis*, or apophysis, is associated with a major muscle attachment and linked to the bone shaft by a physeal plate which, histologically, resembles that of the more common pressure epiphysis. By exerting tension on the physis, the muscles shape not only the apophysis but the bone itself. Outcome measures for injury to this type of physis will be discussed separately at the end of the chapter.
2. *The pressure epiphysis* lies at right angles to the long axis of the bone, joining epiphysis to metaphysis, and is normally subjected to compression forces. It is responsible for longitudinal bone growth.

   Histologically, the physis consists of four main layers: the germinal layer (or resting zone), the proliferative zone, the hypertrophic zone and the zone of calcification. It is surrounded by the perichondrial ring which is contiguous with the articular cartilage and receives the metaphyseal periosteum. This plays a critical rôle in the structural integrity of the immature bone, and by contributing cells to the germinal layer of the physis is responsible, in part, for latitudinal bone growth.

Whilst the growth plate itself is devoid of vascular channels, it receives blood from three sources. *Epiphyseal vessels* nourish the reproductive cells of the germinal layer to these vessels and damage irreparably alters the physeal growth potential. The *periosteal vasculature* supplies the perichondrial ring and the peripheral physis. The *nutrient artery* feeds the metaphyseal side of the central 75% of the physis, damage to these vessels is not considered to affect growth (Bright *et al.*, 1991).

The physis interdigitates with the metaphysis and by increasing its area of contact enhances its resistance to transverse or shear stresses. Early discussions of growth plate injuries described a plane of cleavage through the junctional zone of the physis where the chondrocytes were hypertrophying. The germinal cells responsible for bone growth remained with the epiphysis, their fate being dependent on the state of the epiphyseal vascular supply. However, more recent clinical and pathological evidence suggests that in up to 50% of cases, the cleavage plane may traverse any zone of the plate. This occurs particularly in the adolescent patient as distinct from the infant (Bright *et al.*, 1974) and may account for some of the unpredictable growth disturbances which have been noted.

Assessment of physeal injury

Classification

Classification systems are commonly used in all branches of medicine and applied according to different parameters. In order to be useful a system must: (1) be easy and accurate to apply; (2) facilitate exact communication between physicians and (3) have implications for outcome.

Several systems for classifying growth plate injuries have been proposed, some relating specifically to individual physes. Poland, in his textbook *Traumatic Separation of the Epiphysis*, was one of the first to propose a general classification which defined four broad categories of separation based on the anatomical features of injury (Bright *et al.*, 1991). As interpretation of radiographs improved, further injury patterns were identified and modifications to this classification were developed.

Aitken (1965) described three fracture types and although he felt that deformity secondary to malunion or growth disturbance was rare, he emphasised that a compression injury, whilst difficult to diagnose, could lead to major growth problems. Weber's system (1980) based on fracture line propagation was developed to help the clinician distinguish fractures which had a good prognosis and could be treated closed, from those with a poorer prognosis which required operative treatment.

However, it is the classification system published by Salter and Harris in 1963 which has gained most widespread acceptance. This system was based on the mechanism of injury, the relationship of the fracture line to the germinal cells of the physis and outcome as regards growth disturbance. In general, fracture types 1, 2 and 3, had a good prognosis for growth whilst types 4 and 5 did not. In his book, *The Growth Plate and its Disorders*, Rang (1969) extended the Salter–Harris classification by describing a type 6 injury with localised damage to the perichondrial ring and a significant risk of growth disturbance (Figure 11.1).

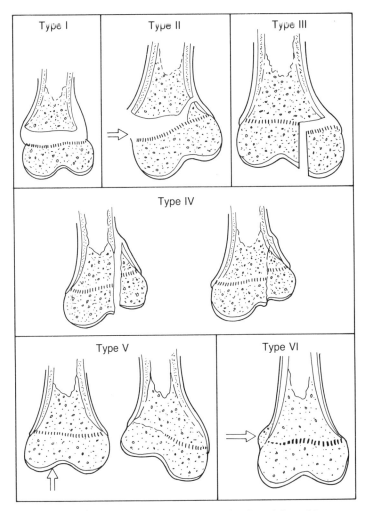

Figure 11.1 Rang's version of the Salter–Harris classification for epiphyseal fractures. (Reproduced from Rockwood *et al.*, 1991)

This classification system is concise and has shown itself to be of diagnostic and clinical importance but certain injury patterns, such as the triplane fracture of the distal tibia, are not readily accommodated by it. Ogden (1981, 1982) detailed specific subgroups which he felt explained the 'unexpected' cases of growth disturbance which were becoming more recognised. His classification system also defines additional fracture patterns (types 7, 8 and 9) which affect areas of the growth mechanism other than the physeal plate (Figure 11.2).

Imaging techniques

Plain radiography is by far the most important imaging tool for the assessment of growth plate injuries and it is always essential that radio-

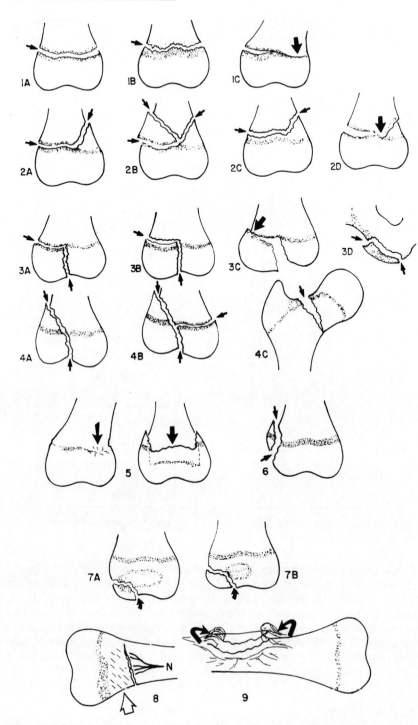

Figure 11.2 Ogden's extensive classification of physeal fractures. (Reproduced from Ogden, 1982)

graphs are of good quality and that two views at 90° to each other are obtained. Growth plate injuries may pose particular problems as the physis is radiolucent, yet accurate interpretation of the radiographic features is a prerequisite for application of the classification systems detailed above. Not all injuries to the developing skeleton are easily seen on standard views and 15–20% of fractures may only be evident on oblique films (Rogers, 1970) and occasionally the actual fracture line may never be discerned. Whenever possible, radiographs should be taken perpendicular to the physis and equivalent views of the contralateral physis are often required for comparison. In the assessment of the injured child, it is important to suspect physeal injury and to understand where the weak points in an immature skeleton lie. A child with a lax knee secondary to trauma is more likely to have a physeal injury than a collateral ligament rupture (Skak *et al.*, 1987) and although the physeal injury may not be apparent on plain radiographs, stress views will define the problem. In such instances, careful review of the radiographs may demonstrate avulsion fractures at the proximal insertion of the lateral collateral ligament; an injury which damages the perichondrial ring and is associated with growth disturbance (Hresko and Kasser, 1989).

In selected cases, modalities such as hypocycloidal motion tomograms (linear tomograms can be misleading), computerised tomograms and magnetic resonance imaging may be helpful in defining the plane of injury and the fracture fragments. Ultrasonography may be useful in evaluating birth injuries (Dias *et al.*, 1988) and arthrography has been of value in young children with elbow injuries (Yates and Sullivan, 1987).

Clinical factors

As with every patient, the importance of taking a history and conducting a clinical examination can not be overemphasised. A detailed account of the exact mechanism of injury including the force involved will help in the assessment of the severity of the physeal damage.

Early assessment of outcome

Once the injury has been defined, its likely outcome can be determined and suitable parameters for measuring this can be identified. In certain respects the outcome measures for growth plate injuries need not differ too greatly from those used to assess other skeletal injuries and factors such as fracture union and malunion, range of movement and deformity can be measured (cf. Chapter 9). However, each of these will be influenced by growth of the immature skeleton and by the child's ability to adapt to handicap.

Fracture union

Fracture union is usually assessed both clinically and radiologically. Radiological union may be difficult to define when fracture lines involve radiolucent plates and its value as an outcome measure is doubtful.

Growth plate injuries unite rapidly but clinical assessment of fracture union is considered to be too subjective to be of scientific value (Radford, 1993). More objective techniques such as those evaluating limb stiffness (Kay *et al.*, 1991) are not yet widely available and may not be easily applicable to a child with a growth plate injury. Non-union of a fracture following injury to a compression physis (as distinct from a tension physis) is extremely rare (Beekman and Sullivan, 1941).

Malunion

There are no generally accepted criteria for measuring the cosmetic or functional effects of residual deformity but, in the child, functional hindrance from a fracture malunion is rare. In the immature skeleton, minor angulatory deformity should remodel with growth (providing the growth plate has not been damaged) but it is widely agreed that angular deformity in excess of 20° will probably not correct especially if the angulation is not in the axis of movement of the adjacent joint (Evans, 1990). Similarly, rotational deformities are unlikely to correct spontaneously. Remodelling is not a reliable phenomenon and there must be at least 2 years of growth remaining, estimated by skeletal age rather than chronological age, if significant correction is to be achieved (Ogden, 1991). Radiographic evaluation of deformity may be useful in an individual case to assess progress with time, but as an outcome measure it is impracticable as the deformity is rarely maximal in the standard radiographic planes and is essentially unique to each case.

Joint incongruity occurs with malunion of physeal injuries which extend onto the articular surface. It will not remodel with time and indeed may progress if growth has been disrupted. The development of osteoarthritis, secondary to joint incongruity, may be used as an outcome measure for growth plate injuries and is discussed in general terms in Chapter 10. There have only been a few long-term follow-up studies of growth plate injuries addressing this issue and most of these reports have many deficiencies (Caterini *et al.*, 1991a, 1991b).

Joint movement

Joint stiffness is an important outcome measure in adult trauma management but clinically range of movement is difficult to measure and to correlate with subjective feelings of stiffness. In the child, post-traumatic stiffness is uncommon unless there is direct damage to the joint. Subjective complaints of stiffness are extremely unusual and restricted movement at one joint is often compensated for, at least initially, by movement in adjacent joints.

Symptoms

There are few data on the subject of symptoms following skeletal injury in the child and, indeed, the evidence to support any objective assessment of such symptoms is also sparse. Pain assessment in children has been documented (McGrath *et al.*, 1986; McGrath, 1989) but evaluating persistent discomfort as distinct from pain is more difficult. A review of 281 wrist injuries (Fodden, 1992) showed that 3 years after injury, seven patients (2.5%) complained of symptoms such as aching, crepitus and weakness. In this study, all three patients who developed premature fusion of the physis were symptomatic although it is interesting to note that only one patient had a recognised physeal injury, the other two having sustained shaft fractures. In contrast, a study of distal ulnar physeal injuries commented that, even with significant growth arrest, the majority of patients were asymptomatic (Golz et al., 1991). It seems unlikely that the presence or absence of symptoms could be used as anything more than a very general measure of outcome. Reflex sympathetic dystrophy is infrequent in childhood and trauma is the precipitating factor in only 50% of cases.

Late assessment of outcome

Skeletal injury in childhood, particularly when the physis is involved, may result in disturbance of the growth mechanisms and in this respect the outcome following fracture differs considerably from that following injury to an adult and thus a unique form of measurement is required.

Growth disturbance

The most feared outcome of physeal injury is growth retardation with formation of a bone bridge across the physis, however this is uncommon. The likely outcome is restoration of normal anatomy with a normal potential for growth. The reported risk for growth disturbance following physeal injury varies considerably from 1.4% to 33% (Smith, 1924; Mizuta et al., 1987), with significant growth disturbance complicating between 0.6% and 10% of cases (Rogers, 1970; Mizuta et al., 1987). This wide variation reflects the lack of adequate follow-up studies to skeletal maturity, the problems of identifying growth arrest and defining 'significant growth disturbance'. Growth arrest is uncommon and recognition of the problem may be difficult unless the clinician maintains a high index of suspicion. Complete physeal closure is usually well seen on plain radiographs but identification of a partial growth arrest is not always straightforward. It is important to emphasise again that careful attention must be paid to the siting and orientation of the radiographs in relation to the physis under investigation and both the epiphysis and the metaphysis must be scrutinised for evidence of disordered bone growth.

Harris Lines

These metaphyseal lines (Harris, 1926) often appear after trauma (Siffert and Katz, 1983; Ogden, 1984) and the presence of such a line parallel to a physeal contour indicates that bone growth has resumed and the risk of physeal damage is minimal. As the lines are often present bilaterally, the rates of growth can be compared in the two limbs. If the metaphyseal line and the physis appear to converge, eccentric physeal damage has occurred. Harris lines are most obvious in regions of rapid growth such as the distal femur and proximal tibia; in areas of slow growth they may be difficult to see and thus, except for specific injuries about the knee and ankle, their appearance is of doubtful value as an outcome measure.

It is important to identify growth arrest early and, if plain radiographs leave any doubt as to whether physeal damage exists, additional imaging techniques such as bone scans and tomograms should be employed. To plan further treatment appropriately, specific delineation of the area of bridge formation is necessary and mapping techniques using hypo-cycloidal or computerised tomograms must be performed (Carlson and Wenger, 1984; Porot et al., 1987). More recently, MRI has been used to determine the presence, nature and extent of the bone bridge and it is hoped that it will allow earlier identification of growth plate arrest (Jara-millo et al., 1990). Occasionally the only method of identifying physeal closure is indirectly, by assessing its overall effect on bone growth. The measurement of limb-length discrepancy remains a problem and clinical methods are still considered by some to be as accurate as the radiological methods (Eastwood and Cole, unpublished data).

Classification of growth arrest

The identification of premature growth arrest following physeal injury is an important outcome measure and a classification system which relates growth arrest to outcome and treatment options is useful.

Complete

Complete growth arrest is uncommon but it usually leads to a progressive limb-length discrepancy (Shapiro, 1982), the clinical effect of which depends on the age at which the arrest occurs, the growth potential of the particular physis involved and whether the involved bone is part of a paired unit. Despite some evidence that loss of growth from one physis will be partially compensated for by accelerated growth from the plate at the opposite end of the bone (Bright, 1991), in Shapiro's study no such tendency was demonstrated.

Partial

Partial growth arrest with bone bridge formation is more common. The size and the location of the physeal tether determines the clinical deform-ity and the age at injury and potential growth remaining define the ultimate severity (Figure 11.3).

TYPE 1 – PERIPHERAL

This type of partial arrest may result in progressive limb-length discrep-ancy but more commonly it is associated with an increasing angulatory deformity.

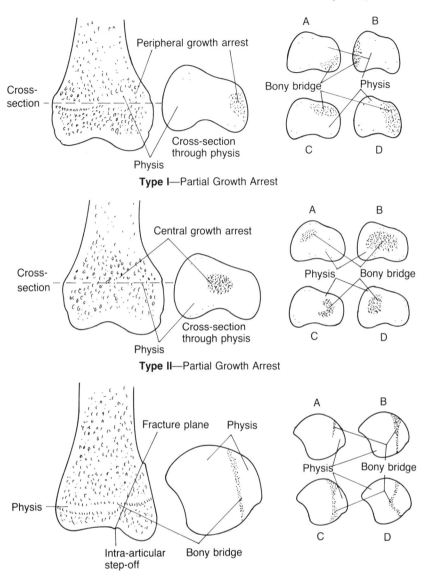

Figure 11.3 Bright's classification of partial growth plate arrest. (Reproduced from Rockwood *et al.*, 1991)

TYPE 2 – CENTRAL

A central partial arrest is less common and, radiographically, is manifested as a tenting of the physis as the peripheral plate continues to grow. Overall, longitudinal growth may be significantly restricted but angulatory deformity is unusual. Significant incongruity may develop at the articular surface secondary to distortion of the physis and epiphysis.

TYPE 3 – COMBINED

This subgroup of partial growth arrest is secondary to malunion of a Salter–Harris type 3 or 4 fracture and again is associated with incongruity of the articular margin.

Occasionally, small bone tethers may be overcome by the germinal forces within the physis but once a substantial tether has developed, progression of deformity has an almost linear relationship with time (Osterman, 1972). Although some bone bridges may be detected within a few weeks of injury, physeal damage may not become evident clinically for some years. If damage occurs when the epiphyseal ossification centre is very small, the bone bridge may not form until the bony centre expands to oppose the area of physeal damage. In such instances, there will be a considerable delay before radiological/clinical deformity is apparent but it may then progress rapidly.

In Bright's series of cases of premature growth arrest treated surgically, 53% were type 1, 33% type 2 and 14% type 3 lesions (Bright, 1991). However, as was discussed earlier, assessment of the type and severity of growth plate arrest can be difficult on plain radiographs and the validity or reproducibility of such assessments has not been confirmed.

Although it is growth retardation following physeal injury which is of most concern to orthopaedic surgeons, growth acceleration may also occur. A fracture adjacent to a physis is known to stimulate growth (Shapiro, 1981; Taylor *et al.*, 1987), although the effect is usually only detectable for the first year postinjury. Physeal injury itself may accelerate growth but the hyperaemic response to injury is short as is any subsequent growth disturbance and the result is rarely of clinical significance. Metallic implants used in the internal fixation of some fractures act as a chronic stimulus for accelerated longitudinal growth in experimental animals (Wilson, 1970; Castle, 1971) but the relevance of this in man has not been fully addressed.

Variables which may affect outcome

The measures discussed above assess early and late outcome following growth plate injury. However, the outcome of any individual physeal injury is highly dependent on a number of variables.

Age

The younger the child is when the growth plate injury occurs, the greater is the potential effect of such an injury on growth. However, the peak age for physeal injury is 12 years and by this age many physes have only a limited growth potential. The Salter–Harris fracture types most associated with growth disturbance are more common in the adolescent patient than in the infant. The size of the physis, its contour and its rate of growth all change with increasing age and each of these factors may influence outcome. The size of the growth arrest does not increase with time but the size of the unaffected physis does, thus a growth arrest affecting 50% of the physis of a 2 year old will represent a smaller proportion of the physis in the same child aged 10 years.

Mechanism of injury

Whilst the Salter–Harris classification system was based partially on mechanism of injury and detailed the shearing, avulsion, splitting and crushing elements which could affect the physis, an understanding of the degree of force applied and how the growing skeleton reacts to it is also required. In the adolescent age group the periosteal/perichondrial sheath, in thickness and in strength, resembles that of the adult and the amount of force required to disrupt the physis is relatively less than that needed to rupture the thicker sheath of the younger child (Riseborough *et al.*, 1983). The force required to fracture certain physes such as those of the distal ulna and metacarpal heads may account for the associated high incidence of growth disturbance (Light and Ogden, 1987; Golz *et al.*, 1991). Sometimes the force applied is sufficient to cause physeal damage without disruption of the periosteum. A history of a glancing blow to a subcutaneous physeal plate such as the proximal tibia, may increase suspicion of a type 6 perichondrial injury and encourage patient follow-up. Repetitive application of subcritical forces may result in fatigue failure of the physis.

Site

Extra-articular epiphyses derive their blood supply from multiple soft tissue attachments remote from the physis, whilst intra-articular epiphyses such as those of the proximal femur and radius are supplied by vessels arising from the periosteal vasculature which penetrate the periphery of the physis (Dale and Harris, 1958). These vessels are often damaged when epiphyseal displacement occurs and growth disturbance is more common when this type of physis is injured.

The growth potentials of physes vary considerably, thus 70% of the final length of the femur is due to growth at the distal physis and 80% of humeral longitudinal growth occurs at the proximal physis. Injuries to the proximal tibia and distal femur represent only 3% of physeal injuries (Peterson and Peterson, 1972; Ogden, 1981) but they are amongst the sites most frequently complicated by physeal arrest. The distal radial physis is the most frequently injured physis and yet growth disturbance at this site has been regarded as extremely uncommon. Recent studies, however, suggest that if these injuries are followed closely to maturity and their outcome evaluated carefully a higher incidence of problems will be identified (Golz *et al.*, 1991; Fodden, 1992). Physeal damage leading to limb-length discrepancy is more likely to be of clinical significance in the lower limb than the upper limb.

Fracture type

Soft tissue damage or contamination may lead to infection or bone bridge formation and will adversely affect the outcome of any physeal injury.

Many fracture classifications have attempted to link outcome with fracture type and although the Salter–Harris system is widely used, it has only been partially successful in this respect.

Type 1

This fracture type, accounting for 6–26% of cases (Rogers, 1970; Oh *et al.*, 1974), occurs in the younger child or as a birth injury (Salter and Harris, 1963). If the plane of cleavage is through the junctional zone of the physis, the outcome should be excellent unless the epiphysis is intra-articular. Occasional cases of growth arrest have been reported but these are usually associated with periosteal rupture and displacement at the fracture site.

Type 2

This injury pattern, occurs in 55–75% of fractures (Rogers, 1970; Oh *et al.*, 1974). Fracture reduction is usually both easy to obtain and maintain and it has long been considered a 'safe' injury as far as preservation of growth potential is concerned. An increasing number of reports suggest that significant growth disturbance does occur following this type of injury (Stephens and Louis, 1974; Kling *et al.*, 1984; Light and Ogden, 1987; Fodden, 1992) and this has been highlighted in the case of injuries to the distal femur (Riseborough *et al.*, 1983). In response to the biomechanical stresses exerted on them, the basic shape of certain physeal plates changes with growth and becomes highly convoluted. In so doing, its susceptibility to fracture changes and a fracture line which would have normally passed transversely through the junctional zone of the physis, may now shear through the physeal projections risking damage to the germinal layer of the physis at certain points. The greater the undulation of the physeal plate, the greater the risk of variable fracture line propagation and the greater the risk of growth plate damage (Alexander, 1976).

Type 3

This fracture type accounts for 6–8% of cases (Rogers, 1970; Mizuta *et al.*, 1987) and occurs towards the end of growth. In outcome terms, both growth disturbance and malalignment at the articular surface must be assessed. To re-establish joint congruity an operative approach is often required (Kling *et al.*, 1984). The outcome will then be good if physeal damage did not occur either at the time of injury or at the time of surgery. The epiphyseal fragment may be rendered avascular if its soft tissue attachments are damaged preoperatively (Bright, 1991).

Type 4

Ten per cent of physeal injuries (Mizuta *et al.*, 1987) fall into this category. If the fracture is not reduced anatomically the chances of a type 3 partial growth arrest are said to be high (Kling *et al.*, 1984). With operative reduction and fixation, a good outcome should be secure if avascular necrosis of the fragment is avoided.

Type 5

This is a compression injury to the physis. The initial radiographs are normal and the injury is rare (Rogers, 1970; Mizuta *et al.*, 1987). Discussion recently has centred on whether this fracture pattern actually exists and if it does whether the aetiology is vascular or mechanical (Peterson and Burkhart, 1981; Keret *et al.*, 1990). A type 5 injury is said to have a poor outcome although it is difficult to accept this statement totally when, due to the difficulty in diagnosis, the incidence of the injury is unknown. Several people comment on unexpected physeal closure or eccentric physeal arrest following trauma to non-physeal areas of the bone (Pappas and Toczylowski, 1984; Hresko and Kasser, 1989) and some suggest that type 5 physeal injuries went unrecognised at the time of injury. Elements of a type 5 pattern may occur in other fracture types, accounting for the unexpected cases of growth disturbance noted in these groups. Type 5 injuries are often eccentric and occur most frequently in joints which move in one plane only (Hresko and Kasser, 1989). Injury is said to be most common just before the physis closes and if this is true, growth disturbance is likely to be less significant.

Type 6

As for the type 5 injury, this is often a diagnosis in retrospect and although the radiographs are often normal, small avulsion fractures involving the perichondrial ring may be seen. Angular deformity secondary to a peripheral growth arrest may manifest itself quite quickly after injury.

Displacement

In the medical literature there seems to be general agreement with the statement, fracture outcome is related to initial displacement, that is the greater the displacement the poorer the outcome. However, in terms of growth plate injuries, little data exists to justify this statement. One paper commenting on injuries to the proximal femur felt that the severity of the initial displacement was of more prognostic value in children and adolescents than in infants (Caterini *et al.*, 1991a). In injuries involving intra-articular epiphyses severe displacement is associated with a high risk of avascular necrosis and growth plate arrest.

Treatment

When assessing the outcome of growth plate injuries it is important to differentiate between the outcome of the injury alone and the outcome of the injury combined with its treatment. A forceful manipulation particularly of a type 2 injury may damage the growth plate as the metaphyseal fragment is re-positioned across the physeal plate. Similarly, whilst it is recognised that intra-articular fractures require anatomical reduction for a good outcome (Salter and Harris, 1963), overzealous clearing of the soft tissues during the operative approach may render the fragment avascular or damage the perichondrial tissues. Direct instrument pressure on the physis may disturb future growth and, if possible, any penetration of the physis with wires or screws should be avoided (Bright *et al.*, 1991).

Fracture outcome is related to adequacy of reduction which in turn is related to severity of the initial displacement, although figures referring to growth plate injuries are difficult to find (Lombardo and Harvey, 1977; Caterini *et al.*, 1991a,b).

The timing of treatment in growth plate injuries is also an important factor. Physeal injuries heal rapidly and treatment instigated after the first few days may adversely affect the outcome particularly if force is used. Delayed primary treatment or repeated attempts to improve outcome must be judged in this light.

Apophyseal injuries

Injuries to the apophyseal physis are caused by direct trauma or by a sudden major muscular contraction which disrupts the integrity of the bone–physis–tendon unit. Cleavage through the growth plate is more likely to occur than tendon avulsion. The physeal vascular supply, via muscle attachments to the apophysis, is usually maintained despite injury. If the blood supply is lost, irreparable damage to the germinal layer of the physis occurs and the plate closes. The exact plane of cleavage through the apophyseal physis has not been documented histologically. It has been suggested that fractures similar to a Salter–Harris type 3 or an Ogden type 7 may occur and be responsible for the development of an apophysitis. There is increasing evidence that the development of an apophysitis such as Osgood–Schlatter disease predisposes the tibial tuberosity to fracture (Ogden *et al.*, 1980; Merloz *et al.*, 1987) and a similar pathological process may occur at other sites.

The outcome of apophyseal plate injuries is dependent on the displacement of the apophysis and its muscular attachments. If this displacement is significant (> 1 cm) there may be a measurable reduction in muscle strength. In such instances, repair is often achieved by abundant callus formation and, both functionally and cosmetically, the outcome may be less than satisfactory. Formal muscle strength testing in both the short- and long-term follow-up of apophyseal avulsion injuries could be used to assess outcome objectively. The other outcome measure is physeal arrest. Closure of the physis is common whether the injury is treated operatively or not. If the injury occurs at an early age, considerable disturbance of bone shape may develop although the exact significance of this is unknown. Most commonly, these injuries, particularly those affecting the tibial tuberosity, occur as the physis is undergoing physiological closure and thus growth disturbance is not a significant problem (Ogden *et al.*, 1980).

Summary

Much has been written on the subject of injury to the growth plate or physis but there is a relative lack of factual information on which to base many of the statements made. Quoted references are often outdated in the light of changing ideas on the histological basis of the fracture patterns, the availability of newer investigative modalities and the improving therapeutic options which exist today. There are few reliable, objective or appropriate measures for assessing outcome of growth plate injuries but the identification of growth disturbance is perhaps the best available. The injury must be clearly defined before the outcome can be predicted and then measured. Accurate diagnosis of both the injury and the growth plate arrest is thus all important.

For ease of application the use of the Salter–Harris fracture classification in routine clinical situations is recommended. Nevertheless, recent work does suggest that outcome is not as closely related to Salter–Harris fracture type as was initially thought, perhaps, for more research-oriented work a somewhat more unwieldy but more specific system such as Ogden's should be adopted.

In assessing outcome following growth plate injury, the major measurement tools available are radiographic. Predictive, process and end-point assessments of outcome can be made.

Predictive

It is impracticable to follow up all physeal injuries radiographically until skeletal maturity is reached. However, a knowledge of the variables which are known to affect outcome will help identify a group of injuries, such as Salter–Harris fracture type 5 and 6 or Salter–Harris type 2 fractures of the distal femur, which are at high risk of developing malunion or growth plate arrest.

Process

Careful assessment of the state of the physis and the presence of Harris lines by either plain radiography or computerised tomography (or MRI in the future) may define cases in which growth retardation is occurring. Some of these may revert spontaneously.

End-point

The tools for measuring end-point growth arrest and malunion are the same as the process tools. Indirect measures of growth plate function such as the measurement of leg-length discrepancy may occasionally be necessary.

References

Aitken AP (1965) Fractures of the epiphysis. *Clin. Orthop. Rel. Res.*; **41**: 19–23

Alexander CJ (1976) Effect of growth rate on the strength of the growth plate–shaft junction. *Skeletal Radiol.*; **1**: 67–76

Beekman F, Sullivan J (1941) Some observations of fractures of long bones in the child. *Am. J. Surg.*; **51**: 722

Bright RW (1991) Physeal injuries. In Rockwood CA, Wilkins KE, King RE (eds) *Fractures in Children*, 3rd edn. Philadelphia: Lippincott, chap. 2, pp. 87–186

Bright RW, Burstein AH, Elmore SM (1974) Epiphyseal-plate cartilage. A biomechanical and histological analysis of failure modes. *J. Bone Joint Surg.*; **56A**: 688–703

Carlson WO, Wenger DR (1984) A mapping method to prepare for surgical excision of a partial physeal arrest. *J. Pediatr. Orthop.*; **4**: 232–238

Castle ME (1971) Epiphyseal stimulation. *J. Bone Joint Surg.*; **53A**: 326–334

Caterini R, Farsetti P, d'Arrigo C, Ippolito E (1991a) Unusual physeal lesions of the lower limb. A report of 16 cases with very long-term follow-up observation. *J. Orthop. Trauma*; **5**: 38–46

Caterini R, Farsetti P, Ippolito E (1991b) Long-term follow-up of physeal injury to the ankle. *Foot Ankle*; **11**: 372–383

Dale GG, Harris WR (1958) Prognosis of epiphyseal separation. *J. Bone Joint Surg.*; **40B**: 117–122

Dias JJ, Lamont AC, Jones JM (1988) Ultrasonic diagnosis of neonatal separation of the distal humeral epiphysis. *J. Bone Joint Surg.*; **70B**: 825–828

Eastwood DM, Cole WG A graphic method for the timing of epiphysiodesis in cases of leg length discrepancy. Unpublished data

Evans GA (1990) Management of disordered growth following physeal injury. *Injury*; **21**: 329–333

Fodden DI (1992) A study of wrist injuries in children: the incidence of various injuries and of premature closure of the distal radial growth plate. *Arch. Emerg. Med.*; **9**: 9–13

Golz RJ, Grogan DP, Greene TL, Belsole RJ, Ogden JA. (1991) Distal ulnar physeal injury. *J. Pediatr. Orthop.*; **11**: 318–326

Harris HA (1926) The growth of long bones in childhood with special reference to certain bony striations of the metaphysis and to the role of vitamins. *Arch. Intern. Med.* **38**: 785–793

Hresko MT, Kasser JR (1989) Physeal arrest about the knee associated with non-physeal fractures in the lower extremity. *J. Bone Joint Surg.*; **71A**: 698–703

Jaramillo D, Shapiro F, Hoffer FA, Winalski CS, Koskinen MF, Frasso R, Johnson A (1990) Posttraumatic growth-plate abnormalities: MR imaging of bony-bridge formation in rabbits. *Radiology*; **175**: 767–773

Johnson RM, Jones WW (1980) Fractures through human growth plates. *Orthop. Trans.*; **4**: 295

Kay P, Freeman AJ, Taktak A, Laycock D, Edwards J (1991) Quantification of Fracture Repair by Direct Stiffness Measurement and Vibrational Analysis. Paper at BOA ASM Cambridge, UK

Keret D, Mendez AA, Harcke HT, MacEwen GD (1990) Type V physeal injury: A case report. *J. Pediatr. Orthop.*; **10**: 545–548

Kling TF, Bright RW, Hensinger RN (1984) Distal tibial physeal fractures in children that may require open reduction. *J. Bone Joint Surg.*; **66A**: 647–657

Light TR, Ogden JA (1987) Metacarpal epiphyseal fractures. *J. Hand Surg.*; **12a**: 460–464

Lombardo SJ, Harvey Jr JP (1977) Fractures of the distal femoral epiphyses. Factors influencing prognosis: a review of thirty-four cases. *J. Bone Joint Surg.*; **59A**: 742–751

McGrath PA (1989) Evaluating a child's pain. *J. Pain Sympt. Manag.*; **4**: 198–214

McGrath PJ, Cunningham SJ, Goodman JT, Unruh A (1986) The clinical measurement of pain in children: A review. *Clin. J. Pain*; **1**: 221–227

Merloz Ph, de Cheveigne C, Butel J, Robb JE. (1987) Case report: bilateral Salter–Harris type II upper tibial epiphyseal fractures. *J. Pediatr. Orthop.*; **7**: 466–467

Mizuta T, Benson WM, Foster BK, Paterson DC, Morris LL (1987) Statistical analysis of the incidence of physeal injuries. *J. Pediatr. Orthop.*; **7**: 518–523

Ogden JA (1981) Injury to the growth mechanisms of the immature skeleton. *Skeletal Radiol.*; **6**: 237–253

Ogden JA (1982) Skeletal growth mechanism injury patterns. *J. Pediatr. Orthop.*; **2**: 371–377

Ogden JA (1984) Growth slowdown and arrest lines. *J. Pediatr. Orthop.*; **4**: 409–415

Ogden JA (1990) *Skeletal Injury in the Child.* Philadelphia: Saunders, pp. 65–174

Ogden JA (1991) In Rockwood CA, Wilkins KE, King RE (eds) *Fractures in Children*, 3rd edn. Philadelphia: Lippincott, chap. 1, pp. 1–86

Ogden JA, Tross RB, Murphy MJ (1980) Fractures of the tibial tuberosity. *J. Bone Joint Surg.*; **62A**: 205–215

Oh WH, Craig C, Banks HH (1974) Epiphyseal injuries. *Pediatr. Clin. North Am.*; **21**: 407–422

Osterman K (1972) Operative elimination of partial premature epiphyseal closure. An experimental study. *Acta Orthop. Scand. Suppl.*; 147

Pappas AM, Toczylowski AM (1984) Asymmetrical arrest of the proximal tibial physis and genu recurvatum deformity. *J. Bone Joint Surg.*; **66A**: 575–581

Peterson HA, Burkhart SS (1981) Compression injury of the epiphyseal growth plate: fact or fiction? *J. Pediatr. Orthop.*; **1**: 377–384

Peterson HA, Peterson CH (1972) Analysis of the incidence of injuries to the epiphyseal growth plate. *J. Trauma*; **12**: 275–281

Porot S, Nyska M, Nyska A, Fields S (1987) Assessment of bony bridge by computed tomography: experimental model in the rabbit and clinical application. *J. Pediatr. Orthop.*; **7**: 155–160

Radford PJ (1993) General outome measures. In Pynsent P, Fairbank J, Carr A (eds) *Outcome Measures in Orthopaedics*. Oxford: Butterworth-Heinemann, chap. 5, pp. 59–80

Rang M (1969) *The Growth Plate and its Disorders*. Baltimore: Williams & Wilkins.

Riseborough EJ, Barrett IR, Shapiro F (1983) Growth disturbances following distal femoral physeal fracture-separations. *J. Bone Joint Surg.*; **65A**: 885–893

Rockwood CA, Wilkins KE, Ring RE (eds) (1991) *Fractures in Children*, 3rd edn. Philadelphia: Lippincott.

Rogers LF (1970) The radiography of epiphyseal injuries. *Radiology*; **96**: 289–299

Salter RB, Harris WR (1963) Injuries involving the epiphyseal plate. *J. Bone Joint Surg.*; **45A**: 587–621

Shapiro F (1981) Fractures of the femoral shaft in children. The overgrowth phenomenum. *Acta Orthop. Scand.*; **52**: 649–655

Shapiro F (1982) Developmental patterns in lower-extremity length discrepancies. *J. Bone Joint Surg.*; **64A**: 639–651

Siffert RS, Katz JF (1983) Growth recovery zones. *J. Pediatr. Orthop.*; **3**: 196–201

Skak SV, Jensen TT, Poulsen TD, Sturup J (1987) Epidemiology of knee injuries in children. *Acta Orthop. Scand.*; **58**: 78–81

Smith MK (1924) The prognosis in epiphyseal line fractures. *Ann. Surg.*; **79**: 273–282

Stephens DC, Louis DS (1974) Traumatic separation of the distal femoral epiphyseal cartilage plate. *J. Bone Joint Surg.*; **56A**: 1383–1390

Taylor JF, Warrell E, Evans RA (1987) Response of the growth plates to tibial osteotomy in rats. *J. Bone Joint Surg.*; **69B**: 664–669

Weber BG (1980) Fracture healing in the growing bone and in the mature skeleton. In Weber BG, Brunner C, Freuler F (eds) *Treatment of Fractures in Children and Adolescents*. New York: Springer-Verlag, pp. 20–57

Wilson CL (1970) Experimental attempts to stimulate bone growth. *J. Bone Joint Surg.*; **52A**: 1033–1040

Yates C, Sullivan JA (1987) Arthrographic diagnosis of elbow injuries in children. *J. Pediatr. Orthop.*; **7**: 54–60

Chapter 12

Complications in the treatment of musculoskeletal trauma

S. P. Frostick and J. B. Hunter

Introduction

Williamson (1971) states:

> One of the most important questions to be asked of any health care system is the following: *Who* needs to learn *what* to most improve health status of the population receiving care? Previous studies have demonstrated first that there is an important relationship between patient care assessment and education that might provide a framework for answering this question and second, that systematic application of this approach requires a priority list of health problems to be studied.

Williamson goes on to demonstrate that there is a link between diagnostic outcomes and therapeutic outcomes and also between these and their process equivalents, the diagnostic and therapeutic process. It may be argued that inaccuracies in either of the process areas will be associated with complications. The problem is not entirely an iatrogenic one as adverse events may be either associated with, or be modified by, pre-existing disease occurring before presentation to a doctor.

Complications in patients who suffer from trauma are common. Some are avoidable or their effect can be lessened, but it is unlikely that all can be eliminated completely. The incidence and effect of complications in trauma may depend upon the following factors:

- The severity of the trauma.
- The age of the patient.
- The physiological status of the patient.
- The pre-injury health of the patient.
- The rapidity of the resuscitation.
- The methods of treatment used.
- The availability and appropriateness of the facilities and medical staff.

Frostick and Hunter have defined complications and have reviewed the concept of severity in relation to complications (Frostick and Hunter, 1993). The authors will use the same definition of complications in this chapter. The working definition is, therefore, any adverse event in a treatment episode, this may be divided into those which can be directly attributed to a pre-existing disease and those arising as a direct consequence of the admission*. Severity is a concept of great importance to the understanding of the risk of developing a complication and to the understanding of the effect of the complication on outcome whenever that might occur. Severity, therefore, must be considered in relation to the pre-admission health status of the patient, to the physiological status of the patient on admission or at the time of the development of the complication and to the extent and effect of the complication itself.

Major and minor are also terms that are used in relation to complications. Frostick and Hunter have previously defined major as 'a complication resulting in a prolongation of hospital stay, results in further treatment or which is life threatening'. It should be added that any complication that results in long-term disability should be regarded as major. An alternative way of distinguishing major and minor would be to define a major complication as one which adversely affects outcome. This definition presupposes that it is possible to estimate when the *level of maximum final impairment* (Williamson, 1971) has been achieved and that it is also possible to define in an individual patient how far from the expected outcome the actual outcome has occurred. It may be possible to establish the level of maximum final impairment for the purposes of a study, though this may be entirely arbitrary†.

Complications and litigation

There is fear from some elements of the medical profession that if there is a public admission that complications do occur then this will lead to an increase in litigation. The fact is that most of the examples cited by the General Medical Council and many cases of medical negligence are associated with complications of treatment. The example of deep vein thrombosis (DVT) and the use of prophylaxis is an example which is important to orthopaedic surgeons. In the recent British Orthopaedic Association survey of the use of prophylaxis in major joint-replacement surgery some 10% of surgeons admitted to never using any form of prophylaxis (Laverick *et al.*, 1991). The use of thrombo-prophylaxis has been put centrally in the public domain by the report of the Thrombo-embolic Risk Factors (THRIFT) Consensus Group (1992). This group have stated that all high risk patients should be properly assessed for their risk of developing a thromboembolic complication and should be treated accordingly. Many different groups of orthopaedic and trauma patients are high risk patients and at present there is little real consensus on who should be given prophylaxis and who should not.

It is important that doctors are seen to admit that they are capable of making mistakes. It is also important to demonstrate that doctors are considering why the mistakes have occurred and that they are examining

---

* The discussion group considered the definition of a complication and suggested that a useful alternative would be 'an adverse event outside the natural progress of a condition or its treatment'.

† The discussion group considered the role of complications in outcome and concluded that adverse events do contribute to outcome but it is very difficult to estimate the proportion compared to other parameters.

the ways of reducing those mistakes to a minimum. Hence it is necessary to recognise complications and to examine each critically to determine the reasons for them happening. Further, if doctors recognise that all surgical procedures are associated with complications, then it is possible to obtain a properly informed consent from the patient who is about to undergo a major operation and to whom the doctors cannot give a cast iron guarantee of success.

Complications and trauma

Complications (especially death and its prevention) occurring in trauma patients have been the stimulus to the examination of the provision of trauma services. This chapter will review some of the work in this field. Death has been the outcome measure that has been studied most frequently, particularly in the area of multiple trauma. There has been a general recognition that other complications, such as DVT and wound infection, do occur in trauma patients but complications have not been used as specific measures of outcome. Age, health status on admission and length of hospital stay have been considered in relation to trauma patient outcome.

Assessment of injury

Many different scores have been devised to determine the severity of injury particularly in the severely injured but the scores are also applicable to less severely injured individuals. These scores have been reviewed in Chapter 1. The main relation to complications is that these scores have been used in calculations of the probability of death/survival. Further, these scores have been used, and are increasingly used, to compare the effectiveness of trauma treatment between trauma hospitals (Moylan *et al.*, 1976; Knaus *et al.*, 1982, 1986).

Death, the ultimate complication of trauma, has been used extensively as an outcome measure (Friesen, 1974; Moore *et al.*, 1991; Bradbury, 1991; Bull, 1975). It can be difficult to determine the true mortality rate and the cause of death after major injuries. For example, in the UK it is not routine to perform radiographs of all bodies of individuals who die at the scene of an accident. In a recent air-crash, for example, it was not possible to determine accurately the causes of death and the types of injuries suffered by those who died on site. Bucholz *et al.* (1979) examined the cervical spine of road-accident fatalities by post-mortem radiographs and found that 24% of the patients had very significant injuries and of these half were occult. Dove *et al.* (1980) studied 108 patients admitted to one trauma centre who died. The patients had an age range of 3–84 years and an injury severity score (ISS) which ranged from 9 to 66. Significant complications had occurred in these patients: sepsis 30%, respiratory failure 15% and renal failure 10%. It is worth noting that the authors deemed that medical care was optimum in only 45% of the patients, in the remaining 55% of patients at least one error of management was found. Lowe *et al.* (1983) concluded that 25% of those who died in their survey did so inappropriately and 16% of the overall outcomes were inappropriate for the severity of the injuries. These authors particularly highlighted the fact that the resuscitation of injured patients was inadequate in the small hospitals studied and resulted in a significant number of unnecessary emergency room deaths. Gilroy (1984) introduced the idea of Class I and Class II deaths. Class I are those in whom the fatal lesion was undiagnosed or inadequately treated and in whom this had no effect on outcome; Class II deaths were those in which the outcome was affected. These patients represent a group of preventable deaths. Another controversial area is that of the transportation of injured patients to hospital (Baxt and Moody, 1983; Gilroy, 1985).

Age and pre-existing disease

Bull (1975) found that increasing age was associated with an increasing probability of death following multiple trauma. Eichelberger *et al.* (1988) compared the outcome of blunt trauma in children compared to adults under the age of 54. Using the TRISS methodology the authors were unable to show any differences in the probability of survival in these groups. Knaus *et al.* (1984) describes five factors that determine outcome following major illness: (1) disease type; (2) the severity of the disease; (3) the patient's age; (4) the prior health status; and (5) the therapy available. Wu *et al.* (1990) retrospectively compared elderly (over 75 years) and patients between the ages of 55 and 65 for the probability of survival following admission to an intensive care unit (ICU). The authors found that the APACHE II scoring system for physiological status was an excellent predictor of mortality but older age did not predict mortality if severity of illness, admitting diagnosis and malignancy were excluded. MacKenzie *et al.* (1989) studied the effect of pre-existing disease upon length of stay. The authors found that the presence of a pre-existing condition increased the length of stay significantly and that the effect was more extensive in young patients. Only 8% of patients admitted to an ICU over the age of 75 had no pre-existing disease process (McClish *et al.*, 1987) and raw mortality data showed that the hospital survival declined with age. However, if severity of illness and prior health were controlled the differences in survival rate disappeared between the groups, indicating that age was not the most important factor. In contradistinction to this, Champion *et al.* (1989) compared 3833 patients over 65 with 42 944 patients under 65 admitted to 111 trauma centres in North America. The patients were controlled for injury severity. However, the older patients had a higher mortality rate and longer hospital stay; this had major cost implications. Similarly, Ridley *et al.* (1990) have shown that long-term survival following admission to an ICU was related both to age and to severity of illness. Mahul *et al.* (1991) have also found that age and previous health status are predictors of early mortality (within 1 year) after discharge from an ICU. A recent Editorial in *The Lancet* (1991) reviewed the literature concerning the relationship of age and survival after ICU treatment, the conclusion was that ageing was necessarily relevant and that impaired physiological reserve may also be important. Grimley-Evans (1984) has shown that in patients with fractures of the proximal femur, the main risk factors are age and mental state. It would seem that age alone may not be a risk factor in trauma but, probably, a combination of age and chronic disease is a factor.

General complications of trauma

Adult respiratory distress syndrome/fat embolism

Fat embolism and long bone fractures are frequently related (Peltier, 1969; Gurd and Wilson, 1974). Riska and Myllynen (1982) suggested that the development of grade 3 fat embolus syndrome can be prevented if patients undergo early internal fixation of fractures. Similarly, Goris et al. (1982) proposed that early fracture fixation and elective postoperative ventilation reduced or prevented the onset of adult respiratory distress syndrome (ARDS) in severely injured patients. Goris and Draaisma (1982) also suggested that the main cause of death more than 7 days after multiple trauma, severe sepsis, could be reduced by adequate early immobilisation of fractures. Fifty-five per cent of late deaths in a group of 359 trauma patients died as a result of sepsis and/or multi-organ failure (Baker et al., 1980). Fein et al. (1983) found that ARDS was a frequent association with septicaemia and increased the chance of death; age, sex, type of septicaemia and other factors were not important. Fife et al. (1983) also found that pneumonia and pulmonary embolus was a major cause of death in a population of injured bicyclists. Allgöwer et al. (1980) emphasised the fact that the pulmonary effects of trauma have been substantially reduced by an elective ventilation policy linked to the early internal fixation of fractures. Seibel et al. (1985) reported a prospective study of the effects of immediate versus delayed internal fixation of fractures and the relationship to developing respiratory complications (particularly pulmonary failure-septic state). The authors reported that those patients who underwent delayed fixation of fractures had a significantly longer ventilation period and higher incidence of respiratory problems; fracture complications also increased with increasing delay in fixation. Johnson et al. (1985) retrospectively studied patients with an injury severity score of 18 or higher, the effect of fracture fixation and the development of ARDS. The authors found that in the most severely injured patients the development of ARDS was particularly affected by early fixation of the fractures. Broos et al. (1987) examined mortality data on 1063 patients and found that the mortality rate was reduced from 13.5% to 1.8% if early internal fixation of fractures was undertaken and that the effect was more pronounced if the fixation was performed within the first 24 hours. More recently, Bone et al. (1989) undertook a prospective study of the effects of early fixation of femoral fractures on the development of pulmonary complications. The study was not ideally organised but indicated that early fixation was associated with less morbidity.

Pulmonary failure after trauma was increasingly recognised during the 1980s as an important source of mortality, morbidity and excess cost. All three of these categories have been used as outcome measures in research papers investigating the role of both early fracture fixation (sometimes termed prophylactic) and ventilatory support. Mortality and cost are easily measured, as is morbidity when confined to duration of hospital stay, or within that length of time spent on intensive care units. However when diagnostic categories are introduced to compare patient groups the position becomes less clear. A possible reason for this is the difficulty in defining the condition of fat embolism.

Fat embolism is a clinical diagnosis and is therefore open to interpretation. The diagnostic criteria advanced by Riska and Myllynen (1982) included:

1. PaO_2 less than 60 mmHg on air.
2. Petechial rash.
3. Disturbance of consciousness.
4. Progressive anaemia.
5. Pyrexia.
6. Tachypnoea.
7. Thrombocytopenia.
8. Requirement for ventilatory support.
9. X-ray showing typical diffuse infiltration.

The syndrome was then divided into three grades:

Grade 1 – petechiae and other mild signs.
Grade 2 – petechiae and other signs, but harmless and not requiring treatment.
Grade 3 – several diagnostic criteria present including need for respiratory support.

In this situation diagnostic criteria and outcome have become hopelessly confused and it is unlikely that the categories are reproducible.

To address this problem pulmonary failure or impairment has been divided into two categories, pulmonary dysfunction and ARDS, on the basis of the following criteria:

- PaO_2 less than 250 mmHg on 100% O_2.
- Pulmonary venoarterial shunt greater than 25%.
- X-ray showing diffuse interstitial oedema.

Dysfunction is defined by one criterion being present, ARDS by two or more. These categories have been shown to have predictive value for mortality and morbidity and have been fairly widely used (e.g. Johnson *et al.*, 1985; Bone *et al.*, 1989).

Sepsis and multiple organ dysfunction

Multiple trauma victims are at risk of a severe generalised response to their insult that has been variously described as 'Progressive or sequential organ failure', 'Multiple organ failure' and 'Multiple systems organ failure'. The symptoms and signs of this condition are very similar to those seen in systemic sepsis, although by no means necessarily caused by infection. Hence there is further confusion of the terminology through the terms 'Sepsis', 'Septicaemia', 'Septic shock', 'Septicaemic shock' and so on. Furthermore, there is clearly distinct overlap with the conditions described above under 'ARDS/fat embolism'.

A Consensus Conference of the American College of Chest Physicians and the Society of Critical Care Medicine published a series of definitions for sepsis and organ failure in June 1992 and the recommended definitions are reproduced below (Consensus Conference of the American College of Chest Physicians and the Society of Critical Care Medicine, 1992a, 1992b). The main recommendations are that the terms septicaemia and multiple organ failure be abandoned, and replaced with Systemic Inflammatory Response Syndrome (SIRS) and Multiple Organ Dysfunction Syndrome (MODS). The former may be termed sepsis when it is proven that the inflammation to which the body is responding is infection.

Some definitions

Infection	Microbial phenomenon characterised by an inflammatory response to the presence of micro-organisms or the invasion of normally sterile host tissue by those organisms.
Bacteraemia	The presence of viable bacteria in the blood.
Systemic Inflammatory Response Syndrome	The response to a variety of severe clinical insults, manifested by two or more of the following conditions:- Temperature $> 38\,°C$ or $< 36\,°C$ Heart rate > 90 beats/min. Respiratory rate > 20 breaths/min or $PaCO_2$ < 32 mmHg (< 4.3 kPa) WBC $> 12\,000$ cells/mm^3, < 4000 cells/mm^3 or $> 10\%$ immature forms.
Sepsis	The systemic response to infection, manifested by two or more of the following conditions *resulting from infection*:- Temperature $> 38\,°C$ or $< 36\,°C$ Heart rate > 90 beats/min Respiratory rate > 20 breaths/min or $PaCO_2$ < 32 mmHg (< 4.3 kPa) WBC $> 12\,000$ cells/mm^3, < 4000 cells/mm^3 or $> 10\%$ immature forms.
Severe sepsis	Sepsis associated with organ dysfunction, hypoperfusion or hypotension. Hypoperfusion and perfusion abnormalities which may include, but are not limited to lactic acidosis, oliguria, or an acute alteration in mental status.
Septic shock	Sepsis with hypotension, despite adequate fluid resuscitation, along with the presence of perfusion abnormalities which may include, but are not limited to lactic acidosis, oliguria, or an acute alteration in mental status. Patients who are on inotropic or vasopressor agents may not be hypotensive at the time that perfusion abnormalities are measured.

Hypotension	A systolic BP of < 90 mmHg or a reduction of > 40 mmHg from baseline in the absence of other causes for hypotension.
Multiple Organ Dysfunction Syndrome	Presence of altered organ function in an acutely ill patient such that homeostasis cannot be maintained without intervention.

Thromboembolism

The discrepancy between the outcome measures used in thrombosis research and clinical reality have been discussed elsewhere (Frostick and Hunter, 1993). The most important outcome is fatal pulmonary embolus (PE). Clinically apparent thromboembolism is normally reflected as increased hospital stay. Embolism diagnosed by ventilation/perfusion scintigraphy should be classified according to the well-validated criteria:

- High probability of PE.
- Intermediate probability of PE.
- Low probability of PE.

Essentially the first and last categories require no further investigation, whilst indeterminate may require pulmonary angiography if the clinical signs are strongly suggestive of embolus.

Similarly venograms need to be reported in a standard fashion, documenting both location and extent of any thrombus. This is particularly important in orthopaedic surgery especially multiple trauma where the benefits of treating thrombosis need to be carefully weighed against the risk of bleeding. The risk of bleeding when arthroplasty patients are fully anticoagulated with heparin is 45% in the first postoperative week and 20% in the second week (Patterson *et al.*, 1989).

Specific complications of fractures

Non-union (see also Chapter 9)

Non-union is the failure of a fracture to unite with radiological signs that the situation is permanent in the absence of intervention. Two radiological categories are recognised:

1. Hypertrophic – abundant bone formation with flaring of the bone at the fracture site, the 'elephant's foot'
2. Atrophic – narrow, rounded, osteoporotic bone ends. At the microscopic level the ends are acellular and frequently avascular.

Malunion

Theoretically healing with any abnormality. In practice defined as union with any anatomical abnormality sufficient to affect function either of the limb or the patient and therefore including cosmetic deformity. Measurement of the malunion takes the form of angulation assessment, loss of movement, and radiographic congruency of intra-articular fractures.

Delayed union

Delayed union is not an outcome measure as it will always proceed to non-union or union. Any analysis of fracture treatment should have sufficient follow-up that delayed union is never the final status.

Infection

Definitions for infection are difficult and confusing. In orthopaedics and trauma there has been a tradition to divide infections into deep and superficial, early and late. These are not particularly helpful or even accurate terms. The Surgical Infection Study Group (SSIG) (1991) has developed a series of definitions of infection and suggested their use in all surgical specialties.

SSIG have defined wound infections as follows: 'a wound infection should have either a purulent discharge in, or exuding from the wound, or a painful, spreading erythema indicative of cellulitis':

Minor: 'discharge of pus from the wound without lymphangitis or deep tissue destruction'.

Major: 'when purulent discharge is accompanied by painful or complete dehiscence of the fascial layers of the wound, or by spreading cellulitis and lymphangitis that requires antibiotic therapy'.

Postoperative infection in bone

Early: 'the presence of pain at rest, a fever greater than 38 °C persisting for more than 48 hours supported by the isolation of bacteria from cultures when available'.

Late: 'indicated by the presence of pain at rest, a persisting elevation of the ESR greater than 30 mm hr^{-1} above the preoperative level, radiological changes in bone indicative of infection and the isolation of bacteria from cultures when available'.

Infection after implant surgery

'Indicated by the presence of one or more of the following: pain, persistent pyrexia greater than 38 °C for 48 hours, local signs of inflammation where the implant is superficial, radiological signs where the implant involves, or is adjacent to bone, an elevated white blood-cell count.'

The main confusion probably lies in not distinguishing (1) infection that affects the wound alone and eventually results in normal wound healing, from (2) those infections that affect the wound only but do not result in normal wound healing, and (3) wounds that heal normally but there is infection surrounding an implant and wounds that do not heal and are associated with infection around an implant. If it could be certain which of these categories is being encountered in an individual patient then relatively simple definitions like those above can be used. The problem, may, therefore, be one of diagnosis and its certainty, rather than definition.

The signs of a wound infection mentioned in the SSIG definitions do occur in orthopaedic and trauma patients. However, some patients appear to 'simply' have serous discharge without any growth on culturing swabs but eventually are diagnosed as having a definite infection. This may be a limitation of the methods of obtaining swabs and the methods of culture used.

Infection around an implant may or may not be associated with any of the symptoms and signs of the SSIG definition; indeed infection around a joint replacement may not be apparent unless an operation is undertaken.

The role of the ESR in many patients is doubtful in the diagnosis of infection, especially in those patients who may have a raised ESR for other reasons (e.g. rheumatoid)*.

Gustilo et al. (1990) have reviewed the management of open fractures. The authors report that the recorded infection rates in the different grades of open fracture range from 0–2% in type I to 25–50% for type IIIC. Type IIIC fractures are associated with the most serious soft tissue damage, that of an arterial lesion affecting the major limb vessels. The other major complications in open fractures are the risk of compartment syndrome and non-union. Gustilo et al. report a 2.7% compartment syndrome rate in open fractures. Blick et al. (1986) have found a 9.1% incidence of compartment syndrome after open fractures. Caudle and Stern (1987) reported a high non-union rate in open fractures of the tibia which was reduced by early free flap soft tissue coverage. In this series 42 type IIIB fractures were reviewed; 15 non-unions occurred 12 of which were associated with deep infection, secondary amputation was performed in seven. Court-Brown et al. (1990b) have reviewed the use of external fixation in type III fractures of the tibia and found an overall infection rate of 17·6%. In type IIIC fractures they found that the time to union was increased with the increasing severity of the injury and there was a high amputation rate. Interlocked nailing of the tibia is still controversial, especially in open fractures, because of the risk of infection (Court-Brown et al., 1990a).

Compartment syndrome and vascular injuries

Holden (1979) has defined two types of vascular injuries:

Type 1 – proximal arterial injury leading to distal ischaemia.
Type 2 – direct injury leading to ischaemia at the site of injury.

Severe ischaemia has three possible outcomes,

1. Recovery.
2. Gangrene.
3. Contracture.

Contracture always occurs as a result of swelling in 'unyielding osseofascial compartments', and this swelling can be the result of either type 1 or type 2 injuries. This is because both set in motion the same vicious cycle of swelling and ischaemia that is compartment syndrome. The final

* Perhaps the CRP (C-reactive protein) level would provide a better measure (Editors).

common pathway is reduction in capillary blood flow due to increased pressure within the compartment. Pain is the predominant symptom, although it may be absent in cases of severe primary nerve injury. Nerve is the tissue most sensitive to ischaemia, so paradoxically to make a clinical diagnosis of a vascular problem the nervous system must be examined as closely as the circulation. The absolute pressure required to impair capillary flow varies between individuals, however a prospective study using a wick catheter showed that fasciotomy could be withheld if the compartment pressure was less than 30 mmHg (Mubarak et al., 1978).

It is known that compartment syndrome occurs particularly in the lower limb and especially after closed fractures, the incidence varies from 3% to 10% (Gershuni et al., 1987). Tischenko and Goodman (1990) have recently shown that compartment syndrome can be induced by closed tibial nailing and that, if pressure studies are performed during the operative procedure, peaks of pressure could be recorded both when the traction is applied and during the actual nailing procedure. Different methods of performing a fasciotomy for compartment syndrome are described; it is important to fully decompress all four compartments. Cohen et al. (1991) have suggested that if the length of the skin incision is not adequate then the decompression will not be properly performed and compartment pressures will remain elevated.

Heterotopic bone formation

Heterotopic bone formation is particularly recognised as a complication of hip and elbow injury and surgery, although it can occur in the soft tissue around any joint. A widely used classification was described by Brooker et al. (1973) (Table 12.1).

McLaren (1990) found that 50% of patients undergoing surgery for acetabular fractures who did not receive indomethacin developed evidence of moderate heterotopic calcification; this was reduced to 5.5% in patients receiving the drug.

Nerve damage

Nerve injuries are common both directly due to the trauma and as a result of the subsequent surgery. In a group of 65 iatrogenic nerve injuries Birch et al. (1991) found 21 that were associated with fracture fixation. There may be medicolegal consequences of these injuries.

Table 12.1 Brooker classification of heterotopic ossification

Grade	Radiographic findings	Movement	Function
0	No heterotopic bone	Normal	Normal
1	Islands of bone	Normal	Normal
2	Bar of bone: gap > 1 cm	Decreased	Minimal loss
3	Bar of bone: gap < 1 cm	Decreased	Moderate loss
4	Bone bridging joint	Ankylosis	Severe loss

Reproduced from Brooker et al., 1973.

Avascular necrosis

Avascular necrosis is a complication of many fractures. In the hip, pathology and radiographic findings are related by the classification of Ficat (1985) which recognises five grades. Outcome is particularly affected by bony collapse, which heralds the onset of osteoarthritis, and denotes the moment when treatment ends and reconstruction starts. Such a classification is not available for other common sites of avascular necrosis.

Osteoarthritis (see also Chapter 10)

The development of secondary osteoarthritis after trauma is a major complication which may be reduced by open reduction and internal fixation of intra-articular fractures. Some patients complain of pain and difficulty with walking after, for example, malunion of ankle fractures (Marti et al., 1990). Jupiter (1991) in his review of distal radial fractures reported that complications including osteoarthritis have been found following Colles' fractures. Upadhay and Moulton (1981) found a high incidence of osteoarthritis of the hip following posterior dislocation of the hip despite prompt reduction. Similarly, Teitz et al. (1980) found that, with malunion of a tibial fracture, patients developed osteoarthritis of the ankle within 2 years of injury. The role of internal fixation in reducing osteoarthritis is still controversial.

Algodystrophy

Algodystrophy is a syndrome of pain, tenderness, loss of mobility and vasomotor changes that can follow a variety of injuries, but is most extensively studied following Colles' fractures. The work of Atkins et al. (1990) shows that a combination of criteria, both objective and subjective, can be used to diagnose the condition (Table 12.2).

The relatively recent appearance of proper diagnostic criteria for this condition means that studies relating them to outcome are still awaited. A follow-up of Colles' fractures from Bristol suggested that a quarter of patients still exhibited these signs at 10 years. Patients whose hand function had deteriorated over the 10 years were more likely to have algodystrophy Field et al. (1992).

Table 12.2 Indices of algodystrophy

Abnormal feature	Sensitivity (%)	Specificity (%)
Pain in the hand	86	100
Dolorimetry ratio	100	97
Hand volume ratio	14	100
Digital circumference	32	94
Skinfold thickness ratio	45	62
Vasomotor instability	100	95
Finger movement	100	95

Reproduced from Atkins et al., 1990, with permission.

Implant removal and timing of surgery

The removal of metalwork may be associated with complications. Forty per cent of a series of 55 patients had significant complications following plate removal from the forearm, the incidence was higher if the plates were removed by a junior surgeon, and there was permanent disability in 50% of the patients (Langkamer and Ackroyd, 1990). Rosson *et al.* (1991) have been able to show that there are definite bone changes in patients in whom plates were removed prematurely and this may be associated with an increase risk of refracture. The timing of operation may have an effect on the overall complication rate following trauma. Carragee *et al.* (1991) have shown that delay in the fixation of displaced ankle fractures is associated with an increased incidence of complications, including failed reduction and infection. These authors found that in patients operated upon within 24 hours of injury the complication rate was 5.3% but those operated upon more than 24 hours after injury had a complication rate of 44%.

Conclusions

This chapter has not sought to be an exhaustive review of complications. Scoring systems for complications are almost non-existent despite the fact that complications may be an important factor in determining outcome, including patient satisfaction. It is important that adequate documentation of complications occurs both in the case records and also for purposes of audit. Complications may be the source of litigation but an acknowledgement of their existence and that attempts are being made to reduce them may to some extent allay the fears of the general public.

References

Allgöwer M, Dürig M, Wolff G (1980) Infection and trauma. *Surg. Clin. North Am.*; **60**: 133–144

Atkins RM, Duckworth T, Kanis JA (1990) Features of algodystrophy after Colles' fracture. *J. Bone Joint Surg.*; **72B**: 105–110

Baker CC, Oppenheimer L, Stephens B, Lewis RF, Trunkey DD (1980) Epidemiology of trauma deaths. *Am. J. Surg.*; **140**: 144–150

Baxt WG, Moody P (1983) The impact of a rotorcraft aeromedical emergency care service on trauma mortality. *JAMA*; **249**: 3047–3051

Birch R, Bonney G, Dowell J, Hollingdale J (1991) Iatrogenic injuries of peripheral nerves. *J. Bone Joint Surg.*; **73B**: 280–282

Blick SS, Brumback RJ, Poka A, Burgess AR, Ebraheim NA (1986) Compartment syndrome in open tibial fractures. *J. Bone Joint Surg.*; **68A**: 1348–1353

Bone LB, Johnson ND, Wiegelt J, Scheinberg R (1989) Early versus delayed stabilization of femoral fractures. A prospective randomized study. *J. Bone Joint Surg.*; **71A**: 336–340

Bradbury A (1991) Pattern and severity of injury sustained by pedestrians in road traffic accidents with particular reference to the effect of alcohol. *Injury*; **22**: 132–134

Brooker AF, Bowerman JW, Robinson RA, Riley LH (1973) Ectopic ossification following total hip replacement. Incidence and a method of classification. *J. Bone Joint Surg.*; **55A**: 1629–1632

Broos PLO, Stappaerts KH, Luiten EJT, Gruwez JA (1987) The importance of early internal fixation in multiply injured patients to prevent late death due to sepsis. *Injury*; **18**: 235–237

Bucholz RW, Burkhead WZ, Graham W, Petty C (1979) Occult cervical spine injuries in fatal traffic accidents. *J. Trauma*; **19**: 768–771

Bull JP (1975) The injury severity score of road traffic casualties in relation to mortality. Time of death, hospital treatment time and disability. *Accid. Anal. Prev.*; **7**: 249–255

Carragee EJ, Csongradi JJ, Bleck EE (1991) Early complications in the operative treatment of ankle fractures – influence of delay before operation. *J. Bone Joint Surg.*; **73B**: 79–82

Caudle RJ, Stern PJ (1987) Severe open fractures of the tibia. *J. Bone Joint Surg.*; **69A**: 801–807

Champion HR, Copes WS, Buyer D, Flanagan ME, Bain L, Sacco WJ (1989) Major trauma in geriatric patients. *Am. J. Public Health*; **79**: 1278–1282

Cohen MS, Garfin SR, Hargens AR, Mubarak SJ (1991) Acute compartment syndrome – effect of dermotomy on fascial decompression in the leg. *J. Bone Joint Surg.*; **73B**: 287–290

Consensus Conference of the American College of Chest Physicians and the Society of Critical Care Medicine (1992a) *Chest*; **101**: 1644–1655

Consensus Conference of the American College of Chest Physicians and the Society of Critical Care Medicine. (1992b) *Crit. Care Med.*; **20**: 864–874

Court-Brown CM, Christie J, McQueen MM (1990a) Closed intramedullary tibial nailing. Its use in closed and type I open fractures. *J. Bone Joint Surg.*; **72B**: 605–611

Court-Brown CM, Wheelwright EF, Christie J, McQueen MM (1990b) External fixation for type III open tibial fractures. *J. Bone Joint Surg.*; **72B**: 801–804

Dove DB, Stahl WM, Del Guercio LRM (1980) A five-year review of deaths following urban trauma. *J. Trauma*; **20**: 760–766

Editorial (1991) Intensive care for the elderly. *Lancet*; **337**: 209–210

Eichelberger MR, Mangubat EA, Sacco WS, Bowman LM, Lowenstein AD (1988) Comparative outcomes of children and adults suffering blunt trauma. *J. Trauma*; **28**: 430–434

Fein M, Lippmann M, Holtzman H, Eliraz A, Goldberg SK (1983) The risk factors, incidence and prognosis of ARDS following septicemia. *Chest*; **83**: 40–42

Ficat RP (1985) Idiopathic bone necrosis of the femoral head – early diagnosis and treatment. *J. Bone Joint Surg.*; **67B**: 3–9

Field J, Warwick D, Bannister GC (1992) Features of algodystrophy ten years after Colles' fracture. *J. Hand Surg.*; **17B**: 318–320

Fife D, Davis J, Tate L, Wells JK, Mohan D, Williams A (1983) Fatal injuries to bicyclists: the experience of Dade County, Florida. *J. Trauma*; **23**: 745–755

Friesen G (1974) Vancouver Island traffic fatalities, 1966–1970. *J. Trauma*; **14**: 791–797

Frostick SP, Hunter JB (1993) Complications. In Pynsent PB, Fairbank J, Carr A (eds) *Outcome Measures in Orthopaedics*. Oxford: Butterworth Heinemann.

Gershuni DH, Mubarak SJ, Yaru NC, Lee Y-F (1987) Fracture of the tibia complicated by acute compartment syndrome. *Clin. Orthop. Rel. Res.*; **217**: 221–227

Gilroy D (1984) Deaths from blunt trauma: a review of 105 cases. *Injury*; **15**: 304–308

Gilroy D (1985) Deaths (144) from road traffic accidents occurring before arrival at hospital. *Injury*; **16**: 141–242

Goris RJA, Draaisma J (1982) Causes of death after blunt trauma. *J. Trauma*; **22**: 141–146

Goris RJA, Gimbrere JSF, Van Niekerk JLM, Schoots FJ, Booy LHD (1982) Early osteosynthesis and prophylactic mechanical ventilation in the multitrauma patient. *J. Trauma*; **22**: 895–903

Grimley-Evans J (1984) Fractured proximal femur in Newcastle-upon-Tyne. *Age Aging*; **6**: 16–24

Gurd AR, Wilson RI (1974) The fat embolism syndrome. *J. Bone Joint Surg.*; **56B**: 400–416

Gustilo RB, Merkow RL, Templeman D (1990) The management of open fractures. *J. Bone Joint Surg.*; **72A**: 299–304

Holden CEA (1979) The pathology and prevention of Volkmann's ischaemic contracture. *J. Bone Joint Surg.*; **61B**: 296–300

Johnson KD, Cadambi A, Seibert GB (1985) Incidence of adult respiratory distress syndrome in patients with multiple musculoskeletal injuries: effect of early operative stabilization of fractures. *J. Trauma*; **25**: 375–384

Jupiter JB (1991) Fractures of the distal end of the radius. *J. Bone Joint Surg.*; **73A**: 461–469

Knaus WA, Wagner DP, Loirat P, Cullen DJ, Glaser P, Mercier P, Nikki P, Snyder JV, Le Gall JR, Draper EA, Campos RA, Kohles MK, Granthil C, Nicolas F, Shin B, Wattel F, Zimmerman JE (1982) A comparison of intensive care in the USA and France. *Lancet*; **i**: 642–647

Knaus WA, Wagner DP, Draper EA (1984) The value of measuring severity of disease in clinical research on acutely ill patients. *J. Chron. Dis.*; **37**: 455–463

Knaus WA, Draper EA, Wagner DP, Zimmerman JE (1986) An evaluation of outcome from intensive care in major medical centers. *Ann. Intern. Med.*; **104**: 410–418

Langkamer VG, Ackroyd CE (1990) Removal of forearm plates – a review of the complications. *J. Bone Joint Surg.*; **72B**: 601–604

Laverick MD, Croal SA, Mollan RAB (1991) Orthopaedic surgeons and thromboprophylaxis. *Br. Med. J.*; **303**: 549–550

Lowe DK, Gately HL, Goss JR, Frey CL, Peterson CG (1983) Patterns of death, complication and error in the management of motor vehicle accident victims: implications for a regional system of trauma care. *J. Trauma*; **23**: 503–509

MacKenzie EJ, Morris JA, Edelstein SL (1989) Effect of pre-existing disease on length of hospital stay in trauma patients. *J. Trauma*; **29**: 757–765

Mahul P, Perrot D, Tempelhoff G, Gaussorgues P, Jospe R, Ducreux JC, Dumont A, Motin J, Auboyer C, Robert D (1991) Short- and long-term prognosis, functional outcome following ICU for elderly. *Intensive Care Med.*; **17**: 7–10

Marti RK, Raaymakers ELFB, Nolte PA (1990) Malunited ankle fractures – the late results of reconstruction. *J. Bone Joint Surg.*; **72B**: 709–713

McClish DK, Powell SH, Montenegro H, Nochomovitz M (1987) The impact of age on utilization of intensive care resources. *J. Am. Geriat. Soc.*; **35**: 983–988

McLaren AC (1990) Prophylaxis with indomethacin for heterotopic bone. *J. Bone Joint Surg.*; **72A**: 245–247

Moore TJ, Wilson JR, Hartman M (1991) Train versus pedestrian accidents. *South. Med. J.*; **84**: 1097–1098

Moylan JA, Detmer DE, Rose J, Schulz R (1976) Evaluation of the quality of hospital care for major trauma. *J. Trauma*; **16**: 517–523

Mubarak SJ, Owen CA, Hargens AR, Garetto LP, Akeson WH (1978) Acute compartment syndromes: diagnosis and treatment with the aid of the wick catheter. *J. Bone Joint Surg.*; **60A**: 1091–1095

Patterson BM, Marchand R, Ranawat C (1989) Complications of heparin therapy after total joint arthroplasty. *J. Bone Joint Surg.*; **71A**: 1130–1134

Peltier LF (1969) Fat embolism: a current concept. *Clin. Orthop. Rel. Res.*; **66**: 241–253

Ridley S, Jackson R, Findlay J, Wallace P (1990) Long term survival after intensive care. *Br. Med. J.*; **301**: 1127–1130

Riska EB, Myllynen P (1982) Fat embolism in patients with multiple injuries. *J. Trauma*; **22**: 891–894

Rosson JW, Petley GW, Shearer JR (1991) Bone structure after removal of internal fixation plates. *J. Bone Joint Surg.*; **73B**: 65–67

Seibel R, Laduca J, Hassett JM, Babikian G, Mills B, Border DO, Border JR (1985) Blunt multiple trauma (ISS 36), femur traction, and the pulmonary failure-septic state. *Ann. Surg.*; **202**: 283–293

Surgical Infection Study Group (1991) Proposed definitions for the audit of postoperative infection: a discussion paper. *Ann. Roy. Coll. Surg. Engl.*; **73**: 385–388

Teitz CC, Carter DR, Frankel VH (1980) Problems associated with tibial fractures with intact fibulae. *J. Bone Joint Surg.*; **62A**: 770–776

Thromboembolic Risk Factors (THRIFT) Consensus Group (1992) Risk of and prophylaxis for venous thromboembolism in hospital patients. *Br. Med. J.*; **336**: 567–574

Tischenko GJ, Goodman SB (1990) Compartment syndrome after intramedullary nailing of the tibia. *J. Bone Joint Surg.*; **72A**: 41–44

Upadhyay SS, Moulton A (1981) The long-term results of traumatic posterior dislocation of the hip. *J. Bone Joint Surg.*; **63B**: 548–551

Williamson JW (1971) Evaluating quality of patient care. *JAMA*; **218**: 564–569

Wu AW, Rubin HR, Rosen MJ (1990) Are elderly people less responsive to intensive care? *J. Am. Geriatr. Soc.*; **38**: 621–627

Chapter 13

Peripheral nerve injuries

D. Marsh

Introduction

A cut peripheral nerve is unique among injuries to musculoskeletal tissues, because it involves transection of the nerve cells themselves. The axons below the level of the lesion, being isolated from the cell body, must inevitably die; so *repair*, in the sense of healing by scar formation, is impossible and nerve function can only be restored by a process of *regeneration*. The regenerative response in primates is poor, and functional loss is further increased by the fact that, if the endoneurial tubes were transected as part of the injury, the chances of a given regenerating axon eventually reaching its original target organ are vanishingly small. Not surprisingly, when the results of nerve repair are examined critically, they are found to be extremely disappointing. However, we stand at the threshold of an era when the poor regenerative response of these highly specialised cells may become open to enhancement by biological adjuvant treatments. Reliable and valid quantitative measures of peripheral nerve function will be greatly needed in the next few years. Unfortunately, they are in short supply.

The bulk of this chapter is a discussion about the validity of various *quantitative* measures of peripheral nerve function following surgical repair of cut nerves. There are many problems associated with all of them and none are suitable for rapid use in the clinic situation. Sensory testing, in particular, requires time and the careful application of rigorous psychophysical methods; otherwise the surgeon is likely to gain false reassurance from highly unreliable, indeed meaningless, pseudoscientific numbers. The surgeon in the clinic should be monitoring outcome by *qualitative* assessment of function of the injured part, distal progress of the regeneration process and the possible development of the various pain syndromes which can follow nerve injury. These are what will affect management.

Quantitative measurement of outcome is only required when a formal process of audit or clinical research is being undertaken. It requires trained personnel, either research workers or hand therapists or, in the case of nerve conduction studies, a clinical neurophysiologist with experience of the low amplitude signals obtained after nerve repair. The available tests are grouped into:

- Quantitative, timed tests of integrated sensorimotor function.

- Tests of motor function, both composite grips and individual muscle observations.
- Sensory tests, subdivided into:
    assessment of sensory modalities;
    tests of spatial discrimination;
    threshold tests.
- Electrophysiological measures.

In each family of tests, the literature concerning reliability and validity is reviewed, and possible pitfalls are identified.

Rapid qualitative evaluation

When following up patients in the clinic after nerve injury and suture, outcome needs to be monitored to guide rehabilitation and possible further surgery. The questions to address are:

- Is function returning? Is the continued functional deficit due to the nerve injury itself or some other problem which could be tackled? Would further functional therapy help? These questions require primarily direct enquiry of the patient, supplemented by observation of the appropriate integrated function. In nerve injuries affecting the hand, this means grip and manipulation; Seddon's coin test is valuable, if closely observed.
- Is there any evidence of reinnervation of muscles known to have been denervated by the injury?
- Does the patient have feeling in areas previously numb? What sort of feeling is it? Vague appreciation of touch may mean no more than that friction on the denervated skin sends vibrations into neighbouring normal territories (often the radial nerve on the dorsum of fingers), where the incredibly sensitive Pacinian system detects them. A report that the quality of feeling is improving and getting less unpleasant is the most encouraging sign.
- Are there symptoms or signs of causalgia, neuroma, algodystrophy or cold intolerance? In particular, does light stroking touch induce a sensation of pain (allodynia)?
- Is axon regeneration proceeding at an acceptable rate? This question is answered by performing the Tinel test, percussing lightly over the course of the nerve from distal to proximal, and *recording* the most distal level at which electric tinglings are felt. Normally there is a lag of 6 weeks or so, followed by progress of 1 mm per day. This test must be done last, even though logically one would wish to know the answer first, since its performance may be uncomfortable and prejudice further examination.

General observations on quantitative testing

Individual peripheral nerve fibres must be either afferent or efferent. However, they form part of a system whose function is highly integrated, whereby muscle activity is controlled by sensory feedback, and sensory information is gathered by active exploration. The true measure of recovery after peripheral nerve injury is really the integrated sensorimotor function of the reinnervated part. None the less, in order to understand *why* integrated function has reached a certain level, we will normally want to analyse separately the sensory and motor components. For tests of integrated function and muscle reinnervation, different approaches must be adopted for upper and lower limbs. For tests of cutaneous sensory reinnervation, the same tests are equally applicable to hand and foot, though more detail is likely to be required in the former.

In addition to the functions of sensorimotor control, normally mediated by large myelinated fibres, complete evaluation after nerve injury must encompass positive symptoms such as pain and paraesthesiae, hypersensitivity and the dystrophic effects of denervation. Thus the evaluation of outcomes after nerve injury must involve a battery of tests, some more quantitative than others. Nerve evaluation, particularly sensibility testing, tends to be regarded as a somewhat tedious job and is often left to hand therapists. Table 13.1 shows the contents of two recent reviews of methods, written by leading modern therapists. These two lists give a similar picture of the current orthodoxy, with a general, qualitative overview of the affected part, followed by quantitative measures of sensibility and function.

Motor, sensory and functional tests all rely on some sort of behavioural response from the patient. There would obviously be advantage in an evaluation which was free of this, and thus potentially more objective. Nerve conduction studies are a candidate for such a test but require especially careful scrutiny from the point of view of validity: do the results correlate with the degree of useful function?

In order to evaluate the efficacy of treatment, measures of injury severity are just as important as measures of outcome. At the very least, these must include the following:

- The grade of nerve damage, described as (Seddon, 1943):
    neuropraxia – conduction block without axonal death below the lesion;
    axononotmesis – death of axons, but intact endoneurial tubes;
    neuronotmesis – death of axons, with transected endoneurial tubes.
- The length of the damaged segment: whether a direct suture was possible or an interposition graft was required.
- The mechanism of injury: clean cut, traction, crush and so on.
- Associated injuries: energy dissipated in the tissues overall.
- Delay between injury and suture.

Since nerve regeneration is a slow process, generally considered not to reach its plateau until something like 4 years after injury, the timing of assessment is critical. In any given study, it is necessary that either all cases are seen 4 years or more after treatment, or that the time between treatment and evaluation is taken into account by multivariate analysis. Similarly, factors such as the age of the patient at the time of injury and treatment may be extremely potent; in particular, children of 13 years or

Table 13.1 Structures of two papers describing sensory evaluation schemes

Callahan (1984)	Waylett-Rendall (1988)
Sympathetic function	Sympathetic function
Tinel	Pain
Modalities	Heat
pinprick	
temperature	
Touch	Touch – threshold
monofilaments	monofilaments
	Touch – discrimination
2PD	static 2PD
localisation	moving 2PD
ridge sensitometer	ridge sensitometer
Function	Pick-up test
pick-up	

less are apt to make enormously better sensory recovery, probably mainly due to the greater plasticity of their central nervous systems.

A further complicating factor, particularly relevant in assessing sensibility, is the interaction between training exercises used in rehabilitation and the tasks set in measuring outcome. Object identification is a challenge frequently used in both contexts. Also, it is common for sensory tests, such as two-point discrimination, to be applied repeatedly during rehabilitation, as a way of monitoring progress and providing encouragement to the patient. Both these practices, laudable though they are in a therapeutic sense, give great problems in the interpretation of test results, because of the powerful practice effects they induce. The information transmitted centrally after nerve repair is effectively scrambled and the business of learning anew what the incoming signals mean is part and parcel of recovery. In studies designed to evaluate regeneration in the periphery, this important factor constitutes noise.

In evaluating the outcome measures available, we need to know four things about them:

Practicality can the test realistically be applied in the setting intended? Does it require equipment 'weighing a ton', 'costing a bomb' or usable only by someone with an engineering degree?

Range is the test sensitive over the range of function likely to be encountered in the subjects under study? Different sensory tests may be needed for evaluating nerve suture or nerve compression

Reliability do you get the same results in the same patient on different days, or when the test is applied by a different examiner?

Validity do the results of the test reflect the degree of useful function to the patient: do they correlate with the results of quantitative tests of integrated function? Do we know what is the neural basis for the test: can we infer anything about the quality or quantity of reinnervation which produced it?

Finally, a clear policy is needed as to how results will be expressed: in absolute terms?; in relation to a bank of 'normal values'?; in relation to the patient's contralateral limb? In the case of the hand, given that traumatic peripheral nerve lesions are usually unilateral, it is much better to express results as a percentage of the score achieved on the unaffected side: variation between individuals is much greater than that between left and right hands in the same individual, except for a small number of highly skilled actions. In the case of lower limb lesions the situation is different, since the main integrated function is walking, which is essentially a bilateral activity.

Measures of integrated sensorimotor function

The safest and most obvious way to compare, for example, the outcomes of treatment in two similar groups of nerve-injured patients is to measure the performance of the hands supplied by the nerves in question. This requires the design of tasks which are as near to everyday activity as possible, while being amenable to some form of quantitative scoring. Provided there are no large systematic differences between the groups with respect to age, intelligence or other (non-neural) damage, differences in performance should reflect differences in nerve function.

The pioneer in the use of functional tests, to evaluate the outcome of peripheral nerve repair in the hand, was Moberg (1958). His test, involving the timed picking up and identification of small objects, a task which stresses median sensory function (indeed Moberg regarded it as a test of sensibility), is still in wide use today. The picking-up test described in that article has been followed by many other functional tests (e.g. see Wynn-Parry, 1981). In some the numerical score is a measure of accuracy, in others of speed of performance of the task. Tasks include manipulating or picking up small objects, identifying shapes and textures.

Functional tests should be tailored to the nerve in question. The picking-up test, for example, is less appropriate for the ulnar nerve than the median. Brink and Mackel (1987) used an 'ulnar grip' test, measuring the thinnest rod that could be gripped by the ring and little fingers. Identification of textures may be applicable to both, providing satisfactory screening-off of neighbouring intact nerves is achieved. Eliminating the contribution of neighbouring intact nerves to the conduct of the task is not easy. Local anaesthetic blocks have the advantage of thoroughness, done properly, but score low on patient acceptability and may cause confusion due to motor paralysis. Masking with cut-down gloves is a realistic alternative (Marsh and Smith, 1986).

The development of functional testing has been accompanied by increasing general awareness of the importance of the functional outcome of any treatment directed at the hand and has occurred in parallel with the establishment of hand therapists as a specialised subset of physiotherapists and occupational therapists, with their own, functionally oriented regimens. This means that many of the tests used to assess outcome are the same as the exercises used in treatment. Caution is needed therefore in interpreting the results, since training effects are prominent.

Certainly in any clinical trial it would be necessary to standardise the rehabilitation regimen just as rigorously as the surgical technique.

Whatever battery of tests is selected for evaluating the outcome of peripheral nerve injuries, it is essential that some functional tests are included, since they score so highly on face validity, as judged against the yardstick of usefulness to the patient.

Measures of motor function

The two most important aspects of the function of reinnervated muscle are the amount of force the muscle can produce and the extent to which that force can be controlled. Traditionally, the assessment of the former has been a fundamentally subjective process, depending heavily on the skill of the observer.

One reason why a skilled observer will always be indispensable is the need to isolate the action of the muscle under scrutiny in each specific case. A rigorous application of anatomical knowledge, as exemplified in the MRC pamphlet *Aids to the Examination of the Peripheral Nervous System* (MRC, 1976), is essential. In the upper limb, special knowledge of trick movements, whereby the normal action of a muscle is achieved in some other way, is also needed (Seddon, 1975; Wynn-Parry, 1981). For example:

- Secondary action of another muscle, as when flexor pollicis brevis extends the interphalangeal joint of the thumb or brachioradialis flexes the elbow.
- Tenodesis effects, as when finger flexion is produced passively by the long finger flexors when the wrist is actively extended.
- Contraction of antagonists followed by relaxation, producing rebound of the passively stretched muscle.
- Gravity, especially at the elbow, if triceps is paralysed.

In addition there are neural pitfalls which may lead to false optimism about the results of nerve repair, because the motor nerve under test was never severed in the first place:

- Incomplete nerve lesions.
- Atypical patterns of motor innervation.
- Atypical routes taken by motor fibres, as when median fibres to the thenar eminence cross over to the ulnar nerve in the forearm (Martin–Gruber anastomosis).

Clarification can often be obtained by the use of electrical stimulation of nerve trunks in addition to voluntary testing. Once the relevant muscles can be isolated, the degree of motor reinnervation is traditionally expressed on 'the MRC Motor Scale'. In fact there are two such scales. The first, of general applicability in assessment of motor function (MRC, 1976), is as shown in Table 13.2.

The second scale (Highet, 1954) was specifically designed for assessment of the outcome of nerve injuries. Like its sensory counterpart, the categories are qualitative, with no attempt to quantify force (Table 13.3).

Table 13.2 The MRC Scale of Motor Power (MRC, 1976)

0   No contraction
1   Flicker or trace of contraction
2   Active movement, with gravity eliminated
3   Active movement against gravity
4   Active movement against gravity and resistance
5   Normal power

Table 13.3 The MRC Scale of Motor Recovery (Highet 1954)

M0   No contraction
M1   Return of perceptible contraction in the proximal muscles
M2   Return of perceptible contraction in the proximal and distal muscles
M3   Return of function in both proximal and distal muscles of such degree that all
     important muscles can act against resistance
M4   Return of function as in stage 3 with the addition that all synergic and independent
     movements are possible
M5   Complete recovery

Neither of the above two scales is particularly helpful in assessing the results of treatment of the typical modern, peacetime median or ulnar nerve injuries at the wrist. The first's emphasis on the ability to overcome gravity is irrelevant in the case of intrinsic hand muscles. The second's distinction between proximal and distal reinnervation is inappropriate for such distal lesions, although the recovery of 'synergic and independent movements' is important. However, their main disadvantage is the fact that they are qualitative and subjective.

Although there have been few reports of the outcome of nerve suture using quantitative force measurements, the techniques are available. Composite grips, such as power and pinch, can be measured by a variety of devices:

- Pneumatic, involving compression of rubber bulbs.
- Hydraulic, such as the Jamar dynamometer.
- Spring-loaded, such as the Preston pinch dynamometer.
- Strain-gauged strips of various configurations.

Mathiowetz *et al.* (1984) showed that there is high interobserver and test-retest reliability for such tests, provided that the patient is tested in a standard anatomical position, with standard verbal instructions and scoring the mean of three trials. These authors stress the need for observers to establish normative data for the particular instruments they use. However, in the case of nerve lesions, almost always unilateral, this problem is obviated by expressing scores obtained as a percentage of the patient's other hand. Using the patient's other hand as the control also has the great advantage of controlling for practice effects if serial observations are taken across time. Smith and Benge (1985) make the point that there are several variations of both power and pinch grips, differing significantly in the combination of muscles used to produce them, and showed that there is great variation between observers as to which is used in routine testing.

Even when this problem is overcome, standard grips, which are easy to measure, involve the combined action of several muscles. To compare cases, therefore, it is necessary that they are similar in the extent of the original motor loss produced by the injury; that the lesions not only involved the same nerve, but also occurred at the same level. Thus Gaul (1968), in comparing measured grip and pinch strength with clinical assessment of power of individual intrinsic muscles after ulnar nerve suture, divided his cases into high and low lesions. He also investigated the effect of the patients' ages and made the fascinating observation that complete ulnar paralysis reduces pinch strength in a young person (with supple joints and hence greater need for muscular stabilisation of the thumb) by 60%, but only by 30–40% in an older person with stiffer joints.

Quantitative measurement of the force output of individual muscles has so far not been reported after nerve suture, although devices for measuring the force of finger abduction in the plane of the palm (abductor digiti minimi and first dorsal interosseous) are available (An et al., 1980) and anaesthetic colleagues (Walts, 1973; Stanec and Stanec, 1983) have developed a range of instruments for monitoring the action of adductor pollicis during neuromuscular blockade.

It could be argued that pinch and grip measurements are more functional in any case and are therefore all that is needed for clinical outcome measures after nerve suture. However there are at least two reasons for wanting to measure the mechanical output of individual muscles:

- A more detailed study of the pattern of motor reinnervation would require the combination of force measurement with electromyography. This could allow, for example, an estimate of the size of individual reinnervated motor units.
- Observations of other muscle parameters, such as fatigue, contraction speed and relaxation time, which could give insight into the processes of reinnervation, would be clearer on individual muscle action, rather than in composite grips, where the output of the reinnervated muscle would be diluted by that of normal synergists.

If evaluation of the power capability of reinnervated muscles has been rather unambitious, attempts to quantify capacity for controlling force output after damage to peripheral nerves have so far been only embryonic (Marsh, 1990). This is a pity, since such measures could form a bridge between measurements of force capacity and those of integrated sensorimotor function, giving insight into the reasons for functional impairment. Further research would be worthwhile.

Measures of sensory function

Tests designed to evaluate cutaneous sensibility derive historically from two different methodologies, clinical neurology and sensory physiology:

- Tests originating in neurological practice tend to be qualitative: they chart the presence or absence of the different sensory modalities in the territory under consideration. Such observations can be rendered quasi-quantitative by describing their distribution in space or time; another way of doing the same thing is embodied in the MRC sensory scale which is considered below.

- Tests derived from sensory physiology can usefully be analysed into two classes, which echo Weber's 150-year-old concepts of Ortsinn and Drucksinn. Tests of spatial discrimination address the issue of 'location sense': for suprathreshold stimuli, what is the accuracy with which cutaneous imprints can be localised, and their spatial features discriminated? Detection threshold tests address one aspect of 'pressure sense': at a given location, what is the minimum perceptible stimulus magnitude?

Sensory modalities

As Moberg (1978) pointed out, the usual aim of clinical neurologists in conducting a sensory examination is not to measure degrees of sensibility but to establish a pattern of sensory impairment which will permit localisation and diagnosis of a (usually central) lesion. When evaluating recovery after peripheral nerve repair, the situation is totally different: the location and nature of the lesion are known; what is needed is a quantitative grading of the dysfunction. The contribution of neurology to the methodology of peripheral nerve assessment might therefore be expected to be small.

However the MRC scale of sensory recovery (Table 13.4), the workhorse of clinical reporting since the Second World War, is a derivative of classical neurology. The scale was designed for use in cases of nerve regeneration and its use in other pathologies, such as entrapment neuropathy, does not make sense. It is essentially a sequence of submodalities of mechanoreception which embodies the progression of recovery described by Head (1920) and Rivers and Head (1908) who, having experienced the division and suture of his own digital nerve, made the distinction between the early, unpleasant, 'protopathic' sensation and the much-delayed, discriminatory, 'epicritic'. In this scale, one can see the expected succession of sensory modalities subserved by C-fibres, then A-∂ and finally A-β.

When recording the progress of an individual patient, there is no doubt about the usefulness of the scale in charting the return of protective sensation and the beginnings of true discriminatory sensibility beyond that. What is in dispute, however, is the usefulness of the scale for

---

Table 13.4 The MRC Scale of Sensory Recovery (Highet 1954)

S0   Absence of sensibility
S1   Recovery of deep cutaneous pain sensibility
S2   Return of some degree of superficial cutaneous pain and tactile sensibility
S3   Return of superficial cutaneous pain and tactile sensibility throughout the autonomous area with disappearance of over-reaction
S4   Return of sensibility as in stage 3 with the addition that there is some recovery of two-point discrimination
S5   Complete recovery

measuring the quality of end-results in a research context. This scale was used for the series which constitutes the British benchmark for peripheral nerve repair: that in H.J. Seddon's book *Surgical Disorders of the Peripheral Nerves* (Seddon, 1975), whose concluding chapter summarises the results of 2930 nerve repairs – some military, some civilian. Comparison between the results of primary and secondary suture, and investigation of the degree of recovery as a function of the patient's age, are made by giving the proportion of sutured nerves reaching each level of recovery for different groups of cases.

If the purely qualitative description of the neurologist (using cotton wool, hat-pin, tuning fork, hot and cold tubes) can provide only a nominal scale, this is a step forward. When applied to cases of nerve regeneration, it is a true ordinal scale: a case attaining a given level on the scale has already attained all lower levels. One can therefore begin to contemplate the use of at least some statistical techniques. As a measure of outcome comparing groups of nerve repairs it can be used in two ways: as a coarse measure of final recovery or, by recording when the various stages are reached, as a means to measure the speed of recovery. Its weakness is in its lack of resolution at the upper end, of particular relevance in the hand, where the need for tests is greatest. The recovery of tactile gnosis, essential for useful hand function, is submerged somewhere between S3+ and S4. The question 'how much tactile gnosis?' does not arise.

However, levels of S3+ and even S4 have been ascribed to many hands whose sensory deficit is such as to result in severely impoverished function. This fact is perhaps better realised now that the vital role of cutaneous feedback in the control of hand movement has been elucidated and become more widely appreciated. Because of this, Moberg (1978) lays at the door of the MRC Sensory Scale the responsibility for much surgical complacency and regards it as 'a serious deterrent to progress'.

Spatial discrimination

For practical purposes, this group comprises the two-point discrimination (2PD) test and the rest. Two factors combine to make the former the most important quantitative test currently in use, requiring particular attention:

- It is the only test for which studies have purported to show correlation with integrated hand function.
- It is a *de facto* standard, currently applied whenever a quantitative measure is required.

Two-point discrimination

Weber (1834) believed that his 2PD test, in charting differences in acuity between different body regions, provides an index of the richness of cutaneous innervation. Microneurography has proved him correct (Vallbo and Johansson, 1978). Not surprisingly, the test was seized upon by clinicians wishing to estimate the richness of *reinnervation*. As early as 1872, Mitchell used it in reporting the results of nerve injuries sustained in the American Civil War. Modern advocates are led by Moberg and Dellon.

However, the fact that it would be wonderful if a simple test, which can be carried out at an outpatient consultation with a paper clip, gave a numerical index of such an important parameter of reinnervation does not mean that it does. In the situation following nerve division and suture, this test requires great rigour if spurious results are to be avoided.

The reason for this lies in the inherent difficulty of the psychophysical task. Even in a person with normal nerves, the application of the two-alternative forced choice paradigm with acceptable levels of both rigour and economy is not easy. In patients with malfunctioning peripheral nerves, the complexity is enormously greater because the threshold is so much less clear-cut. The patient is asked to choose between only two alternatives – even if the hand is completely numb, 50% of the responses will be correct, yet 70% correct is taken as a positive result.

The situation is ripe for false-positive results to be caused by the inadvertent passage of cues. If two points are applied in such a way that the total force is greater than when one is applied, a discrimination based on force rather than spatial acuity is possible. If two points are applied not quite simultaneously, a temporal discrimination can be made. This is not to mention the myriad cues which may be conveyed via other senses from the mind of the examiner to that of the subject. It only has to happen once or twice in ten trials!

One cannot help being highly suspicious of reports giving 2PD thresholds for patients following nerve repair when, almost without exception, the papers do not mention either who did the test or which psychophysical method was used to set threshold. One is inclined to agree with Moberg that there is a tendency for junior doctors or hand therapists administering the tests to 'press harder until the boss is satisfied'. It is instructive that in spatial discrimination tests which do not rely on the two-alternative forced choice paradigm, such as the letter test (Porter, 1966, see below) or the wheel aesthesiometer (Marsh, 1986), scores tend to be much lower.

A detailed description of a rigorous application of the 2PD test is given in Moberg (1990). Moberg is certain, after many years of experience with the test before and after reconstructive surgery, that 2PD, properly measured, is a valid predictor of useful hand function. He is supported in this by several other authors (Dellon and Kallman, 1983; Novack *et al.*, 1992). Marsh (1990b) questions this, on the basis that age at suture is such a powerful determinant of recovery of both 2PD and function, and could produce a spurious correlation.

Although there is quite good evidence that 2PD correlates with integrated hand function, there is no evidence that it does so because it is measuring the density of reinnervation. Jabaley *et al.* (1976) performed the Weber 2PD test (among others) in 23 previously denervated fingertips after nerve sutures, mainly at wrist level. Skin biopsies from the same sites were examined for the presence of reinnervated Meissner corpuscles. There was no correlation.

Moving two-point discrimination

Mindful of the classification of low-threshold mechanoreceptors by sensory physiologists into slowly and rapidly adapting groups, Dellon reasoned that the Weber 2PD test would reflect the innervation density of slowly adapting receptors because, once applied, the points are held stationary. He described the moving two-point discrimination test (m2PD; Dellon, 1978) in which the two (or one) points are stroked lightly over the skin in the territory under test. This, he argues, measures the innervation density of small-receptive-field, rapidly adapting receptors, namely Meissners' corpuscles, RAI receptors.

Dellon has developed this idea with great thoroughness. He has correlated the findings of both static and moving 2PD tests with both histological (Dellon and Munger, 1983) and functional (Dellon and Kallman, 1983) evaluations in patients after nerve suture, demonstrated test-retest reliability (Dellon *et al.*, 1987) and built the test, and the underlying theory, into an integrated therapeutic philosophy (Dellon, 1981), in which sensory tests guide the progress of sensory re-education.

Nevertheless, the theory that slowly adapting receptors do not contribute to the perception of a moving two-point stimulus is inherently implausible. There is no evidence that SAI receptors fail to respond to a brief touch: they are slowly adapting, not slowly responding. Nor is there any evidence that RAI receptors do not assist in the Weber 'static' test: the initial application of the points constitutes a moving stimulus and, in most cases, the examiners' hand tremor produces continuing movement well above threshold for RAI receptors (Bell and Buford, 1982). It seems likely that differences in results between static and moving 2PD tests (the latter usually show lower thresholds) are due to the fact that, with a moving stimulus, greater areas of skin are stimulated, so the brain has more afferent information to work on.

As with static 2PD, reasonable correlation between m2PD and integrated function has been observed, not only by Dellon and Kallman (1983), but also by (Novak *et al.*, 1992). Again, the evidence for a correlation with the density of reinnervation, as confirmed histologically is non-existent: Dellon and Munger's (1983) study consisted of only three cases and Maiorana *et al.* (1987), with 14 cases of reimplanted digits, performing moving 2PD tests on each case before taking biopsies, found no correlation between m2PD results and the density of reinnervated Meissner's corpuscles.

Conclusions about two-point discrimination

- The thesis that 2PD is a measure of the density of reinnervation must be regarded as totally unproven. The further thesis, that moving and static versions of the test estimate the densities of separate receptor populations, is not only unproven but also inherently implausible. Yet it is frequently quoted as established fact (e.g. Waylett-Rendall, 1988). However, the thesis that 2PD is a predictor of useful function, irrespective of the underlying neurophysiological basis, does have some evidence in its favour.

- The two-alternative, forced choice test paradigm is a demanding one. Results should be viewed critically, in the light of the care and rigour used in obtaining them.
- The situation is complicated by the fact that powerful prior variables – the age of the patient and time elapsed since nerve suture – may produce covariance of 2PD and useful function.

Other spatial discrimination tests

Localisation of a single-point (suprathreshold) touch stimulus depends on the same parameters of nerve regeneration as does 2PD: density of touch-sensitive nerve endings and accuracy of fibre projection. The part to be tested is divided up into zones and, with vision eliminated, each zone in turn is touched with a firm but well-localised, though not sharp, stimulus. The patient indicates where the sensation was felt and the distance between the actual and perceived sites is scored in some way. The size of the zones may need to be altered for different body regions and comparison made between normal and abnormal sides. Marsh (1990a), in a multivariate analysis of results after median and ulnar nerve suture, taking into account both the age of the patients at suture and the follow-up time between suture and assessment, found that localisation scores were better predictors of integrated hand function than moving 2PD. It may be that localisation is a simpler sensory task than 2PD and further study of its usefulness is warranted.

Renfrew (1969) described a device for testing sensibility in the finger, which is probably best classified as a test of spatial discrimination. A small rectangular plastic plate has, on one surface, a 2-mm wide ridge which rises up gradually to a maximum height of 1 mm (1.5 or 2 mm in later versions). The examiner slides the ridge in its long axis along the fingertip; the patient indicates when he begins to feel the ridge; the height of the ridge at this point is the result yielded by the test, although what is often actually recorded is the distance along the ridge.

Although this instrument was originally conceived for use by neurologists, some hand surgeons use it. Much of its popularity stems from its easy portability and speed of application: it uses the method of limits, rather than the two-alternative forced choice method which should be employed with 2PD, and is therefore much faster. In a study of the results of digital nerve suture (Poppen et al., 1979), results obtained with this device were found to correlate with results of the Weber 2PD test, but not with those of applying Semmes–Weinstein monofilaments (see below). This tends to substantiate the classification as a test of spatial discrimination, albeit in a plane at right angles to that used in 2PD. No studies validating this test against hand function have been done.

Porter (1966) reported the use of a test of sensibility in 51 fingertips which had had either skin graft or flap. This was to score the number (out of 5) of raised letters that could be identified by palpation. The letters were 1 cm by 0.8 cm; their height was not given, but looks about 1 mm in the photograph. All five letters used were symmetrical: H O U V Y. The letters were first given into the normal hand for leisurely examination, before being applied to the tested finger pulp, by the patient himself.

Incorrect identification, or failure to identify the letter after 30 seconds, scored nought. The results obtained were correlated with 2PD, measured both longitudinally and transversely and, in 22 cases, with the qualitative, yes/no version of Moberg's picking-up test. In an inversion of the logic of this chapter, the letter test is, for its author, vindicated by its correlation with 2PD and the imperfect scores in the group who were able to perform the picking-up test are evidence of 'false-positives' in the latter.

Porter's letter test has one great advantage over 2PD as a test of spatial discrimination. This is that the patient with no discriminatory sensibility has only a 1 in 5 chance of guessing correctly, compared to 1 in 2 for 2PD. This must greatly reduce the risks of false-positive results. If other symmetrical letters, such as A I M T W X, were included, this advantage could be amplified and the resolution of the scoring scale increased.

A similar test, in daily use for rapid screening purposes, is Seddon's coin test, where the patient is asked to identify whatever coins there happen to be in the examiner's pocket at the time. Although very informative in a qualitative sense, particularly if the palpating action of the patient is closely observed, it is rarely used in any standardised way with numerical scoring.

Sensory threshold tests

If the tests described in the previous section measure some combination of the number of regenerated sensory fibres and the degree of accuracy of their central projection, the tests of detection threshold, it may be hoped, provide an index of the efficiency of transduction of mechanical stimuli by the receptors or free nerve endings.

In attempting to correlate receptor morphology with sensibility Max von Frey had need of instruments for applying precisely graded force to small areas of skin. He developed many such devices, of which the 'von Frey hair' is the best known. The principle of its operation is that, when it is applied perpendicular to the skin surface, the hair buckles and exerts a force which remains constant in spite of variation in the exact distance between the holder and the skin surface. A range of hairs is used and the psychophysical task is to establish which is the smallest force perceivable.

The modern version is the Semmes–Weinstein monofilament (Semmes *et al.*, 1960), a set of nylon 'hairs', marked with figures representing $4 + \log_{10}$ of the force they exert. The mode of use is to map out the territory of the nerve under scrutiny, in zones according to the lightest monofilament perceived. The range of forces applied is designed to cover painful as well as light touch stimuli.

Mapping of this sort is used for predicting high-risk areas in diabetic feet and many hand therapists use the pattern of returning sensitivity after nerve suture to guide their rehabilitation (Bell, 1986). However, as the descriptive terms in the leftmost column of Table 13.5 indicate, used in this way the test produces results comparable to the MRC Sensory Scale: essentially qualitative. Can the potentially higher resolution of the mono-filaments be used to provide a quantitative index of receptor function?

So far, studies which have addressed this question have produced confusing answers. Moberg (1962) interpreted his findings as showing that

Table 13.5 Interpretation of monofilament thresholds

Interpretation	Filament marking	Force (g)
Normal	1.65–2.83	0.0045–0.068
Diminished light touch	3.22–3.61	0.166–0.408
Diminished protective sensation	3.84–4.31	0.697–2.06
Loss of protective sensation	4.56–6.65	3.63–447
Untestable	> 6.65	> 447

Reprinted by permission from Semmes *et al.*, 1960. (© Harvard University Press.

pressure threshold measurements did not predict function as well as 2PD, but the opposite conclusion is also supported by his data (Marsh, 1990a). Similarly, Dellon and Kallman (1983), already discussed, actually showed that pressure thresholds do predict function, although the main line of argument in the paper is that 2PD, both 'static' and 'moving', is better. As Table 13.6 shows, when the results of Semmes–Weinstein testing were compared with the object–recognition scores, they performed very similarly to the results of the Weber 'static' test.

Yet another study which concludes that 2PD is the best measure of the functional value of sensibility, but contains data showing that pressure threshold is as good or better, is the classic by Onne (1962). He studied 30 patients who had suture of complete median nerve divisions, using 2PD, von Frey hairs, object recognition and picking up tests. The von Frey hairs were criticised for not correlating well with 2PD; neither sensory test was correlated with the functional tests. When this is done from the raw data given in the paper (Marsh, 1990a) and the ages of the patients are taken into account by multivariate analysis, touch threshold correlated more strongly than 2PD.

Critical analysis of published evidence therefore suggests that it would be premature to write off tests of detection threshold as potential providers of valid indices of sensory function. A further reason for not doing so is that they are open to considerable refinement. Although the von Frey hair is capable of indenting the skin with accurately controlled force, there is no control over the time-course of the indentation. Since the various populations of low-threshold mechanoreceptors differ in their responses to the rate of indentation and in their adaptation to sustained application of pressure, it is possible that a more selective assessment of sensitivity could be achieved by controlling the time-varying aspects of the stimulus.

Table 13.6 Correlations (r) and associated P-values between 2PD, pressure threshold and object recognition

	Number of objects recognised		Mean recognition time	
	r	P	r	P
Static 2PD	−0.356	0.147	0.777	< 0.001
Moving 2PD	−0.873	< 0.001	0.446	0.036
Semmes–Weinstein	−0.377	0.120	0.722	< 0.001

Reproduced from Dellon and Kallman, 1983.

Dellon (1983) used the 'Biothesiometer', which gives a measurement of threshold amplitude. He found it was no more sensitive to the presence of compression neuropathy than the tuning forks and argued in favour of the latter's cheapness and simplicity. However, in this paper the vibrometer results are only given as 'normal' or 'abnormal', so its potential for providing a quantitative assessment is not explored. Moreover, the Biothesiometer operates at a fixed frequency of 120 Hz and uses a 13-mm diameter contactor with no static surround. This means that this particular instrument is adequately testing only the Pacinian system. Szabo *et al.* (1984) report a trial of various sensibility tests in an experimental study in which localised pressure was applied to the carpal tunnel in normal subjects. Using the same fixed-frequency (120 Hz) vibrometer, they showed that thresholds for the detection of vibration were elevated much sooner than those for detection of pressure or discrimination of two points. Lundborg *et al.* (1986) report the use of a variable-frequency vibrotactile stimulator to produce 'digital vibrograms' analogous to the audiograms produced by a Bekesy audiometer. These too are a sensitive early indicator of carpal tunnel compression.

Marsh (1990a) used a variable-frequency vibrometer to measure the outcome of carpal tunnel decompression. The mean level of the thresholds at various frequencies between 15 and 350 Hz was a powerful predictor of performance on a battery of functional tests, far better than a spatial discrimination test. However, the differences in threshold, as a function of frequency, did not appear to contain extra information.

In such neuropathy, with axons in continuity, the projection of fibres from receptor locations in the skin to locations within the CNS remains undisturbed and the distortion of signals is presumably due to non-uniform slowing of conduction times. Therefore it is not surprising that a test utilising a strongly time-varying stimulus shows up abnormality better than one demanding spatial discrimination. Caution is needed, however, because of the normal effects of age. Many authors have described impairment of vibrotactile sensibility with advancing age (e.g. Verrillo, 1980). Thus the normal processes of ageing mimic the effects of nerve compression. Any use of the vibrogram for diagnostic purposes must take this into account. Comparison with the other side is of course the ideal where it is possible.

The use of a vibrometer for assessment of sensibility after median nerve repair was reported by McQuillan *et al.* (1971) (see also Neilson *et al.*, 1969). The apparatus was capable of frequency variation, but was only used at frequencies of 60 Hz and above, thus effectively limiting the assessment to the Pacinian system. It was used with a 7-mm contactor and rigid surround, which is probably a good arrangement since the contactor is big enough to stimulate the Pacinian corpuscles sufficiently, while the surround would prevent the transmission of vibration along the skin surface and stimulating remote receptors (innervated by different nerves). Other good features of the apparatus are that it was counterbalanced to provide a controlled force of 10 g and that it was modified to deliver short bursts of vibration, rather than a continuous stimulus, so avoiding errors due to adaptation. The degree of vibrotactile sensibility was expressed by comparing the vibrograms from the normal and uninjured hands. A score, consisting of the area between the two curves, was calculated. This was found to be repeatable in serial examinations of both normal and abnormal cases, and to improve with the passage of time since suture. In advocating the use of vibrometry after nerve suture, the authors stress its objectivity and the fact that it yields a quantitative measure. However, there was no attempt to correlate the results with functional tests.

Dellon (Dellon *et al.*, 1972; Dellon, 1980) has also reported the use of vibratory test stimuli after nerve repair. Applying the neurophysiological discoveries of Mountcastle *et al.* (1967), he used tuning forks of 30 Hz and 256 Hz with the explicit intention of testing Meissner and Pacinian afferents respectively. However, there was no measurement of amplitude, the ability to perceive the vibration at all was tested; the only quantitative aspect of the results was the time after suture, at which the perception of the two stimuli returned. Perception of 30 Hz was found to recover well ahead of perception of 256 Hz. Jabaley *et al.* (1976) and Gelberman *et al.* (1978) reported similar findings. In a later study, Dellon (1983) evaluated the fixed-frequency Biothesiometer after nerve suture. He found no correlation between threshold amplitude and moving two-point discrimination, although it must be remembered that this vibrometer only gives information about the Pacinian system. He concluded that the vibrometer offered little practical advantage over tuning forks.

Mansat *et al.* (1981) report the use of a variable-frequency vibrometer after nerve suture. This is capable of stimulating at any frequency between 20 and 400 Hz, although 30 Hz and 256 Hz are the two frequencies most frequently used. Accurate thresholds are measured, relative to the normal hand. These authors also report the relatively early return of sensitivity to 30 Hz stimuli and use this as an indication to commence sensory re-education. They regard the test as a valuable form of training in its own right, the patients constantly striving for lower thresholds.

Morley *et al.* (1988) studied vibrotactile thresholds in the territory of the radial digital nerve of an index finger after it had been divided and sutured, using a vibrating probe in the absence of a static surround. Although thresholds for perception of low frequency vibration were elevated 15-fold, thresholds for perception of 80–250 Hz, in the Pacinian range, were normal. This, they suggest, was due to the spread of higher frequency vibrations through the skin to normally innervated territory and indeed this result was predictable on the basis of the known properties of low-threshold mechanoreceptors, in particular the very wide receptive fields of Pacinian corpuscles. This study underlines the importance of using low frequencies, if vibrotactile testing is undertaken in the context of peripheral nerve injuries. The fixed, high frequency of the Biothesiometer render it and similar instruments totally inappropriate for this purpose. The fact that McQuillan *et al.* (1971) did find elevation of high-frequency thresholds in their patients was undoubtedly due to the fact that they used a static surround, thus limiting the spread of high-frequency vibrations across the skin. A static surround is necessary for Pacinian assessment, and the Biothesiometer fails on this count also.

The study which is really needed is one which applies the available neurophysiological knowledge about low-threshold mechanoreceptors in designing the spatial and temporal aspects of the stimulus and correlates the results with functional tests. This has not yet been reported.

Electrophysiological tests

These have the great advantage that they do not require a behavioural response from the patient. In the absence of any possibility of biopsy in surgical disorders of peripheral nerves, clinical neurophysiology offers the only direct route to measurement of the neural parameters underlying hand function. Well-established techniques for recording compound nerve and muscle action potentials have recently been supplemented by methods for observing the activity of single units. However, one must acknowledge the crudity of the measurements currently possible, relative to the complexity of neural information transmission.

Observing activity in motor nerves is easier than in sensory fibres, since in the former case the small electrical signals produced by action potentials in the nerve are amplified by the muscle action potential itself. A historical review (Kimura, 1983, chap. 5) shows that the first estimation of motor conduction velocity based on observation of the latter was reported as early as 1909, whereas recording of nerve action potentials was not achieved until 1936. The recording of pure sensory action potentials had to await the arrival of the technique of electronic averaging, which allows the signal to be separated from the noise, and was first achieved in 1956.

The modern method of measuring motor conduction velocity was described by Hodes *et al.* (1948). It eliminates the uncertain element of neuromuscular transmission time by stimulating proximal and distal to the nerve segment of interest and measuring the difference in conduction times to the muscle. Corresponding techniques are now in routine use for mixed nerve and sensory action potentials also, often using antidromic stimulation. The measurement of velocity can be quite precise, because the only electrical signal required is a recognisable point of onset of the muscle or nerve action potential; the velocity is derived from external measurements of time and distance. However, it must be recognised that the value obtained relates only to the fastest fibres in the nerve, which may be few in number.

The converse is true of measurements of the amplitude of nerve and muscle action potentials. All the fibres contribute to the signal, but the magnitude of that signal is more ambiguous, because the value obtained depends on the impedance between nerve and recording electrode. In fact the situation is more complicated because the issues of conduction velocity and amplitude of the compound action potential (CAP) are intimately related. When a sufficiently strong electrical stimulus is applied to a nerve, all the fibres are depolarised simultaneously. The CAP at that point will have the same waveform as a single-fibre action potential and its magnitude will reflect the number of fibres contributing to it. However, at points progressively more remote from the site of stimulation, the contribution of each fibre to the CAP being timed according to its own conduction velocity, the CAP will be more or less dispersed. Since this is bound to cause the coincidence of negative peaks from some fibres with positive peaks from others, the peak-to-peak amplitude of the CAP will be progressively reduced, and its duration increased.

What is needed, in order to extract the maximum information from the

CAP after nerve suture, is a method for measuring the distribution of conduction velocities. Current attempts to achieve this are based on making two recordings of activity in the nerve, either two CAPs dispersed over different distances, or one whose shape approximates to that of a single fibre action potential (e.g. a CAP recorded at very short remove from the site of stimulation) and one a dispersed CAP at a known distance from the site of stimulation. To these two waveforms, various mathematical techniques, all computationally very demanding, may be applied (for review, see Dorfmann *et al.*, 1981) to deduce the distribution of conduction velocities among the constituent fibres of the nerve. This reveals the amplitude of the signal from each subpopulation of fibres, and thus at least a relative estimate of the number of fibres with a given conduction velocity.

An entirely different strategy for electrical examination of peripheral nerve is to measure its excitability. This approach is based on the concept of the strength-duration curve, which applies to all excitable tissues: the shorter the duration of an electrical stimulus, the greater the amplitude needed for depolarisation. For a given tissue (nerve vs muscle, or large diameter vs small diameter nerve fibres), there is a minimum stimulus duration, below which no excitation can be obtained, however high the amplitude. Similarly, there is a minimum intensity of stimulation – the rheobase – below which no excitation occurs, however prolonged the application.

Seddon (1975, chap. 4) describes the use of strength-duration curve measurement in muscle, where it can distinguish direct electrical activation of the muscle from nerve-mediated activation and thus index reinnervation after injury. Smith and Mott (1986) describe an application of the same principle to sensory nerves, where 10 μs pulses, too brief to stimulate any but the large Aβ fibres, are applied to the injured finger after nerve suture and can indicate the time at which regenerated Aβ fibres appear in the distal segment by the production of a sensation of touch.

That these methods can give accurate quantitative information about excitability of nerve and muscle is not in dispute, although Seddon warns of the precautions which must be taken in practice to get comparable measurements. However, it has yet to be shown that the values obtained correlate with the functional capabilities of the nerve or the hand it supplies.

Validity of whole-nerve and muscle observations

This is perhaps one area where validity in the sense of correlation with neural parameters can realistically be evaluated. The reason is that, since no psychophysical testing is involved, animal work is possible; one may reasonably expect that relationships between the morphology and electrophysiology of nerve fibres may not be so different in laboratory animals and man. In the situation after nerve suture, one would expect that fastest conduction velocity gives an index of maturation of at least the best of the regenerated nerve fibres and the amplitude of the CAP gives an index of their number. Of the many studies which have addressed the relationship between histological and electrophysiological measures of outcome of nerve suture in experimental animals, two are particularly seminal and will serve to illustrate the findings:

1. *Velocity and maturation*. Sanders and Whitteridge (1946) studied rabbit peroneal nerves. They correlated fastest conduction velocity with the morphology of the largest nerve fibre present in the specimen. Their method of analysis is hard to follow but, re-analysing the data from 38 cases in their appendix, a multiple regression analysis, with conduction velocity as the dependent variable, and axonal diameter and myelin thickness as the predictors produces the following, in agreement with their own conclusions:
   - 90% of the variance in conduction velocity is explained.
   - The standardised regression coefficient, β, for axonal diameter is 0.23, that for myelin thickness is 0.77 (both statistically significant).
   Thus, both axonal diameter and myelin thickness are important for conduction velocity, but myelin thickness much more so.

2. *Amplitude and axon numbers*. Other animal studies, such as that by Davis *et al.* (1978), have shown correlation between the cumulative, or integrated, amplitude of the CAP (the area under the curve) and the number of regenerated axons. However, one must have reservations as to whether the lengths of the segments over which these were recorded in experimental animals were sufficient to reproduce the degree of dispersion, and hence attenuation, of the CAP that would obtain in humans.

Of course, no whole-nerve electrophysiological observation can hope to estimate the degree of somatotopic disorganisation at the site of suture. But there is at least some indication that amplitude and velocity measurements do index the number of regenerated axons and the degree of maturation of at least the best of them. This is a start. What about validity, as judged by correlation with functional outcome? Unfortunately, no study has yet been published which correlates electrophysiological results with the results of tests of integrated hand function. A number have correlated electrical findings with 2PD or the MRC Sensory Scale, but these beg the question as to the latters' validity.

Almquist and Eeg-Olofsson (1970) compared sensory conduction velocity and electrical stimulation threshold with 2PD in 19 patients who were at least 5 years from median or ulnar nerve suture; their ages ranged from 10 to 35 years. They found that the electrical parameters did not correlate with age or 2PD, but 2PD correlated strongly with age. From this they concluded that maturation of regenerated fibres was not the reason for the better results in children, but some other factor such as CNS adaptability. This conclusion assumes that 2PD is a valid index of the functional result.

Tackmann *et al.* (1983) studied a group of patients in the 5 years following median or ulnar nerve repair or graft, correlating electrophysiological and clinical measures of outcome. They used a near-nerve needle electrode and averaged up to 4000 responses, obtaining a detailed sensory action potential (SAP) with many (between 8 and 48) components; this was quantified as the height of the maximum peak-to-peak deflection and also as the algebraic sum of the components, as well as maximum conduction velocity. Clinically, they graded the sensory result on the MRC S0–4 scale, measured 2PD by the method of Weber and measured thresholds for detection of 100 Hz vibration, using a 13-mm wide probe with no static surround. They did not give results of any functional assessment. No correlation was found between fastest conduction velocity and the clinical measures of sensibility. SAP amplitude measurements, especially the cumulative amplitude expressed as a percentage of the normal side, correlated strongly with both the sensibility score and 2PD, but not with the vibration threshold. In the absence of the raw data, especially the ages of the patients, it is not possible to exclude the possibility that these correlations are spurious.

Marsh (1990a), in the multivariate analysis of outcome of median and ulnar nerve suture already referred to, found that the sensory conduction velocity and a measure of the dispersion of the CAP were strong predictors of integrated hand function. The amplitude of the SAP did not predict function.

Other electrophysiological studies after nerve suture, such as those by Ballantyne and Campbell (1973) and Buchtal and Kuhl (1979), are mainly concerned with the time-course of recovery of electrical parameters after suture and do not contain any data which would allow an assessment of their validity.

Single unit studies

The application of the technique of microneurography to nerves after suture can potentially shed light on at least two questions which CAP analysis can never address. First, it is possible to quantify the degree of somatotopic disorganisation by comparing the location of receptive fields versus projected fields for individual units, or fascicular aggregations of units. Secondly, it is possibly to study the stimulus-response functions of individual afferent units and thus estimate the extent to which functional reconnections have been re-established with the specialised, low-threshold mechanoreceptors so important for hand function. Unfortunately, the skills needed to perform microneurography are not widespread and such studies are few.

Hallin et al. (1981) report the results of microneurography in 11 patients at least 5 years after median nerve suture. This paper demonstrates graphically the basis for faulty localisation and impaired spatial discrimination. Multi-unit recordings in normal nerves show overlapping of projected and receptive fields in contiguous patches of skin. The same observations in patients after nerve suture show dispersal of the receptive fields into several discrete patches and a dissociation from projected fields.

Mackel (1985) sampled 140 primary afferent fibres from 34 patients at various stages after nerve repair. By recording their responses to mechanical stimulation, each unit could be identified as being one of the four established low-threshold types, or a deep-lying, high-threshold mechanoreceptor. Table 13.7 shows the distribution found. Most notable are the absence of PC reinnervation and the high proportion of 'deep' receptors, which are presumed to be regenerated axons which have failed to make

Table 13.7 Proportions of single units of different types in glabrous skin of human hand, normal and after suture

	Re-innervated (%)	Normal (%)
Pacinian (RA II)	0	8
Meissner (RA I)	27	40
Merkels (SA I)	23	27
Ruffini (SA II)	16	20
Deep nerve endings	34	5

Reproduced from Mackel, 1985.

functional connections with specialised receptors. Equally important was the finding that the distribution of units in space was inverted, compared to the normal: greater numbers appeared in the palm as compared to the fingertips.

As yet there have been no published reports attempting to correlate single-unit recordings with functional outcome. Brink and Mackel (1987) state there was no obvious association in 13 of the above group of patients who performed pick-up, identification and ulnar-grip tasks. However, no quantitative analysis was given.

Obviously there must be reservations about a relatively invasive technique such as microneurography after nerve suture. The main role of microneurography up to now seems to be to give qualitative insight into the neural basis for function after nerve suture. However, it is likely that powerful quantitative methods will emerge and be validated before too long.

References

Almquist E, Eeg-Olofsson O (1970) Sensory-Nerve-Conduction Velocity and Two-point Discrimination in Sutured Nerves. *J. Bone Joint Surg.*; **52A**: 791–796

An KN, Chao EYS, Askew LJ (1980) Hand strength measurement instruments. *Arch. Phys. Med. Rehabil*; **61**: 366–368

Ballantyne JP, Campbell MJ (1973) Electrophysiological study after surgical repair of sectioned human peripheral nerves. *J. Neurol. Neurosurg. Psychiat.*; **36**: 797–805

Bell JA (1986) Light touch–deep pressure testing using Semmes–Weinstein monofilaments. In Hunter JM, Schneider LH, Mackin EJ, Bell AD (eds) *Rehabilitation of the Hand*. St Louis: CV Mosby.

Bell JA and Buford WL (1982) The Force/Time Relationship of Clinically Used Sensory Testing Instruments. Presented at the Thirty-seventh Annual Meeting of the American Society for the Surgery of the Hand, New Orleans, 1982

Brink EE, Mackel R (1987) Sensorimotor performance of the hand during peripheral nerve regeneration. *J. Neurol. Sci.*; **77**: 249–266

Buchtal F, Kuhl V (1979) Nerve conduction, tactile sensibility and the electromyogram after suture or compression of peripheral nerve: a longitudinal study in man. *J. Neurol. Neurosurg. Psychiat.*; **42**: 436–451

Callahan AD (1984) Sensibility testing: clinical methods. In Hunter, Schneider, Masker, Callahan (eds) *Rehabilitation of the Hand*, 2nd edn. St Louis: CV Mosby, chap. 36, pp. 407–431

Davis LA, Gorden T, Moffer JA *et al.* (1978) Compound action potentials recorded from mammalian peripheral nerves following ligation or suturing. *J. Physiol.*; **285**: 543–558

Dellon AL (1978) The moving two-point discrimination test: clinical evaluation of the quickly-adapting fiber receptor system. *J. Hand Surg.*; **3**: 474–481

Dellon AL (1980) Clinical use of vibratory stimuli to evaluate peripheral nerve injury and compression neuropathy. *Plast. Reconstr. Surg.*; **65**: 466–470

Dellon AL (1981) *Evaluation of Sensibility and Re-education of Sensation in the Hand.* Baltimore: Williams and Wilkins

Dellon AL (1983) The vibrometer. *Plast. Reconstr. Surg.*; **71**: 427–431

Dellon AL, Kallman CH (1983) Evaluation of functional sensation in the hand. *J. Hand Surg.*; **8**: 865–870

Dellon AL, Munger BL (1983) Correlation of histology and sensibility after nerve repair. *J. Hand Surg.*; **8**: 871–875

Dellon AL, Mackinnon SE, Crosby PM (1987) Reliability of two-point discrimination measurements. *J. Hand Surg.*; **12A**: 693–696

Dellon AL, Curtis RM, Egerton MT (1972) Evaluating recovery of sensation in the hand following nerve injury. *Johns Hopkins Med. J.*; **130**: 235–243

Dorfman LJ, Cummins KL, Leifer LJ (1981) *Conduction Velocity Distributions.* New York: Alan R Liss

Gaul JS (1968) Intrinsic motor recovery – a long-term study of ulnar nerve repair. *J. Hand Surg.*; **7**: 502–508

Gelberman RH, Urbaniak JR, Bright DS, Levin LS (1978) Digital sensibility following replantation. *J. Hand Surg.*; **3**: 313–319

Hallin RG, Wiesenfeld Z, Lindblom U (1981) Neurophysiological studies on patients with sutured median nerve: faulty sensory localisation after nerve regeneration. Physiological correlates. *Exp. Neurol.*; **73**: 90–106

Head H (1920) *Studies in Neurology.* London: Henry Frowde and Hodder and Stoughton

Highet WB (1954) Grading of motor and sensory recovery in nerve injuries. In: Seddon HJ (ed) *Peripheral Nerve Injuries*, MRC Special Report No 282. London: HMSO

Hodes R, Larrabee MG, German W (1948) The human electromyogram in response to nerve stimulation and the conduction velocity of motor axons. Study on normal and on injured peripheral nerves. *Arch. Neurol. Psychiat.*; **60**: 340–365

Jabaley ME, Burns JE, Orcutt BS, Bryant WM (1976) Comparison of histologic and functional recovery after peripheral nerve repair. *J. Hand Surg.*; **1**: 119–130

Kimura J (1983) *Electrodiagnosis in Diseases of Nerve and Muscle.* Philadelphia, SA Davis

Lundborg G, Lie-Stenstrom AK, Sollerman C, Stromberg T, Pyykko J (1986) Digital vibrogram: a new diagnostic tool for sensory testing in compression neuropathy. *J. Hand Surg.*; **11A**: 693–699

Mackel R (1985) Human cutaneous mechanoreceptors during regeneration: physiology and interpretation. *Ann. Neurol.*; **18**: 165–172

Maiorana A, Nigrisoli E, Fano RA, De Benedittis A, Pederzini L, De Luca S (1987) Meissner's corpuscles in reimplanted fingers. *Ital. J. Orthop. Traumatol.*; **13**: 99–103

Mansat M, Delprat J, Delprat JM (1981) The vibrometer. An electromagnetic transducer as an attempt to examine sensibility of the hand in quantitative terms. *Hand*; **13**: 202–210

Marsh D (1986) Use of a wheel aesthesiometer for testing sensibility in the hand: results in carpal tunnel syndrome. *J. Hand Surg.*; **11B**: 182–186

Marsh D (1990a) The Measurement of Peripheral Nerve Function in the Upper Limb. MD Thesis, University of Cambridge.

Marsh D (1990b) The validation of measures of outcome following suture of divided peripheral nerves supplying the hand. *J. Hand Surg.*; **15B**: 25–34

Marsh D, Smith B (1986) Timed functional tests to evaluate sensory recovery in sutured nerves. *Br. J. Occup. Ther.*; **49**: 79–82

Mathiowetz V, Weber K, Volland G, Kashman N (1984) Reliability and validity of grip and pinch strength evaluations. *J. Hand Surg.*; **9A**: 222–226

McQuillan WM, Neilson JMM, Boardman AK, Hay RL (1971) Sensory evaluation after median nerve repair. *Hand*; **3**: 101–111

Mitchell SW (1872) *Injuries of Nerves*. Philadelphia: Lippincott

Moberg E (1958) Objective methods of determining the functional value of sensibility in the hand. *J. Bone Joint Surg.*; **40B**: 454–466

Moberg E (1962) Criticism and study of methods for examining sensibility in the hand. *Neurology*; **12**: 8–19

Moberg E (1978) Sensibility in reconstructive limb surgery. In Fredericks S, Brody GS (eds) *Symposium on the Neurologic Aspects of Plastic Surgery*. St Louis: CV Mosby, pp. 30–35

Moberg E (1990) Two-point discrimination test. *Scand. J. Rehabil. Med.*; **22**: 127–134

Morley JW, Hawken MJ, Burge PD (1988) Vibratory detection thresholds following a digital nerve lesion. *Exp. Brain Res.*; **72**: 215–218

Mountcastle VCB, Talbot WH, Darian-Smith I, Kornhuber HH (1967) Neural basis of the sense of flutter-vibration. *Science*; **155**: 597–600

MRC (1976) Memorandum 45 *Aids to the Examination of the Peripheral Nervous System*. London: HMSO

Neilson JMM, Boardman AK, McQuillan WM, Smith DN, Hay RL, Anthony JKF (1969) Measurement of vibrotactile threshold in peripheral nerve injury. *Lancet*; Sep 27: 669–71

Novak CB, Kelly L, Mackinnon SE (1992) Sensory recovery after median nerve grafting. *J. Hand Surg. (Am.).*; **17**: 59–68

Onne L (1962) Recovery of sensibility and sudomotor activity in the hand after nerve suture. *Acta Chir. Scand. Suppl.*; 300

Poppen NK, McCarroll HR, Doyle JR, Niebauer JJ (1979) Recovery of sensibility after suture of digital nerves. *J. Hand Surg.*; **4**: 212–226

Porter RW (1966) New test for fingertip sensation. *Br. Med. J.*; **2**: 927–928

Renfrew S (1969) Fingertip sensation: a routine neurological test. *Lancet*; **i**: 369–370

Rivers WHR, Head H (1908) A human experiment in nerve division. *Brain*; **31**: 323–450

Sanders FK, Whitteridge D (1946) Conduction velocity and myelin thickness in regenerating nerve fibres. *J. Physiol.*; **105**: 152–174

Seddon HJ (1943) Three types of nerve injury. *Brain*; **66**: 237

Seddon H (1975) *Surgical Disorders of the Peripheral Nerves*. Edinburgh: Churchill Livingstone

Semmes J, Weinstein S, Ghent L, Teuber H-L (1960) *Somatosensory Changes after Penetrating Brain Wounds in Man*. Cambridge, MA: Harvard University Press

Smith PJ, Mott G (1986) Sensory threshold and conductance testing in nerve injuries. *J. Hand Surg.*; **11B**: 157–162

Smith RO, Benge MW (1985) Pinch and grasp strength: standardisation of terminology and protocol. *Am. J. Occup. Ther.*; **39**: 531–535

Stanec A, Stanec G (1983) The adductor pollicis monitor – apparatus and method for the quantitative measurement of the isometric contraction of the adductor pollicis muscle. *Anaesth. Analg.*; **62**: 602–605

Szabo RM, Gelberman RH, Dimick MP (1984) Sensibility testing in patients with carpal tunnel syndrome. *J. Bone Joint Surg.*; **66A**: 60–64

Tackmann W, Brennwald J and Nigst H (1983) Sensory electroneurographic parameters and clinical recovery in sutured human nerves. *J. Neurol.*; **229**: 195–206

Vallbo AB, Johansson RS (1978) Active touch. In Gordon G (ed) *The Tactile Sensory Innervation of the Glabrous Skin of the Human Hand*. Oxford: Pergamon Press

Verrillo RT (1980) Age related changes in the sensitivity to vibration. *J. Gerontol.*; **35**: 185–193

Walts LF (1973) The 'Boomerang' – a method of recording adductor pollicis tension. *Can. Anaesth. Soc. J.*; **20**: 706–708

Waylett-Rendall J (1988) Sensibility evaluation and rehabilitation. *Orthop. Clin. North Am.*; **19**: 43–56

Weber EH (1834) *De Tacto. The Sense of Touch*. A translation by HE Ross (1978). London: Academic Press

Wynn-Parry CB (1981) *Rehabilitation of the Hand*, 4th end. London: Butterworth

Chapter 14

Vascular trauma

N. C. Hickey and M. H. Simms

Introduction

The application of comparative audit to therapeutic interventions for
vascular trauma presents an interesting challenge because of the random
and heterogeneous nature of the insult.

A penetrating wound of the femoral artery, for example, could result in
fatal haemorrhage or acute limb ischaemia according to the precise nature
of the injury. Successful repair might be complicated by a compartment
syndrome whilst spontaneous recovery might be followed by the development of a false aneurysm or arteriovenous fistula. Involvement of the
adjacent veins could produce acute venous insufficiency or deep venous
thrombosis, leading to the late disability associated with a postphlebitic
limb. In a child the long-term effects of arterial stenosis could lead to limb
growth retardation.

A similar catalogue of complications can follow closed arterial trauma
connected with long bone fracture when associated injuries to nerves,
muscles and other soft tissues may profoundly influence recovery.

The aim of treatment following vascular injury is to save life and limb
and to maintain or restore form and function. Because of the heterogeneity of the topic and the unpredictability of outcome, publications on
vascular trauma tend to address broad categories based on site of injury
or treatment modality, with outcome measures based on mortality, amputation rates and recovery time. Very few studies consider the complete-
ness of restoration of form and function to the injured part and full ability
to the individual.

Physiological measurement of the circulation forms an increasingly
important part of vascular surgical practice but has yet to be incorporated
into the evaluation of functional outcome following vascular trauma.
Although there is scope for the objective measurement of function after
vascular repair, such information cannot be used to compare different
treatment strategies as no two series can ever achieve a comparable
clinical mix.

A more comprehensive approach to the study of outcome would undoubtedly provide useful data on rehabilitation after vascular injury and
on the prevalence of subclinical morbidity. The main impetus for the
development of more sophisticated outcome measurement, however, will

probably come from the medicolegal sphere, where the evaluation of compensation claims is a major issue.

In order that the measurement of outcome should be valid, it is important that the assessment of the original injury be accurate and comprehensive. This account will therefore review methods of diagnosis and perioperative assessment before considering outcome in terms of complications, restoration of limb form and function and the overall recovery of the individual.

Initial assessment of vascular injury

Vascular injury is characterised by a high incidence of secondary phenomena resulting from manifestations of reperfusion injury, occurring both locally (compartment syndrome) and systemically (adult respiratory distress syndrome, renal failure). Prompt and adequate initial assessment of the injured patient should enable such complications to be anticipated and, it is hoped, mitigated. The presence of venous injury or the development of a compartment syndrome should always be considered in addition to examination of the arterial tree.

The unpredictable incidence of vascular trauma and the need for a rapid and comprehensive appraisal of the extent of injury dictates that assessment techniques are quick, simple and repeatable, in order to monitor progress stage by stage. A careful history (if obtainable) is obviously vital in establishing the timing and nature of the injury, the latter allowing broad categorisation of the trauma as open (gunshot wounds, stabbings, lacerations and compound fractures) or closed (long bone fractures, crush injury and iatrogenic dissections or injections). The patient's age, premorbid physical status and the extent of associated injuries are the other major variables that will influence the outcome.

The peripheral circulation of the injured patient should be compared with the central circulatory status and, when possible, with uninjured areas. For example, coldness and pallor of a limb would be unremarkable in a patient suffering from hypovolaemia or exposure, whereas the same findings in a single limb of an otherwise well-perfused patient would be significant. Clinical evidence of hypovolaemia combined with signs of distal ischaemia (coldness, pallor, absent pulses, paraesthesia and paralysis) suggests significant vascular injury (Perry, 1987). Palpation of the peripheral pulses must be performed in all four limbs and all the findings recorded. This should then be repeated in the injured limb at 2-hourly intervals for the first 12 hours as pulses present on admission may subsequently disappear (Simms, 1988). The absence of pulses suggests arterial injury but provides no information on the severity of tissue ischaemia or the adequacy of the collateral circulation and does not necessarily mean that exploration is required (O'Gorman et al., 1984). Furthermore, palpable peripheral pulses do not reliably exclude proximal arterial injury (Gelberman et al., 1980). Clinical examination should therefore be augmented by the use of a portable Doppler blood flow detector. Insonation with a 8–10 MHz probe offers a sensitive and objective method of pulse detection and combined with sphygmomanometry permits a measurement of peripheral perfusion pressure which can be compared to values obtained from unaffected limbs (Yao *et al.*, 1969).

When acute peripheral ischaemia is profound, Doppler signals may be unobtainable. In this 'sub-Doppler' range, quantifications of the severity of ischaemia must rely on clinical parameters. Transcutaneous oxygen monitoring may be of use (Kram and Shoemaker, 1984) but is time consuming, requires a skilled operator and is not generally available. The estimation of skin perfusion by temperature or pulse oximetry becomes insensitive in severe ischaemia and clinical parameters such as the extent of sensory loss and paralysis are more helpful, providing nerve injury does not co-exist. Muscle tenderness on passive stretching suggests ischaemia of sufficient severity to incur subsequent reperfusion injury; fixed mottling of skin with plasticity of underlying muscle indicates irreversible tissue death.

The place of angiography in the management of vascular trauma is limited, since the location of an arterial occlusion can usually be deduced clinically and contrast does not easily flow into an acutely ischaemic tissue bed (Slaney and Ashton, 1971). However, angiography may be imperative when vascular injury is suspected in the absence of signs of limb ischaemia. Examples include traumatic rupture of the thoracic aorta and penetrating injury passing close to a major vessel without producing signs of haemorrhage or ischaemia. In these circumstances arteriography may assist injury classification but will not provide a parameter of severity that is helpful in the audit of therapeutic interventions. When surgical exploration of arterial injury is performed, single-shot on-table angiography after proximal vessel control (Pearce, 1985) may provide useful information. The use of the same technique on completion of arterial reconstruction should reveal any technical defects.

The final factor in damage estimation concerns associated injury to bones, joints and soft tissues. These may completely override the vascular injury in importance; a good example being brachial plexus avulsion injury accompanying a subclavian artery disruption, when successful arterial repair may be followed by elective amputation of the denervated and useless limb. Conversely, arterial insufficiency may delay fracture union following combined vascular and bony trauma.

Venous injury is notoriously difficult to assess in acute limb trauma. Associated arterial injury usually ensures that the diminished venous return is insufficient to produce the swelling and cyanosis that normally accompanies venous occlusion. Unfortunately, the late sequelae of venous injury are permanent and disabling. An anatomical description of the injury provides a guide to prognosis but secondary complications such as thrombosis and valvular incompetence are common and may require serial assessment according to the clinical picture.

Outcome

Outcome after vascular trauma is dependent on the severity of the vascular injury, associated soft tissue and bony injury and the effectiveness of management, both early and late.

Mortality

The worst possible outcome is death, which requires no measurement. It may be possible, however, to categorise death into:

1. Vascular injury the most important factor causing death.
2. Vascular injury significantly contributing to death.
3. Vascular injury probably insignificant.

In some cases, post-mortem examination and review of carefully written notes may allow external observers to assess whether death was likely to have been preventable or not and if any treatment (appropriate or inappropriate) actively contributed to it (the CEPOD (1993) approach).

Morbidity

Outcome in a live patient can be divided into six broad groups, according to residual arterial or venous damage or disability resulting from the initial vascular insult:

1. Asymptomatic, with vascular tree restored to normal.
2. Asymptomatic, but with residual vascular damage.
3. Viable limb, asymptomatic at rest but symptoms on exercise.
4. Painful or ulcerated limb (potentially correctable).
5. Limb with permanent morphological change and/or functional disability.
6. Amputated limb.

It should be possible to categorise patients into one of these six groups and attempt to quantify disability within each group. Then it would be desirable to relate outcome to the severity of the injury at presentation.

A normal limb

When the arterial supply of a limb has been fully restored it will be a normal colour and temperature. A normal complement of peripheral pulses will be present and Doppler-measured pressures should be the same as those found in the contralateral limb, with no fall in pressure after exercise. If this is so, then any symptoms experienced by the patient (such as pain) are extremely unlikely to be due to ischaemia. Confirmation of a normal arterial tree may very occasionally require arteriography, when an intravenous digital subtraction angiogram (IV-DSA) is preferable as it is less invasive than conventional angiography.

Normal venous anatomy and function can be assumed if the limb is not swollen or discoloured but non-invasive imaging techniques are available if necessary.

An asymptomatic but abnormal limb

It is quite possible that trauma may result in permanent vascular damage that remains asymptomatic when the patient is reviewed after discharge from hospital. Although there are few indications for intervention in the absence of symptoms, this does not mean that subclinical injury is irrelevant, as it could progress or present with symptoms subsequently. For example, a leg will normally survive after ligation of an iliac artery, but the patient may later complain of intermittent claudication as he or she becomes more mobile; or a vein-graft stenosis may remain asymptomatic until sudden thrombosis leads to acute limb-threatening ischaemia. Subclavian artery stenosis may provide the source of platelet emboli to the digits. Loss of a single tibial vessel in the calf should not compromise limb perfusion, although it is probably an underestimated complication of tibial fracture (Ellis, 1958). In our experience, however, fracture-induced vascular injury may exacerbate the effects of peripheral vascular disease and compromise femorodistal bypass performed for limb salvage many years later.

An impalpable pulse may alert the clinician to asymptomatic vascular injury but examination of the peripheral pulses may be unreliable (Brearley et al., 1992). An absent or damped Doppler signal or reduced Doppler pressure at the ankle or wrist provide confirmation of vessel damage. A mild proximal stenosis may be associated with normal peripheral pressures at rest but a drop in pressure will follow limb exercise.

Vein graft stenosis is a significant cause of graft occlusion in the first 2 years following reconstruction. Grafts should therefore be regularly screened for asymptomatic stenoses, allowing early treatment by balloon angioplasty. A Duplex scanner (incorporating ultrasound and Doppler modalities) is ideal for this purpose, allowing quantification of the stenosis itself and also the resulting changes in blood flow (Moody et al., 1990).

A limb with symptoms on exercise

The symptom of intermittent claudication suggests a moderately compromised limb blood supply that is able to maintain adequate tissue perfusion at rest but is unable to respond to the increased metabolic demands of exercise. Claudication might be expected following ligation of the iliac or subclavian arteries, or late occlusion of a femoropopliteal bypass graft.

Clinical examination may reveal absent or reduced peripheral pulses and resting Doppler pressures are usually lower than those taken from a normal limb. For example, in the case of claudication, a significant perfusion deficit is indicated by an ankle-brachial pressure index (ABPI) of less than 0.8. Resting measurements are, however, unreliable but sensitivity is increased if repeated after a stress-test such as exercise. A standard technique involves measuring ankle systolic blood pressure before and immediately after a 1-minute, 3 km/hour walk on a treadmill inclined at 10° (Laing and Greenhalgh, 1980). A fall of greater than 30 mmHg is significant.

Claudication is difficult to quantify. The commonest investigation employed is a treadmill exercise test to assess pain-free and maximum walking distances (Boyd et al., 1949), but it is subjective, poorly reproducible and may improve spontaneously without a corresponding change in limb perfusion (Larsen and Lassen, 1966). The time taken for ankle pressures to return to resting levels after a standard exercise test – the ankle pressure recovery time (PRT) – is reproducible, correlates with limb transcutaneous oxygen pressure (Shearman *et al.*, 1988) and relates to limb blood flow (Sumner and Strandness, 1969). PRT remains, though, a haemodynamic stress test rather than a direct measurement of muscle ischaemia.

Venous claudication is less common but is suggested by classic symptoms, normal arterial investigations and limb swelling.

A painful or ulcerated limb

Critical ischaemia implies that limb viability is threatened in the absence of successful intervention. The patient complains of pain at rest and signs of ischaemia are evident on examination, possibly including ulceration and gangrene. Doppler pressures will usually be less than 50 mmHg, though tissue induration or arterial calcification may falsely lead to high cuff readings. Angiography is required to plan treatment. The possibility of venous injury should also be considered.

Ischaemia may be quantified by sophisticated laboratory techniques such as transcutaneous oxygen tension ($TcPO_2$, measuring skin oxygenation) or laser Doppler flowmetry (estimating erythrocyte flux in the skin microcirculation), but they have a limited role in routine clinical practice. Pulse oximetry, however, is readily available, simple to use and oxygen saturation levels may reflect the degree of ischaemia and provide an estimation of transcutaneous oxygen pressure (Joyce *et al.*, 1990).

For audit purposes, it is convenient to define levels of ischaemia according to symptoms, by the Fontaine classification:

Stage I – no clinical symptoms.
Stage II – intermittent claudication.
Stage III – ischaemic rest pain.
Stage IV – ischaemic ulcer, gangrene.

This classification can be correlated with ABPI (Yao, 1970) and stage III may be subdivided into: IIIA, an ankle pressure > 50 mmHg; IIIB, an ankle pressure < 50 mmHg (Norgren, 1989). Thus, critical ischaemia includes patients from stages IIIB and IV.

Venous damage producing a postphlebitic limb may be responsible for severe disability including gross limb swelling, pain and ulceration. Deep venous patency can be assessed non-invasively by duplex scanning or, traditionally, by venography. A semiquantitative analysis of venous insufficiency may be obtained by photoplethysmography, measuring venous refilling time of the foot after exercise or cuff occlusion. These laboratory tests do not determine extent of disability. Gross swelling and ulceration may be resistant to treatment and require re-classification into group five below.

A limb with permanent functional and/or morphological disability

A limb that survives major vascular injury with residual ischaemia may be amenable to further elective surgery designed to restore normal function. Far more serious for the patient is the limb that is left with irreversible functional disability. This group, therefore, is the most important in terms of outcome measurement but, unfortunately, is also the most difficult to quantify.

Functional impairment may result from loss of tissue. This could range from the minor inconvenience of the loss of a single toe to the major disablement resulting from amputation of the thumb of the dominant hand. Devascularisation may also result in loss of muscle or soft tissues with both cosmetic and functional implications.

A compartment syndrome that is not rapidly relieved by fasciotomy will progress to muscle necrosis, scarring and Volkman's ischaemic contracture which may be associated with severe handicap. Symptoms are exacerbated when concomitant neural ischaemia results in sympathetic neurodystrophy or painful causalgia.

There is no specific scoring system available that has proved to be a reliable measure of outcome in patients suffering from functional impairment after vascular trauma but general health measurement scales could be applied to these patients to obtain a semiquantitative assessment of their disability. The quality of life index (Spitzer et al., 1981) applies a numerical scoring system (0–2) to five areas – involvement in own occupation, activities of daily living, perception of own health, support of family and friends and outlook on life – but includes social variables over which the trauma surgeon has no control. The Nottingham Health Profile (Hunt et al., 1985) attempts to measure a patient's physical, social and emotional health status, but again has a limited role in comparative audit due to social variables*.

Residual arterial or venous damage, whether symptomatic or not, can be diagnosed and quantified in the vascular laboratory. In contrast, it may be very difficulty to reliably attribute symptoms to transient vascular insufficiency or a subclinical (or undiagnosed) compartment syndrome that has subsequently resolved but resulted in permanent soft tissue injury. It may, however, be possible in the future to demonstrate areas of muscle necrosis or relative ischaemia by the application of radio-nucleotide imaging, magnetic resonance spectroscopy or PET scanning techniques.

Amputation

Limb amputation may be perceived as treatment failure but, after trauma, may be necessary due to the extent of associated tissue injury or to preserve life. Outcome after lower-limb amputation concerns the success of rehabilitation and may be assessed by questionnaires on mobility

---

*These scales are discussed in Chapters 4 and 5 of the first volume of this series.

and use of prostheses (Houghton *et al.*, 1992) and correlated with a more specific scoring system based on walking patterns and level of limb preservation.

Outcome is more favourable for young amputees following trauma than that for elderly patients undergoing amputation for vascular diseases (Purry and Hannon, 1989), and for below-knee compared to above-knee amputees. Upper-limb amputation results in greater disability. Delayed wound healing, psychological problems related to altered body image and phantom pains all contribute to a poor outcome and a badly constructed stump that causes difficulty with prosthesis fitment represents an avoidable technical failure.

Whether amputation represents success or failure depends on whether it might have been avoided, the technical quality of the operation and upon the success of rehabilitation.

Conclusions

No single system exists with which to measure outcome reliably following vascular trauma. It is possible, however, to evaluate the arterial and venous performance of a limb in physiological terms with a high degree of accuracy. Similarly, an individual's disability can be estimated by a questionnaire or scoring system concerned with performance in the activities of daily living. The major difficulty in developing reliable outcome measures lies in relating final outcome with the severity of the initial injury. When this can be achieved then some value might be attached to the therapeutic interventions undertaken. It is suggested that patients may be assigned to one of the six groups outlined above and the extent of disability scored within each group. For primary ischaemic symptoms the Fontaine classification is appropriate and may also be adapted to accommodate venous disability. Permanent functional impairment or morphological change, including amputation, is difficult to quantify but a quality of life score may provide some estimate of outcome. Finally, outcome must be appraised with respect to the extent of injury at presentation. If an accurate and comprehensive vascular assessment is made on admission, it should be possible to evaluate whether the eventual outcome will be excellent, good, acceptable, unacceptable or poor. Ideally, desired (optimal) outcome could be predicted at the time of the initial assessment and eventual outcome subsequently measured against this goal.

References

Boyd AM, Ratcliffe AH, Jepson RP, James GWH (1949) Intermittent claudication: a clinical study. *J. Bone Joint Surg.*; **31B**: 325–355

Brearley S, Shearman CP, Simms MH (1992) Peripheral pulse palpation: an unreliable physical sign. *Ann. R. Coll. Surg. Engl.*; **74**: 169–171

CEPOD (1993) The report of the national enquiry into perioperative deaths 1991/1992. Royal College of Surgeons, London

Ellis H (1958) Disabilities after tibial shaft fractures. *J. Bone Joint Surg.*; **40**: 190–192

Gelberman RH, Menon J, Fronek A (1980) The peripheral pulse following arterial injury. *J. Trauma*; **20**: 948–953

Houghton AD, Taylor PR, Thurlow S, Rootes E, Mcoll I (1992) Success rates for rehabilitation of vascular amputees: implications for preoperative assessment and amputation level. *Br. J. Surg.*; **79**: 753–755

Hunt SM, McEwan J, McKenna SP (1985) Measuring health status: a new tool for clinicians and epidemiologists. *J. R. Coll. Gen. Pract.*; **35**: 185–188

Joyce WP, Walsh K, Gough DB, Gorey TF, Fitzpatrick JM (1990) Pulse oximetry: a new non-invasive assessment of peripheral arterial occlusive disease. *Br. J. Surg.*; **77**: 1115–1117

Kram HB, Shoemaker WC (1984) Diagnosis of major peripheral arterial trauma by transcutaneous oxygen monitoring. *Am. J. Surg.*; **147**: 776–780

Laing SP, Greenhalgh RM (1980) Standard exercise test to assess peripheral arterial disease. *Br. Med. J.*; **280**: 13–16

Larsen OA, Lassen NA (1966) Effect of daily muscular exercise in patients with intermittent claudication. *Lancet*; **ii**: 1093–1095

Moody P, Gould DA, Harris PL (1990) Vein graft stenosis improves patency in femoro-popliteal bypass. *Eur. J. Vasc. Surg.*; **4**: 117–123

Norgren L (1990) Definition, incidence, aetiology. In: Dormandy JA, Stock G (eds) *Critical Leg Ischaemia: its pathophysiology and management*. Berlin: Springer-Verlag, pp. 7–13

O'Gorman RB, Feliciano DV, Bitondo CG, Mattox KL, Burch JM, Jordon GL (1984) Emergency centre arteriography in the evaluation of suspected peripheral vascular injuries. *Arch. Surg.*; **119**: 568–573

Pearce WH (1985) Intra-operative arteriography. In Kempczinski RF (ed) *The Ischaemic Leg*. Chicago: Year Book Publishers, p. 173

Perry MO (1987) Penetrating trauma to the extremities. In Bergan JJ, Yao ST (eds) *Vascular Surgical Emergencies*. Orlando: Grune and Stratton, p. 165

Purry N, Hannon M (1989) How successful is below knee amputation for injury? *Injury*; **20**: 32–36

Shearman CP, Gwynn BR Simms MH (1988) The assessment of intermittent claudication. A role for transcutaneous oxygen measurement? In Price R, Evans JA (eds) *Blood Flow Measurements in Clinical Diagnosis*. London: Biological Engineering Society, pp. 40–43

Simms MH (1988) Management of vascular injuries. In Alpar EK, Owen R (eds) *Paediatric Trauma*. Tunbridge Wells: Castle House Publications Ltd, p. 107

Slaney G, Ashton FA (1971) Arterial injuries and their management. *Postgrad. Med. J.*; **47**: 257–261

Spitzer WO, Dobson AJ, Hall J, Chersterman E, Levi J, Shepherd R, Battista RN, Catchlove BR (1981) Measuring the quality of life of cancer patients: a concise QL-index for use by physicians. *J. Chron. Dis.*; **434**: 585–597

Sumner DS, Strandness DE (1969) The relationship between calf blood flow and ankle pressure in patients with intermittent claudication. *Surgery*; **65**: 763–771

Yao ST (1970) Haemodynamic studies in peripheral arterial disease. *Br. J. Surg.*; **57**: 761–766

Yao ST, Hobbs JT, Irvine WT (1969) Ankle systolic pressure measurements in arterial disease affecting the lower extremities. *Br. J. Surg.*; **56**: 676–679

Chapter 15

Spine and spinal cord injury*

P. Sett

Introduction

Improvement in the quality of life following spinal injury has become increasingly important in health care. Evaluation of the quality of care using outcome measures and performance indicators is also receiving attention.

Spinal injury not only affects the spinal column and spinal cord, but through the involvement of the spinal cord most of the functions of the body. The disabilities and handicaps that result from the injury have enormous implications on the subjects' psychological, emotional, social and recreational health.

Outcome is usually referred to an end-stage assessment. In this chapter assessment and measures in the acute stage of spinal injury which have relevance to the final outcome have been included in the discussion. 'Final' outcome is always relative, as it changes with time from the injury and with ageing of the patient.

The musculoskeletal and neurological systems are the most obviously affected by spinal cord injury, but it is the consequent urological and psychology injury that most affects the patient.

Musculoskeletal outcome

In the majority of spinal injuries there is trauma to the spinal column. The aspects of skeletal damage which are required to be measured in the outcome are stability and deformity.

Stability (or instability) is a much abused term. Instability may be defined in three ways: (a) Postural (difficulty in extending the spine from a fixed position), not often seen in spinal injured patients; (b) abnormal movement/displacement at the site of injury to the spine; and (c) progressive late deformity, developing some time after the injury once the patient has started to mobilise. Methods of measuring these are shown in Table 15.1. Achieving a stable spine is extremely important, the aim in

---

* Editor's note: Outcome measures in spine fractures and soft tissue injuries are also discussed by Thomas in Chapter 7 of the first volume of this series, *Outcome Measures in Orthopaedics*.

Table 15.1 Methods for measuring stability (or instability) and deformity of the spine.

	Methods to measure instability
Plain X-rays	To define bony union or callus formation
Flexion/extension views	To identify abnormal mobility (including 30-minute views)
Tomograms	To detect the same. Particularly useful in cervicothoracic and upper thoracic injuries where X-ray pictures are usually of very poor quality
CT scan	May be required where both the above are non-informative. Possibly 2-D and 3-D reconstruction useful
	Methods to measure deformity
A. Scoliosis	
i. Radiological	Erect AP film Cobb angle (Cobb, 1948; Whittle, 1979)
ii. directly	Height of patient (Aldegheri and Agostini, 1993); scoliometer (Bunnel, 1984); measuring rib deformity (Thulborne, 1986; Punn *et al.*, 1987)
iv. optical method	e.g. ISIS System (Weisz, 1988)
B. Kyphosis	
i. directly	Height of patient (Aldegheri and Agostini, 1993); kyphometer (Ohlen, 1984)
ii. Radiological	Erect lateral X-rays to measure angle angle of kyphos and loss of vertebral body height
iii. Optical (e.g. ISIS)	To measure surface deformity (Carr *et al.*, 1989)
C. Rotational deformity	
i. Radiological	AP X-rays, CT scan

the early management is directed towards this. Instability may not only result in further neurological deterioration but also lead to progression of deformity. This in turn can influence neurological function, rehabilitation, posture and balance. Malalignment of the spinal column can give rise to chronic pain.

Both plain X-rays and dynamic views are used to measure instability and the degree of deformity. The scoliometer, kyphometer and ISIS techniques are not generally used in spinal cord injured patients.

Certain injuries are prone to develop late instability and deformity. These are atlanto-axial injuries, fracture-dislocations of the dorsal spine, particularly those associated with sternal fractures, burst fractures and fracture dislocations of the thoracolumbar junction. In such cases more sophisticated investigation may have to be used to establish instability. McSweeney (1992) is of the opinion that plain X-rays are uninformative in detecting delayed instability at the atlanto-axial region. He recommends the use of flexion/extension cine-radiography or CT scan for assessing the problem. In the thoracic and thoracolumbar region Silver and Henderson (1992) have indicated that plain X-rays and dynamic views are of little benefit in detecting delayed instability. In such cases timed dynamic views (30 minutes in flexion and 30 minutes in extension) may reveal substantial movement. Special investigations in the chronic stage, particularly in these types of injury, can be very useful and may help to prevent poor outcome (this refers to the practice in the National Spinal Injuries Centre (NSIC) of assessing instability of the spine 12 weeks after injury, and would not be appropriate where internal fixation has been used to stabilise the spine).

Neurological outcome

Spinal injury results in varying degrees of spinal cord damage. The neurological deficit is not always proportional to the degree of skeletal injury. Recovery from cord injury is usually slow and may take place over months and even in some case over years. It is therefore important to make repeated and regular assessment to detect any change in neurological outcome.

Neurological outcome can be measured by:

1. Clinical methods.
2. Neurophysiological studies.
3. Magnetic resonance imaging.

Clinical methods

It is of paramount importance to perform a thorough neurological examination and record the findings in a systematic manner. This helps in understanding the extent of cord damage, helps to monitor neurological deterioration or improvement and helps in making a prognosis. In forming an accurate baseline, it is not only important to note the motor and sensory deficit but also to record the level of injury, the nature of the reflexes and the extent of bladder and bowel involvement.

Level of injury

This term refers to the most caudal spinal cord segment which is normal. It may be different for motor and sensory function and it may also be different on each side. It is now the recommended practice to clinically determine the side and the level of neurological deficit as R-motor, L-motor and R-sensory and L-sensory. These should be recorded separately. Clear understanding is required in determining motor level. The motor level in the limbs can be determined by testing designated key muscles and recording their muscle grade on the MRC scale (see below). The American Spinal Injuries Association (ASIA) has identified ten such key muscles as listed in Table 15.2.

Motor assessment

Traditionally it has been the practice to test individual muscles on both sides of the body and grade them according to the MRC grading system (MRC, 1943). In this system muscle strength is graded on a 6-point scale (0–5) (Table 15.3).

Sensory assessment

Conventionally three modalities of sensation are tested separately: pin prick, light touch and temperature. Each modality is tested over 29 dermatomes from C2 to S5 separately on both sides. Sensation is recorded as normal, increased or decreased. Joint position sense and vibratory sense are tested in the toes and fingers and recorded in a similar

Table 15.2 ASIA Motor Assessment: 'key' muscles

C5 – elbow flexors	L2 – hip flexors
C6 – wrist extensors	L3 – knee extensors
C7 – elbow extensors	L4 – ankle dorsiflexors
C8 – finger flexors	L5 – long toe extensors
T1 – finger abductor	S1 – ankle plantar flexors

A muscle with grade 3 power is deemed to have its rostral nerve supply intact. Applying this convention, therefore, as an example, if a key muscle like finger flexors (C8) has grade 3 power and the more rostral key muscle the elbow extensor (C7) has grade 4 or 5 power then the motor level should be designated as C8.

Table 15.3 The MRC grading of motor weakness

0 = Total paralysis
1 = Palpable or visible contraction
2 = Active movement, full ROM with gravity eliminated
3 = Active movement, full ROM against gravity
4 = Active movement, full ROM against active resistance
5 = Normal

ROM = range of movement.

manner. Many believe at least the first examination should include all these details.

Zone of partial preservation (ZPP)

In cases of complete injuries it is possible to have partial preservation of function in a few segments below the level of injury. This zone is termed as ZPP and, if present, should be recorded and its extent noted. If the ZPP extends beyond three levels then the lesion should be termed as incomplete rather than complete.

Complete or incomplete

In spinal cord injury the degree of spinal cord damage has significant relevance to prognosis. Only a small percentage (2%) of patients who have complete lesions at the time of injury then go on to show any further recovery. On the other hand, the extent of recovery is variable in those with incomplete injury.

Cord syndromes

In certain circumstances, damage to the spinal cord produces a particular combination of clinical features to produce special syndromes.

CENTRAL CORD SYNDROME

Usually seen in elderly subjects who have had associated spondylosis prior to cervical injury. The clinical findings are characterised by motor weakness of the hands being much greater than that in the lower limbs. Sacral sensation is spared.

BROWN-SEQUARD SYNDROME

This syndrome gives rise to ipsilateral motor impairment together with ipsilateral loss of posterior column sensation and contralateral loss of pin-prick sensation.

ANTERIOR CORD SYNDROME

Motor impairment is associated with variable amount of impairment of pin-prick sensation. Posterior column sensation remains intact.

CONUS MEDULLARIS SYNDROME

Injury to the conus results in paralysed and areflexic lower limbs. The bladder and rectum are also atonic. In high conus lesions the visceral reflexes, such as the micturition reflex and bulbocavernosus reflex, may be preserved.

CAUDA EQUINA SYNDROME

Damage is to the nerve roots of the cauda equina, this results in an areflexic bladder and rectum and flaccid lower limbs.

Discussion

Clinical findings are often not sufficiently clear cut for patients to be grouped into clinical syndromes. It is, therefore, not always possible to categorise patients into these various groups. Guttman (1973) has pointed out the deficiencies of trying to use the syndrome as a grading system. However, if a patient does have the particular characteristic to fit into one syndrome or another, then it is useful to record this. Each syndrome immediately conveys a particular pattern of injury and prognosis. For example, an elderly person with central cord syndrome is likely to be more disabled compared to another tetraplegic with the same degree of lower limb function. The former would have poorer hand function and, therefore, be more severely handicapped. In Brown-Sequard syndrome there may be varying degrees of recovery. In cauda equina lesion, as the damage is to the nerve roots, a remarkable degree of neurological recovery may occur.

Neurological grading

Frankel *et al.* (1969) were the first to attempt a grading system to define the severity of neurological injury. This is outlined in Table 15.4. The Frankel grading system has been widely used to measure neurological deficit. It can be applied in a variety of conditions to measure neurological change. The advantage of clear-cut grades makes the instrument robust as an outcome measure. The disadvantage of the system lies in its inability to detect and define those who show changes in their neurological function within the defined group.

Table 15.4 The Frankel Grading System

Grade A – complete injury, no motor or sensory function below the level of injury

Grade B – sensation only, some preserved function below the level of injury, this does not apply to a slight discrepancy between the motor and sensory level, but does apply to sacral sparing

Grade C – motor function useless, preserved motor function below the level of injury, but it is of no practical use to the patient

Grade D – motor function useful, preserved useful motor function below the level of injury, patients in this group can walk with or without aids

Grade E – recovery, normal motor and sensory function, abnormal reflexes may be present

Tator (1982) attempted to expand the Frankel system and introduced the Sunnybrook Cord Injury Scale to assess the degree of neurological injury and recovery. The Sunnybrook Scale used 10 grades to define severity of injury. Grade 1 was complete motor and sensory loss and Grade 10 represented normal (Table 15.5). The system has not proved popular in Europe.

ASIA has recently modified the Frankel grading to the one shown in Table 15.6.

Motor and sensory scoring systems

The first attempt at motor scoring was made by Lucas and Ducker (1979). They proposed a Neurotrauma Motor Index. In this index the maximum

Table 15.5 The Sunnybrook Cord Injury Scale

Grade	Description	Corresponding Frankel grade
1	Complete motor loss: complete sensory loss	A
2	Complete motor loss: incomplete sensory loss	B
3	Incomplete motor useless: complete sensory loss	C
4	Incomplete motor useless: incomplete sensory loss	C
5	Incomplete motor useless: normal sensory	C
6	Incomplete motor useful: complete sensory loss	D
7	Incomplete motor useful: incomplete sensory loss	D
8	Incomplete motor useful: normal sensory	D
9	Normal motor: incomplete sensory loss	D
10	Normal motor: normal sensory	E

Reproduced from Tator, 1982.

Table 15.6 The ASIA Neurological Impairment Scale

A = complete. No sensory or motor function is preserved in the sacral segments S4 and S5

B = Incomplete. Sensory function is preserved below the neurological level and extends through the sacral segments S4 and S5

C = Incomplete. Motor function is preserved below the neurological level, and the majority of key muscles below the neurological level have muscle grade less than 3

D = Incomplete. Motor function is preserved below the neurological level, and the majority of key muscles below the neurological level have a muscle grade greater than or equal to 3

E = Normal. Sensory and motor function normal

score was 100. The system graded muscles on a scale 0–5 according to function (0 = absent, 1 = trace, 2 = poor, 3 = fair, 4 = functional and 5 = normal). This grading was then applied to 14 muscles to give the motor index as shown in Table 15.7. This system is self-evidently subject-ive and attempts to add an ordinal scale which contravenes basic statist-ical techniques. The scale has been used by Bondurant *et al.* (1990) and Cotler *et al.* (1990).

Manabe Scale

In order to overcome the deficiencies of the Frankel grading system and that of the Motor Index Score, Manabe *et al.* (1989) combined the two to produce their own grading. This is shown in Table 15.8. The Manabe scale has not been used by spinal injury units. It has been recently employed in a multicentre spine fracture study carried out by the Scoliosis Research Society (Gertzbein, 1992) in the USA.

In the second National Acute Spinal Cord Injury Study (NASCIS II), Bracken *et al.* (1990) used the ASIA motor and sensory scoring systems as outcome measures. For sensory scoring, 29 segments from C2 to S5 were tested bilaterally for pin-prick and light touch. Sensation was scored as: absent = 1, decreased = 2 and normal = 3. Sensory score on one side = 87 and total score = 174. The motor score utilised the MRC grad-ing system (see below) and applied this to test 14 muscles on each side to

Table 15.7 The Neurotrauma Motor Index

Muscle	Right	Midline	Left
Diaphragm		2	
Deltoid	5		5
Biceps	5		5
Triceps	5		5
Flexor digitorum	5		5
Abductor			
Digiti minimi	5		5
Intercostals		2	
Upper abdominals		2	
Lower abdominals		2	
Iliopsoas	5		5
Quadriceps	5		5
Extensor digiti	5		5
Gastrocnemius	5		5
Anal		2	

Each muscle is graded according to a functional grade (0–5), and these grades summated. The grades are as follows: 0 = absent, 1 = trace, 2 = poor, 3 = fair, 4 = functional and 5 = normal.
Normal = 100.

Table 15.8 The Manabe Scale of change of Frankel Grading

Grade I	Excellent	Improvement by more than one Frankel Grade
Grade II	Good	Improvement by only one Frankel Grade
Grade III	Fair	Improvement of function within the same Frankel Grade
Grade IV	No change	No change in Frankel Grade or Motor Score
Grade V	Poor	Deterioration of Frankel Grade or Motor Score

give a total motor score = 140. The NASCIS II trial showed that there was improvement in the motor score by 7 points at the end of 1 year in patients who were given high-dose steroids (a significant improvement in this outcome measure).

ASIA scoring system

ASIA has now combined and modified these two systems and issued a revised motor and sensory scoring system. This is clarified in the ASIA classification (Table 15.9). For sensory scoring ASIA have reduced the number of sensory dermatomes to 28 by combining S4 and S5 into one segment. The scoring is altered to: 0 = absent, 1 = impaired and 2 = normal. Pin-prick and light touch are separately tested and scored. The maximum score for both pin-prick (both sides) and for light touch (both sides) is 112 (Table 15.9 and Figure 15.1).

ASIA recommends that sensation in each dermatome be tested at key sensory points for that dermatome as described by Austin (1972). These points are shown as black dots over each dermatome in Figure 15.1.

Discussion

There has been the need to standardise and simplify neurological examination and scoring in spinal cord injury and the recent revised edition of the ASIA classification (Figure 15.1) is simple and practical. It is hoped that various spinal units and other related specialities like orthopaedics and neurosurgery will use it to grade their patients. Motor and sensory scoring on the ASIA system is now widely practised in the USA and has been helpful in standardising neurological examination. The use of this system by all who are involved in the care of spinal injured subjects may well be beneficial.

Neurophysiological studies

Neurophysiological studies are based on establishing intact fibre tracts within the damaged cord. Motor and sensory evoked studies have shown conclusively that a patient with a clinically complete lesion could still have intact motor and sensory conducting pathways. Such investigations can help in assessment and in prognosis of spinal injury. Much of this work has been done by Dimitrijevic (1988).

Table 15.9 Revised motor and sensory score (ASIA classification, 1992)

ASIA Motor Score:
ASIA motor score uses the MRC grades (0–5) and extends this to the 10 key muscles already mentioned (Table 15.2) to give a maximum score of 50 on one side and a total of 100

Sensory Score:
For sensory scoring ASIA have reduced the number of sensory dermatomes to 28 by combining S4 and S5 into one segment. The scoring is altered to: 0 = absent, 1 = impaired and 2 = normal. Pin-prick and light touch are separately tested and scored. The maximum score for both pin prick (both sides) and for light touch (both sides) is 112

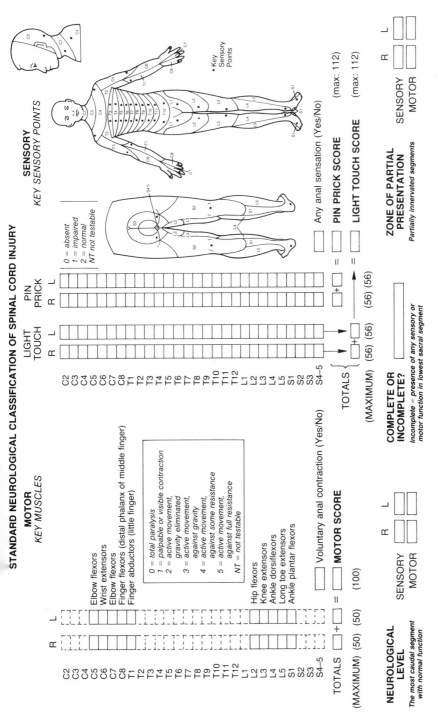

Figure 15.1 ASIA Classification (1992)

Tsubokawa (1987) has evaluated the role of evoked potential in spinal cord injuries and has found it useful in localising and determining the extent of cord injury and in prognosis. Motor responses evoked by magnetic stimulation (Magstim 200, Magstim) in spinal cord injury are being intensely studied. It is likely that this technique will have a substantial role in neurophysiological studies in the future.

Magnetic resonance imaging (MRI)

MRI has made it possible for the first time to visualise the spinal cord directly. It is certainly able to show the structural damage sustained and can help to establish whether the cord has been transected or not. It can play a rôle in defining prognosis. The rôle of MRI in spinal injuries has been elucidated by Sett and Crockard (1991). At the NSIC, where MRI is now routinely used on all spinal injury patients, the incidence of post-traumatic syrinx has been demonstrated in 20% of cases. MRI can also be used to demonstrate disc degeneration adjacent to fractured vertebrae as well as compression of the spinal cord, conus or cauda equina (Levitt and Flanders, 1991; Wilberger, 1991).

Discussion

The measure of neurological outcome is still mainly clinical. With the simplified scoring system of the ASIA classification it is expected that most clinicians will now grade and score spinal injury patients. It will then be possible to measure outcome and prognosis. The neurophysiological studies are improving continuously and will probably have a greater role to play in the future. At the present time, the ASIA classification is used mainly in cases where controversy exists regarding the degree of cord transection, which is in the acute stage in those who have a very high lesion and are on ventilators.

The value of MRI lies in its ability to give an entire picture of the damage, that is to bone, soft tissue and neurological structures. This can help in defining management and outcome. The main rôle of MRI, however, lies in detecting and measuring the progress of post-traumatic syringomyelia. It is now well established from experience at the NSIC that the incidence of asymptomatic syrinxes is far more common than hitherto believed. Symptoms of a developing syrinx can be protean, and may precede neurological change by months or years. In order to plan treatment and measure outcome regular MRI is necessary. Shunting procedures to relieve syrinx must be followed up regularly with MRI scans, Sett and Crockard (1991).

Interrelationship between skeletal outcome and neurological outcome

It has been a matter of great debate over the years whether management of the skeletal injury influences the neurological outcome. Donovan et al. (1992) in their series of 113 cervical patients found no difference in neurological outcome between the operated and the non-operated groups. However, the study showed that patients achieved earlier stability, less deformity and less callus formation in those who were operated upon. Hospitalisation was also marginally reduced in the operated group. In a multicentre study of spinal injury, Gertzbein (1992) found that anterior surgery was more effective than posterior in improving neurological function in the lower limb and bladder. This improvement was shown using the Manabe Scale. The improvement, however, was not statistically significant. Pain was reduced in the patients treated with surgical stabilisation compared with those treated non-operatively. There are obvious advantages in the early mobilisation of patients whose spine has been stabilised surgically.

The degree of vertebral displacement may have influence on outcome. Gertzbein (1992) measured displacement as the percentage to which one vertebra had translated over another when compared to the width of the verterbra. Dickson et al. (1978) graded deformity taking into consideration both angulation and canal encroachment.

Canal stenosis may have relevance to outcome. In clinical practice subjects with previous cervical spondylosis or congenital canal stenosis have been observed to have more profound cord damage when related to the degree of violence. CT scan combined with software packages (Scriptel SDP series, Columbus, Ohio, USA) and (Sigma-Scan, Jandel Scientific, Corte Madera, California, USA) have been used by Gertzbein (1992) in the Scoliosis Research Society (SRS) study to measure canal stenosis and encroachment. Frankel et al. (1987) have shown that complete lesions are more common in injuries from T1 to T10 (81%) compared to the thoracolumbar region (61%). The latter showed a greater improvement when compared to the former by one Frankel grade.

Outcome measures in children

Fortunately childhood injuries to the spine and spinal cord are few in number. This particular group deserves a separate discussion as some of the features in children are unique. It is important to realise that children are more likely to have Spinal Cord Injury without Radiological Abnormalities (SCIWORA). This term was coined by Pang and Wilberger (1982). SCIWORA has considerable significance to outcome. Children with SCIWORA are likely to be inadequately or inappropriately treated leading to poor outcome. It is also known that following spinal injury in children, particularly in those in the SCIWORA group, delayed neurological deterioration can occur. In children with spinal injury, it is important to determine accurately any neurological symptoms present at the time of injury. If there is any such history or evidence of minor neurological deficit, significant injury to the spinal cord should be suspected and the child observed regularly. Serial dynamic views at weekly intervals may be required to assess stability. (Short et al., 1992). In patients who have SCIWORA, CT and MRI scans should be utilised to determine degree of skeletal and cord injury and management planned accordingly.

In the chronic stage, children left with neurological deficit are prone to develop spinal deformity (scoliosis and kyphosis). Spinal deformity needs to be monitored closely. Short *et al.* (1992) suggest that children are followed up three times a year, in order to detect early changes in the joints and spine. These can then be appropriately treated. At the NSIC, it is the practice to photograph any deformity in the sitting and passively corrected postures. In those who have scoliosis, the photographs are taken after marking the spinous processes with ink. Long X-rays of the entire spine are also taken routinely. When scoliosis is present, long films should be taken in both the sitting and corrected posture. Progression of any deformity can be assessed by referring to photographs and X-rays and comparing these to previous records. Treatment can be rationalised accordingly and outcome optimised. ISIS provides an alternative and quantitative optical method of measuring deformity (Weisz *et al.*, 1988).

Urological outcome

Urological dysfunction has substantial and significant influence on the quality of life of a spinal-injured subject. This outcome is best discussed in two stages, early and late. In the early stage following spinal cord injury, detrusor function can be extremely variable. Bladder management has to be based on a clear understanding of detrusor behaviour. This is best done with the help of urodynamic studies. The importance of urodynamics in the management of the neuropathic bladder has been emphasised by McGuire and Sarastano (1985) and Lloyd (1986). Recent studies indicate that video-urodynamics associated with measurement of the maximum urethral pressure gradient (MUPG) are essential for proper assessment of the patient. In the later stages it is essential to determine renal function, which may be compromised by the neuropathic bladder.

Whiteneck *et al.* (1992) in a wide-ranging investigation into the morbidity and mortality of spine-injured patients have confirmed that problems associated with the genitourinary system have the most profound effect on long-term health. It is necessary to be vigilant in detecting any such problem and treating it promptly.

This can only be done by regular follow-up. The tests commonly carried out are:

1. Routine testing of mid-stream urine or catheter specimen urine.
2. Biochemical profile particularly urea and creatinine.
3. Regular intravenous pyelogram or ultrasound and kidney, ureter, bladder X-ray.
4. Cystometrogram and/or urodynamic study.

There is evidence that deterioration of renal function is best prevented by avoiding urinary tract infections (UTI) and renal tract dilatation. Regular IVP or ultrasound examination is essential. The incidence of UTI might be used as an outcome measure.

Plain X-rays and ultrasound are the main methods of assessing patients in the long term. In the event of repeated infections or hydronephrosis a cysto-urethrogram may be necessary, with or without urodynamics. The object is to identify the primary fault with the existing bladder management in order to define the correct treatment. The value of urodynamic studies in predicting who is likely to develop upper tract problems has been discussed by Killorin *et al.* (1992). Further discussion on urological outcome measures can be found in Chapter 6.

Outcome measures of hand function

In the tetraplegic, the quality of life depends upon the degree to which the particular individual can use his upper limb, especially the hands. In the early stages, measurement by motor index scoring or the more conventional MRC grading helps to assess improvement in hand function. Hand function is a complex and highly integrated movement. Subtle changes in function can only be tested by specific tests, such as Sollerman's test discussed below.

It is important to re-examine the hands of tetraplegics at 18 months postinjury in order to assess the rôle of upper limb reconstructive surgery. Tendon transplantation can be used to improve key grip and grasp or help in extension of the elbow. Moberg's (1976) grouping is a good classification and assessment system in those who are severely affected and where tendon transfer is contemplated. The classification is based on the presence or absence of two-point discrimination at the pulp of the thumb and the number of muscles available for transfer below the elbow. This has been modified by McDowell *et al.* (1986). This system is now widely used. Other systems for classification are the Lamb (Lamb, 1987) classification and the Zancolli classification (Zancolli, 1987).

Sollerman's test

This test was devised in the Goteberg Unit of upper limb reconstructive surgery, Sweden (Jacobson-Sollerman and Sperling, 1977). It is now widely used to measure hand function in various conditions. The test requires the subject to carry out 20 Activity of Daily Living (ADL) tasks, where all the seven types of hand grip are tested. The speed at which these tasks are performed is timed.

Grip strength and endurance can be measured by the Grip Analysis System (Medical Research Limited). In this system a device containing a pressure transducer is linked to a software package which shows graphically the strength and endurance of the subject's grip. It is rarely used in practice but could form a useful measuring device for research purposes. Grip and pinch strength can also be measured by the Jamar grip and pinch gauge. Further discussion on these instruments can be found in Chapter 20.

A hand assessment protocol is now being used at NSIC incorporating muscle testing, Sollerman's test, grip and pinch strength, sensory testing and measuring range of motion*.

The modified Moberg's classification is now widely accepted and is being used by those involved in upper limb reconstructive surgery. The

---

* Further information can be obtained from Michael Curtin, Occupational Therapy Department, NSIC.

Sollerman's test in its original version or in slightly modified form is also popular.

Rehabilitation outcome measures

Rehabilitation of the spine-injured patient starts from the very moment the patient is admitted to the hospital. In the early stages it should continue side by side with medical management. Early start of rehabilitation, such as exercises, passive movement to the joints, chest physiotherapy and psychological support may prevent the development of serious medical and emotional complications and have substantial impact on the final outcome and the quality of life of the injured patient. Hitherto each spinal unit has tended to use their own methods to measure the rehabilitation outcomes. The Southport Professional Rehabilitation Programme (Fraser, 1990) is the first published attempt to assess outcome. Rehabilitation outcome measures can be grouped under several headings.

Physical rehabilitation

Standard methods for measuring this have been lacking. At the NSIC, the Physiotherapy Progression Chart (PPC) (Figure 15.2) is used to measure progress. The PPC addresses five key activities: wheelchair manoeuvre, matwork, transfers, standing and gait re-education. These activities are then broken down into several items. A programme is laid out for the subject and it is noted when each was started and when completed. For those who use callipers, the calliper training progression chart is used to measure improvement (Figure 15.3). The system is far from ideal but does allow some outcome to be measured. There is need for a more scientific system.

Southport system

Physiotherapeutic outcome in subjects at the Southport Spinal Unit is being studied by the Southport Professional Rehabilitation Programme (Fraser and Holmes, 1990). This is a combination of assessment charts and a computerised database. Activities assessed are the maintenance of joint mobility, trunkal balance, sitting posture in a chair, matwork, pressure lifts, transfers, wheelchair activities, wheelchair mobility and sports activities. Each of these activities is divided into several items. For a particular level of injury there is a predetermined time at which full independence to a particular item of activity should be achieved. A particular subject's achievement is recorded every 2 weeks and also the time at which full independence is reached. According to the time at which a subject reaches the target time, scores are given. A 2-weekly record of each subject is entered into a computer database, from this progress can be measured and performance compared with the expected progress. Subjects with skeletal level injury from C3 to C8 each have a different target time. Those with lesion T1 are grouped with C8. The next group includes those with T2 to T5 lesions. The target time for this group

PARAPLEGIC PATIENTS PHYSIOTHERAPY PROGRESS CHART

Chair Manoeuvres	Date Started	Date Completed
Push and turn wheelchair etc.		
Relieve pressure in chair		
BWB		
Kerbs		
Stairs		
Matwork		
Rolling		
Lying to sitting		
Lift		
Turn self in bed with pillows		
Turn self prone in bed with pillows		
Transfers		
Plinth T/F legs up		
Bed T/F		
Car T/F		
Toilet T/F		
Shower chair T/F		
Chair into car		
Bath T/F		
Easy chair T/F		
Standing		
Frame independent		
Gait Re-education		
Sit to stand with crutches		
Stand to sit with crutches		
Swing to with crutches		
Swing through with crutches		
4 point with crutches		
Stairs		
Kerbs		
Car T/F with crutches		
Rough ground with crutches		
Slopes with crutches		
Open–close doors with crutches		

Figure 15.2 NSIC physiotherapy progression chart

CALLIPER TRAINING – PROGRESSION CHART

NAME:		LEVEL:			DOB				DOI		

STARTING DATE: FINISHING DATE:

TYPE OF CALLIPER: DATE MEASURED FOR CALLIPER:

DATE FIRST FITTING: DATE CALLIPER DELIVERED:

DATE											
EX'S IN BARS:											
DON											
DOFF											
WALK (FLAT HARD SURF.)											
SITTING DOWN											
STANDING UP											
WALK ON CARPET											
NEGOTIATE DOOR											
" WEIGHTED DOOR											
" AUTOMATIC DOOR											
" LIFT											
WALK UPSTAIRS											
" DOWNSTAIRS											
" BACKWARDS											
" OUTDOORS (EVEN)											
" " (UNEVEN)											
" " SLOPE											
UP KERB											
DOWN KERB											
INTO CAR											
OUT OF CAR											
GETTING UP FROM FLOOR											

Figure 15.3 NSIC calliper training progression chart

is different to the next group which includes those with T6 to T12 injury. The last group are those with L1 to L5 injury and below. An example for a C7 tetraplegic is shown in (Figure 15.4). This system is comprehensive and is also in use at the Mersey Regional Spinal Unit, Southport. The result of the evaluation of this system is awaited.

Timed walking tests

In subjects who can ambulate, measurement of walking ability should be carried out. In most spinal units this is done by a video recording of the gait. The timed walking test is a simple and very practical and easy method of measuring walking ability. This was initially used by Butland *et al.* (1982) to assess ambulation in patients with respiratory disease. Bradstater *et al.* (1983) used the method to study hemiplegic gait. The test can be used to study either speed or endurance. It has not been evaluated in spine-injured patients.

The tests are usually self paced and require the patient to walk as far as possible in either two, six or twelve minutes (Butland *et al.*, 1982). However, these protocols have no standardised pace or incremental facility which limits their sensitivity. A standardised and externally paced shuttle walking test has been developed and evaluated by Singh *et al.* (1992) to assess patients with chronic airways obstruction. It incorporates an incremental and progressive structure which requires the patient to walk for as long as possible, up and down a ten metre walkway, at a speed dictated by a tape cassette. The test has shown to be a simple and reliable method of assessing walking capacity for patients with chronic low back pain and may be a useful outcome measure for other spinal and lower limb disabilities.

Energy costs of ambulation

The metabolic energy costs of ambulation can be measured by collecting and analysing expired gases (Waters and Lunsford, 1985). This method has been recently used by Yakura *et al.* (1990) to assess the outcome of rehabilitation to locomotion. It has been used by Roberts and Carnes (1990) to measure the energy requirements when using different walking aids and of patients with large prosthetic implants following tumour surgery.

Spasticity

In a substantial proportion of spine-injured patients spasticity may affect their functional ability. Difficulties arise from either muscle spasms or increased muscle tone. Measurement of spasticity can therefore be an important outcome measure. Spasticity can be graded by the Modified Ashworth Scale (Table 15.10). Grade 0 indicates normal tone while Grade 5 depicts a rigid limb (Bohnannon and Smith, 1987). This scale has been used by Penn and Kroin (1987) and Coffey *et al.* (1993).

Relief of spasticity can be achieved by medications such as baclofen or

PHYSIOTHERAPY ASSESSMENT CHART (REHABILITATION STAGE)
LESION LEVEL C7

Number of Weeks to Full Independence

MAINTAIN JOINT ROM

b.　independently

TRUNKAL BALANCE

a.　on bed
b.　in chair with sides
c.　in chair without sides
d.　unsupported

SITTING POSTURE IN CHAIR

b.　self achievement

MAT WORK

a.　rolling to right
b.　rolling to left
c.　lying to sitting
d.　self position of pillows
e.　a,b,c,d on mattress

PRESSURE LIFT

b.　on mat
c.　in chair
d.　on mattress

TRANSFERS

b.　move bottom forward in chair
c.　lift feet off footplates
d.　lift feet from chair to floor
e.　lift feet from floor to chair
f.　transfer bottom from chair to bed
g.　transfer bottom from bed to chair
h.　lift legs onto bed
i.　lift legs off bed
j.　transfer bottom from chair to toilet

TRANSFERS (cont.)

k. transfer bottom from toilet to
    chair
l. lift high to low
m. lift low to high
n. lift bottom from chair to chair

o. lift bottom into bath
p. lift bottom out of bath
q. lift legs into bath
r. lift legs out of bath
s. lift legs into car
t. transfer bottom into car
u. lift bottom out of car
v. lift legs out of car
w. lower bottom to floor
x. lift from floor to chair
y. 180 degree transfer

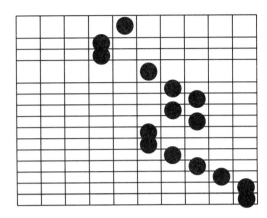

WHEELCHAIR ACTIVITIES

a. sit in upright chair
d. apply brakes
e. remove brakes
f. remove sides
g. replace sides

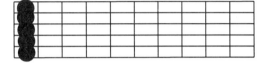

WHEELCHAIR MOBILITY

b. push ministry chair
c. push lightweight chair
d. push forwards
e. push backwards
f. turn to right
g. turn to left
h. push indoors
i. push on carpet
j. push outdoors
k. negotiate tight spaces
l. push up incline
m. control down incline
n. BWB
o. kerbs
p. verbal commands for pushers

r. wheelchair in and out of car
s. wheelchair maintenance

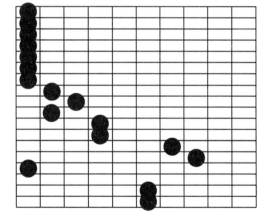

STANDING

q. use of standing frame

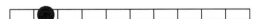

PARTICIPATION IN SPORT

yes

Figure 15.4 Example from Southport Professional rehabilitation programme (1990). Dark spots indicate target times for a C7 lesion

Table 15.10 Ashworth Scale for hypertonicity/spasticity

0 = No spasm
1 = Mild spasm induced by stimulation
2 = Infrequent full spasms occurring less than once per hour
3 = Spasms occurring more than once per hour
4 = Spasms occurring more than 10 times per hour
5 = Rigid limb

dantrolene. The former can be administered orally or intrathecally. Outcome of these treatments has been measured by Penn (1988) using his own scale. Strictly speaking this is a 'spasm' scale. This scale was applied by the same author in another study (Penn *et al.*, 1989), and in comparison with the Ashworth scale by Coffey *et al.* (1993). Spasticity can also be measured by the use of surface EMG. Kanaka (1990) has used this method to assess the effectiveness of dorsal column stimulation to overcome severe and resistant spasticity. A more elaborate and informative method is to record the EMG over a 24-hour period using a portable monitor. This method has been used by Kanamura *et al.* (1989) and Teparac (1992) to evaluate spasms occurring after cervical injury.

Measurement of Activities of Daily Living (ADL)

Most spinal injuries units use some form of the standard scales that are available to measure ADL activity, each one according to their own particular preference.

Katz ADL Index

This is a system where the activities assessed are bathing, dressing, toileting, transfer, continence and feeding. Each item has a score of 0–2. The scores are then divided into eight categories, A to G and O. This may be used again in modified form but is being replaced by the Barthel system (Katz and Lyerly, 1963).

Barthel ADL Index

This a standard scoring system for ADL activities and has been used by various disciplines (Wade and Collins, 1988). The activities studied are management of bladder and bowel, grooming, toilet use, feeding, transfers, mobility, dressing, stairs and bathing. 0 indicates when subject is unable to perform the task and the highest score is 2, when he is independent. The total score is 20. This is used with various modifications in many spinal units. There is probably a need to standardise this scale to the requirement of spinal patients.

Southport System

There is also an occupational therapy assessment and progression chart used in the Mersey Regional Spinal Injuries Centre, similar to the Southport physiotherapy system described earlier. Full independence to 13 activities is measured including communication, environmental control, driving, and sports and recreation. Similar to the physiotherapy assessment system, each injury level or group has designated target times against which performance is measured and scored. The computer database is used to monitor progress. This is not illustrated here in full because of its length. This system is comprehensive and is expected to pave the way to future rehabilitation outcome measurement for spine-injured patients. It has yet to be fully validated.

Functional Independence Measure (FIM)

ASIA recommends the Functional Independence Measure (FIM) to assess the outcome of rehabilitation (Figure 15.5). This system divides subjects into three categories: (a) complete independence; (b) modified independence and (c) complete dependence. Various activities like self-care, sphincter control, mobility, locomotion, communication and social skills and cognition are scored at admission and discharge and compared to give the final outcome. This is a simple method devised for the spine-injured patients and should be tried in spinal units in the UK. It is widely used in the USA.

Measurement of quality of life

The ultimate goal of the care of the spinal injured must be to improve the quality of life for the subject. Some instruments to measure this are listed below. Further descriptions of these and other instruments can be found in Fitzpatrick (1993). Measurement tools recommended for spinal injury patients are:

Sickness Impact Profile (SIP) – This is a well-tried and accepted measure to assess disability (Bergner *et al.*, 1981). It is a time-consuming and thorough system which uses 138 questions. It covers 12 functional areas and the scores are weighted.

Hospital Anxiety and Depression Scale (HADS) – The subjects are asked seven questions on anxiety and seven on depression. Each question can have four answers giving a score 0 to 3. The total score is therefore 21; 0–7 is normal, 8–10 is borderline normal and 11–21 is abnormal (Zigmond and Snaith, 1983).

Siosteen *et al.* (1990) have carried out a study on the quality of life in spinal cord injured subjects in Sweden, using SIP and HADS together with a self-care and mobility index, mood adjective checklist and quality of life rating. Such a comprehensive study on subjects in the UK is not available.

Glass (1992) in the UK has investigated the quality of life of ventilator-dependent spine-injured subjects using the Family Environment Scale (FES) (Moos and Moos, 1986), and the Irritability, Depression and Anxiety Scale (Snaith *et al.*, 1978). The FES is a 100-item measuring system which is divided into 10 subscales. This system deals with the perceptions of individual family members to the social and environmental

Functional Independence Measure (FIM)

L E V E L S	7 Complete Independence (Timely, Safely) 6 Modified Independence (Device)		No Helper
	Modified Dependence 5 Supervision 4 Minimal Assist (Subject = 75%+) 3 Moderate Assist (Subject = 50%+) **Complete Dependence** 2 Maximal Assist (Subject = 25%+) 1 Total Assist (Subject = 0%+)		Helper

	ADMIT	DISCH
Self Care A. Eating B. Grooming C. Bathing D. Dressing-Upper Body E. Dressing-Lower Body F. Toileting	☐	☐
Sphincter Control G. Bladder Management H. Bowel Management	☐	☐
Mobility Transfer: I. Bed, Chair, Wheelchair J. Toilet K. Tub. Shower	☐	☐
Locomotion L. Walk/wheelchair W ☐ C ☐ M. Stairs	☐	W ☐ C ☐ ☐
Communication N. Comprehension A ☐ V ☐ V ☐ N ☐ O. Expression	☐	A ☐ V ☐ V ☐ N ☐ ☐
Social Cognition P. Social Interaction Q. Problem Solving R. Memory	☐	☐
Total FIM	☐	☐

NOTE: Leave no blanks: enter 1 if patient not
testable due to risk.

Figure 15.5 Functional Independence Measure (FIM) (Hamilton and Fuhrer, 1987)

aspects of the family. The subscales attempt to assess three factors: (i) relationship; (ii) personal growth and (iii) system maintenance.

The Irritability, Depression and Anxiety Scale is used to measure the affective state of the subject. It attempts to gauge levels of anxiety, depression, outwardly directed irritability and inwardly directed irritability. Eighteen items are tested with 0–3 scores for each item. Social integration into the community has been studied by the Craig Handicap Assessment and Reporting Technique (CHART) (Whiteneck *et al.*, 1993). Physical dependency, mobility, occupation, social integration and economic self-sufficiency are taken into consideration in a scoring system. This system together with the Sickness Impact Profile, Index of Psychological Well-Being and Individual Needs Questionnaire was used in the study.

Conclusions

The final outcome of a subject with spinal injury is dependent on various factors. In the early stage it is imperative that management is directed at preventing secondary injury to the damaged cord. Surgery to the spinal column must be evaluated critically by those experienced in this specialty weighing the risks of the possibility of further damage to the cord with the long-term advantages. Timing of the operation is extremely important. If any stabilisation procedure is attempted this must be carried out over the smallest segment possible in order not to jeopardise the flexibility of the spine. The range of movement of the spine following injury has considerable bearing on ADL activities and the quality of life. Final measure of outcome is how well the subject has been integrated back into the community. Once integrated, it is essential for the spine-injured subject to be maintained in good health. This can only be done by regular follow-up. Outcome measures in the field of spinal injury are developing. There is a need for standardisation of these measures as they develop. In the future, use of these methods will play a major role in the care of patients with spinal injury.

Group discussion

Skeletal deformity and instability

The group discussed the question of the definitions of instability. They recognised three main forms of instability, using a combination of symptoms and mechanics. The first of these is postural (the patient has difficulty extending the spine from a flexed position), this is a symptom not normally associated with spinal cord injury. The second is abnormal displacement following a spinal injury. The third is progressive late deformity which may often occur years after an injury, and is particularly relevant to thoracolumbar fractures. The time of assessment of instability should be at 3 months, 1 year and 2 years following injury. Late displacement may be seen at the much longer periods of time.

The group felt it was important to measure loss of height of a vertebral body as well as change in angulation. Rotation was considered to be an unimportant deformity following spinal injury.

The 30-minute dynamic flexion-extension method was not familiar to the group. It is only applicable to spinal fractures treated non-operatively.

Motor and sensory outcome measures

Most of the published systems fail tests of validation, reliability and validation. No published reliability studies have been performed on the ASIA method of measuring motor function but in principal it seems a good approach. The group was not aware of reliability studies of the widely used MRC grading, even though this system was published 50 years ago. Similarly, no reliability studies were known to have been performed in the area of sensory assessment.

Unfortunately no reliability studies are available for the well-established and widely used Frankel system. It is important that these are done, as the group felt that this was probably the most useful outcome system available for audit purposes and probably for clinical research. The modifications should be investigated in the same way. They may well prove to be insufficiently robust for clinical research purposes.

The ASIA modification of the Frankel system may be ambiguous because of difficulties in establishing, with precision, the anatomical sites of dermatomes S_4 and S_5. There may also be problems in the reliability of MRC Grade 3, and with what is meant by 'majority of key muscles'.

There are serious methodological problems with the use of an ordinal scale such as the MRC grade in the Neuro Trauma Motor Index, as well as doubts about interobserver reliability.

The ASIA Revised Motor and Sensory Scoring System presents considerable methodological problems, both of observer reliability and repeatability and also of the difficulty in combining ordinal scales. It is by no means certain that even a skilled observer can identify dermatomes with sufficient reliability, as dermatomes are seldom defined as precisely as the anatomy texts would have us believe. The reliability of these new ASIA systems needs urgent investigation, as they have been used as outcome measures in clinical trials of considerable relevance to the early management of spinal injuries.

It was not clear whether the ASIA impairment scale had any advantages over the Frankel scale. The neuro-trauma scale appeared to be considerably flawed by difficulties of reliability and repeatability of measurement although, as far as the group was aware, this had not been tested. The sensory ASIA score was flawed because of difficulty in finding the dermatomes.

Other 'objective' systems

Neurophysiological outcome measures remain experimental. Magnetic resonance scans may be used to assess cord compression and intervertebral disc degeneration, although it is recognised that the latter may occur spontaneously and may, or may not, be symptomatic.

The disability measures included in the chapter relate to various activities as well as activities of daily living. It is desirable to validate these. The group found the goal-related Southport Score attractive, although it was felt this was too complicated and too many goals were available.

References

Aldegrini R, Agostini S (1993) A chart of anthropometric values. *J. Bone Joint Surg.*; **75B**: 86–88

ASIA Classification (1992) In Ditunno JF (ed) *Standards for Neurological and Functional Classification of Spinal Cord Injury*. Chicago, Illinois: American Spinal Injuries Association.

Austin GM (1972) *The Spinal Cord: basic aspects and surgical considerations*. Spingfield, IL: Thomas, p. 762

Bergner M, Bobbit RA, Carter WB, Gibson BS (1981) The Sickness Impact Profile: development and final revision of a health status measure. *Med. Care*; **19**: 787–805

Bohnannon RW, Smith MB (1987) Inter-rater reliability of a modified Ashworth scale of muscle spasticity. *Phys. Ther.*; **67**: 206–207

Bondurant FJ, Cotler HS, Kulkarni MV *et al.* (1990) Acute spinal cord injury – a study using physical examination and magnetic resonance imaging. *Spine*; **15**: 161–168

Bracken MB, Shepard MJ, Collins WF, Holford TR, Young W, Baskin DS, Eisenberg HM, Flamm E, Leo-Summers L, Maroon J, Marshall LF, Perot PL, Piepmeier J, Sonntag VKH, Wagner FC, Wilberger JE, Winn RE (1990) A randomised, controlled trial of methyl prednisolone or naloxone in the treatment of acute spinal-cord injury. Results of the Second National Acute Spinal-Cord Injury Study. *New Engl. J. Med.*; **322**: 1405–1411

Bradstater ME, de Bruin H, Gowland C, Clarke BM (1983) Hemiplegic gait: analysis of temporal variables. *Arch. Phys. Med. Rehabil.*; **64**: 583–587

Bunnel WP (1984) An objective criterion for scoliosis screening. *J. Bone Joint Surg.*; **66A**: 1381–1387

Butland RJA, Pang J, Gross ER, Woodcock AA, Geddes DM (1982) Two, six, and twelve minute walking test in respiratory disease. *Br. Med. J.*; **284**: 1604–1608

Carr AJ, Jefferson RJ, Turner-Smith AR, Weisz I, Thomas DC, Stavrakis T, Houghton GR (1989) Surface stereophotogrammetry of thoracic kyphosis. *Acta Orthop. Scand.*; **60**: 177–180

Cobb JR (1948) Outline for the study of scoliosis. In *Instructional Course Lectures. The American Academy of Orthopaedic Surgeons*, Vol. 5. Ann Arbor: JW Edwards, pp. 261–275

Coffey RJ, Cahill D, Steers W, Park TS *et al.* (1993) Intrathecal baclofen for intractable spasticity of spinal origin – results of long term multicentre study. *J. Neurosurg.*; **66**: 181–185

Cotler HB, Cotler JM, Alder ME *et al.* (1990) The medical and economic impact of closed cervical spine dislocation. *Spine*; **15**: 448–452

Dickson JH, Harrington PR, Erwin WD (1978) Results of reduction and stabilisation of the severely fractured thoracic and lumbar spine. *J. Bone Joint Surg.*; **60A**: 799–805

Dimitrijevic MR (1988) Clinical neurophysiological evaluation of motor and sensory functions in chronic spinal cord injury patient. In: Illis LS (ed) *Spinal Cord Dysfunction*. Oxford: Oxford University Press, pp. 274–286

Donovan WH, Cifu DX, Schotte DE (1992) Neurological and skeletal outcomes in 113 patients with closed injuries to the cervical spinal cord. *Paraplegia*; **30**: 533–542

Fitzpatrick R (1993) Patient satisfaction and quality of life measures. In: Pynsent PB, Fairbank JCT, Carr AJ Eds, Outcome measures in orthopaedics. Butterworth Heinemann, Oxford, 45–58

Frankel HL, Hancock DO, Hyslop G (1969) The value of postural reduction in the initial management of closed injuries of the spine with paraplegia and tetraplegia. *Paraplegia*; **7**: 179–192

Frankel HL, El Masri WS, Ravichandran G (1987) *Non Operative Treatment – Rehabilitation and Outcome. Thoracic and Lumbar Spine & Spinal Cord Injuries*. Vienna: Springer Verlag

Fraser MH, Holmes T (1990) The Southport professional rehabilitation programme. 2nd

International Meeting of Robotics and Handicap. *Revue Europeenne de Technologie Biomedicinale*; **12**: 301–302

Gertzbein SD (1992) Scoliosis Research Society: Multicentre Spine Fracture Study. *Spine*; **17**: 528–540

Glass CA (1992) The impact of home based ventilator dependence on the family life. *Paraplegia*; **30**: 360–368

Guttmann L (1973) *Spinal Cord Injuries: comprehensive management and research*. Oxford: Blackwell Scientific Publications

Hamilton BB, Fuhrer MJ (1987) *Rehabilitation Outcomes: analysis and measurement*. Baltimore: Brooks, pp. 137–147

Jacobson-Sollerman C, Sperling I (1977) Grip function of the healthy hand in standardised hand function test. *Scand. J. Rehabil. Med.*; **9**: 123–129

Kanaka TS, Kumar MS (1990) Neural stimulation for spinal spasticity. *Paraplegia*; **28**: 399–405

Kanamura J, Ise M, Iagumi M (1989) The clinical features of spasms in patients with a cervical cord injury. *Paraplegia*; **27**: 222–226

Katz MM, Lyerly SB (1963) Methods for measuring adjustment and social behaviour in the community: 1. Rational, description, discriminative validity and scale development. *Psych. Rep.*; **13**: 503–535

Killorin W, Gray M, Bennet JK, Green BG (1992) The value of urodynamics and bladder management in predicting upper urinary tract complications in male spinal cord injury patients. *Paraplegia*; **30**: 437–441

Lamb DW (1987) The upper limb and hand in traumatic paraplegia. In *The Paralysed Hand*, Lamb DW (ed). Edinburgh: Churchill Livingstone, pp. 136–152

Levitt MA, Flanders AE (1991) Diagnostic capabilities of magnetic resonance imaging and computed tomography in acute cervical spinal column injury. *Am. J. Emerg. Med.*; **9**: 131–135

Lloyd LK (1986) New trends in urologic management of spinal cord injured patients. *Centr. Nerv. Syst. Trauma*; **3**: 3

Lucas JT, Ducker TB (1979) Motor classification of spinal cord injuries with mobility, morbidity and recovery indices. *Am. J. Surg.*; **45**: 13–20

Manabe S, Tateishi, Abe M, Ohno T (1989) Surgical treatment of metastatic tumors of the spine. *Spine*; **14**: 41–47

McDowell, Moberg EA, House JN (1986) The second international conference on surgical rehabilitation of the upper limb in tetraplegia (quadriplegia). *J. Hand Surg.*; **11A**: 604–608

McGuire EJ, Savastano JA (1985) Urodynamics and management of the neuropathic bladder in spinal cord injury patients. *J. Am. Paraplegia Soc.*; **8**: 28

McSweeney T (1992) Injuries to the upper cervical spine. In Findlay G, Owen R (eds) *Surgery of the spine – a combined orthopaedic and neurological approach*. Oxford: Blackwell Scientific Publications, pp. 1051–1071

Moberg E (1976) Reconstructive hand surgery in tetraplegia, stroke and cerebral palsy. Some basic concepts in physiology and neurology. *J. Hand Surg.*; **1**: 29–34

Moos R, Moos BS (1986) *Family Environmental Scale*. Palo Alto, CA: Consulting Psychologists Press.

MRC (1943) *Aids to Investigation of Peripheral Nerve Injuries. Medical Research Council War Memorandum*, 2nd edn, revised. London: HMSO

Ohlen G, Spangfort E, Tingvall C (1989) The measurement of spinal sagittal configuration and mobility with Debrunner's kyphometer. *Spine*; **14**: 580–583

Pang D, Wilberger JE (1982) Spinal cord injury without radiographic abnormalities in children. *J. Neurosurg*; **57**: 114–129

Penn RD (1988) Intrathecal baclofen for severe spasticity. *Ann. N.Y. Acad. Sci.*; **531**: 157–166

Penn RD, Kroin JB (1987) Intrathecal baclofen for spasticity. *J. Neurosurg.*; **66**: 181–185

Penn RD, Savoy SM, Corcos D (1989) Intrathecal baclofen for severe spinal spasticity. *New*

Engl. J. Med.; **320**: 1517

Punn WK, Luk KDK, Lee W, Leong JCY (1987) A simple method to estimate rib hump in scoliosis. *Spine*; **12**: 342–345

Roberts P, Carnes S (1990) The orthopaedic scooter. An energy saving device for assisted ambulation. *J. Bone Joint Surg.*; **72B**: 620–621

Sett P, Crockard HA (1991) The value of magnetic resonance imaging (MRI) in the follow-up management of spinal injury. *Paraplegia*; **29**: 396–410

Short DJ, Frankel HL, Bergstrom MK (1992) Injuries of the spinal cord in children. In Frankel H (ed) *Handbook of Clinical Neurology: spinal cord trauma*, Vol. 17: 61: 233–252

Silver JR, Henderson NJ (1992) Conservative management of spinal injuries. In Findlay G, Owen R (eds) *Surgery of the Spine – a combined orthopaedic and neurosurgical approach.* Oxford: Blackwell Scientific Publications, pp. 1073–1097

Singh SJ, Morgan MDL, Scott S, Walters D, Hardman AE (1992) Development of a shuttle walking test of disability in patients with chronic airways obstruction. *Thorax*; **47**: 1019–1024

Siosteen A, Lundquist C, Blomstrand, Sullivan L, Sulivan M (1990) The quality of life of three functional spinal cord injury subgroups in a Swedish community. *Paraplegia*; **28**: 476–488

Snaith RP, Constantopoulos AA, Jardine MY, McGuffin P (1978) A clinical scale for the self assessment of irritability. *Br. J. Psychiatry*; **132**: 164–178

Stenehjen J, Swenson JR, Grange TS (1987) *Spasticity Evaluation by Ambulatory EMG. Advances in external control of human extremities IX*. Belgrade, pp. 385–392

Tator CH (1982) *Early Management of Acute Spinal Cord Injury*. New York: Raven

Teperac D, Svenson JR, Stenehjem J, Sarjanovic I, Popovic D (1992) Microcomputer-based portable long-term spasticity recording system. *IEEE-Trans Biomed. Engng*; **39**: 426–431

Tsubokawa T (1987) Clinical value of multimodality spinal cord evoked potential in the prognosis of spinal cord injuries. In: Harris P (ed) *Thoracic and Lumbar Spine and Spinal Cord Injuries*. Wein: Springer Verlag.

Thulborne T, Gillespie R (1976) The rib hump in idiopathic scoliosis. *J. Bone Joint Surg.*; **58B**: 64–71

Wade DT, Collin C (1988) The Barthel ADL index: a standard measure of physical disability? *Int. Disabil. Stud.*; **10**: 64–67

Waters RL, Lunsford B (1985) Energy cost of paraplegic locomotion. *J. Bone Joint Surg.*; **67A**: 1245–1250

Weisz I, Jefferson RJ, Turner-Smith AR, Houghton GR, Harris JD (1988) ISIS scanning: a useful assessment technique in the management of scoliosis. *Spine*; **13**: 405–408

Whiteneck GG, Charlifue SW, Frankel HL, Fraser MH, Gardner BP (1992) Mortality, morbidity, and psychological outcomes of persons spinal cord injured more than 20 years ago. *Paraplegia*; **30**: 617–630

Whiteneck GG, Charlifue SW, Gerhart KA, Overholser, Richardson GN (1993) Qualifying handicap: a new measure of long-term rehabilitation outcome. *Arch. Phys. Med. Rehabil.*; **73**: 519–526

Whittle MW (1979) Instrument for measuring Cobb angle in scoliosis. *Lancet*; **i**: 414

Wilberger JE (1991) Diagnosis and management of spinal cord trauma. *J. Neurotrauma*; **8**: suppl 1, S21–28, and discussion S29–30

Yakura JS, Waters RL, Adkins RH (1990) Changes in ambulation parameters in spinal cord injury individuals following rehabilitation. *Paraplegia*; **28**: 364–370

Zancolli E (1979) *Structural and Dynamic Basis of Hand Surgery*, 2nd edn. Philadelphia Lippincott, pp. 229–262

Zigmund AS, Snaith RP (1983) The Hospital Anxiety and Depression scale. *Acta Psychiatr. Scand.*; **67**: 361–370

Chapter 16

The pelvis and acetabulum

R. B. C. Treacy

A surgeon in his own work must rely on clinical impressions, and when deciding on the type of operation to be performed in a certain case, he must take into account his own preference. This preference may be founded on many factors, including his own experience, his feeling of rightness and suitability in a particular case, and even hero worship for a teacher, as well as a scientific knowledge of the facts. But when he reads a paper to increase this knowledge, it is important that it should convey more precise scientific truth. This depends not only on clinical observation and careful recording but on statistical accuracy, when description gives place to measurement and calculation replaces debate. These measurements and calculations should be available to the surgeon to help him assess methods of treatment, and to discriminate amongst them. An impersonal method of asessment that is comprehensive, generally applicable, and reliable is essential (Sheperd, 1954).

The acetabulum is an integral part of the pelvis and is formed from the confluence of the three pelvic bones. The pelvis supports, protects and transmits the vessels and organs of digestion, excretion, reproduction and ambulation. Disruption of the pelvis may result not only in the loss of local structural stability but may jeopardise structures contained within its volume. In addition, disruption of the pelvic ring with its associated vascular bed may result in catastrophic haemorrhage and remote organ sequelae.

Established outcome measures for trauma to the pelvis and acetabulum reflect the difference in anatomical function of these two structures. Teleologically, the acetabulum is designed to enclose the femoral head providing stability whilst permitting a sufficient range of movement for the lower limb. There are presently a number of methods available for assessing hip function and these may be applicable in assessing some aspects of outcome following acetabular injury.

Outcome measures following pelvic trauma are less clearly defined, these are reviewed first and considered separately from acetabular injuries.

Outcome following pelvic trauma

Mortality

Death is an unequivocal endpoint. It is often used as a method of measuring outcome. However, its use in comparing the results of different treatments may not necessarily be reliable. Major pelvic fractures yield a mortality of about 10% (McMurtry et al., 1980; Goldstein et al., 1986). However, if pelvic fracture is part of a multiple injury then subsequent mortality may result from a variety of unrelated causes. This has not deterred authors from using mortality as an outcome measure. In some studies (Goldstein et al., 1986), this error has been compounded by making a comparison between the mortalities of two different treatment groups using comparable trauma scores as a 'control'. A similar trauma score does not necessarily imply a comparable anatomical or physiological derangement, thus the use of mortality as an outcome measure in this situation may be unsatisfactory. Rothenberger et al. reviewed 604 patients who were admitted to hospital with multiple injuries, including pelvic fractures. Of these, 60% of the deaths were in some way attributable to the pelvic fracture; in 35% of the total, death was wholly due to the pelvic fracture (Rothenberger et al., 1978). Burgess et al. (1990) reviewed 210 patients with high energy pelvic fractures. He investigated the role of the pelvic fractures as a predictor of other injuries. The overall early mortality in this series was 8.6% of which less than 50% were considered to be attributable to the pelvic fracture. Anterior–posterior injuries were three times more likely to be associated with death than lateral injuries. There is evidence that in the haemodynamically unstable patient with a pelvic fracture the outcome can be altered by stabilisation of the fracture (K. Willett, personal communication).

Current debate in the management of pelvic fractures centres on the issue of internal fixation – to fix or not to fix? and if so when? Tile (1988) suggests that only vertically unstable (type 'C') or occasionally rotationally unstable (type 'B') disruptions require fixation. It is necessary to compare the outcomes from isolated fractures to assess the effect of these interventions on the natural history of such injuries. In reality solitary injuries of this nature are rare and comparison of the outcome of individuals with similar trauma scores must be made.

Radiology

Radiological assessment provides an objective measurement but unfortunately often correlates poorly with the clinical outcome (Neer et al., 1967). Plain X-rays can be used to assesss malunion and non-union, whilst CT scanning may provide a three-dimensional anatomical reconstruction and an assessment of rotatory malunion. Radiological assessment provides an outcome measure. It is difficult to measure displacement on radiographs.

Vertical malunion

Pennal has written extensively on pelvic fractures. He reports that antero-posterior (AP) views of the pelvis are most useful for assessment. Three views are taken; straight AP, a 35° caudad (brim) and a 35° cephalad (inlet) view. These provide information on pelvic anatomy and relative migration of fracture fragments. Oblique views are difficult to obtain in the injured patient and often difficult to interpret (Pennal *et al.*, 1980).

Slatis and Karaaharju (1980) described an undisplaced sacroiliac joint as an excellent result, 5–10 mm of displacement as a fair result and greater than 10 mm as a poor result. Henderson (1989) describes measurements made in 26 patients following major anterior–posterior pelvic disruption, taken from standard AP views of the pelvis from inlet views. He describes these measurements as 'crude' and it is clear that there are a number of errors which may arise in making these measurements from films which are vulnerable to rotational variance.

Non-union and malunion

Rotatory malunion is difficult to assess on plain radiographs although measurements can be made from CT scans. Diastasis of the pubic symphysis can be measured from AP films. More than 25 mm separation in follow-up is associated with a poor clinical result (Tile, 1984). Pennal and Massiah (1980) have reported the entity of delayed union or non-union of fractures of the pelvis. In addition to the AP radiographs, tangential views, stress radiographs and tomograms may be required to elucidate non or delayed union.

Employment

Holdsworth (1948) first used inability to return to work as an indication of disability. Time to return to work has been used as an outcome measure by a number of authors (Slatis and Karaaharju, 1980; Richardson *et al.*, 1982). This is an attempt to use a temporal index as an objective measurement of recovery and is clearly flawed. At the outset, this measurement assumes that the patient was employed at the time of injury. The requirements of individuals' jobs are quite different. Patients have different thresholds for returning to work. Attendance at work may not reflect the patient's ability to work and may well be affected by litigation.

Pennal *et al.* (1980) describes a Final Disability Assessment. This is graded as return to pre-injury occupation, return to sedentary occupation, 50% permanent disability and total permanent disability. In an effort to improve upon this index, Majeed (1989) has devised a scale to describe performance at work. This rates as one-fifth of the total available points in his scoring system; return to the same job with the same level of performance yields 20 points, return to work at reduced performance scores 16 points, change of job 12 points, light work 8 points and no regular work 0–4 points. Again this is flawed by many of the inadequacies of the temporal index but allows a comparison with preoperative activity. Henderson (1989) used a scale weighted in terms of work capability, ranging from no disability, able to work full time but at a lower level, able to work only part time and at a lower level and unable to work at all. In his series 80% of those patients with unstable pelvic injuries reported some degree of disability, compared with only 13% with stable disruption.

Pain (see Chapter 2)

Pain is an important factor in the outcome of pelvic fractures, however it is subjective and is assigned arbitrary values. It is included in most assessments. Several authors (e.g. Monahan and Taylor, 1974; Slatis and Karaaharju, 1980) have reported the incidence of persistent disabling back pain following pelvic fractures, but have made no attempt to grade the pain. Raf (1966) graded pain into moderate to severe and severe. Majeed (1989) assigns 30% of his total score to pain and subdivides pain into six classifications: continuous at rest, 0–5 points; intense with activity, 10 points; tolerable limiting activity, 15 points; abolished by rest, 20 points; mild, 25 points; no pain, 30 points. Henderson (1989) used pain diagrams for patients to report symptoms. He found that 85% of his patients had some low back pain following pelvic fractures. Of these, 80% of patients with 'unstable' fractures had pain, as did 30% of those with 'stable' injury. He also found a correlation between the degree of pain and the amount of vertical displacement of the fracture (see above).

Neurological injuries

Minor neurological injuries are common following pelvic fractures. Localised distal dysaesthesia was present in 46% of Henderson's series (Henderson, 1989) and objective neurological deficit in 42%. Most nerve injuries involve the L5 nerve root as it crosses the pelvis. In Henderson's series objective motor weakness in lower limbs was found in 21% and one-third had evidence of deep tendon reflex abnormalities in either the knee or ankle. These were seen in patients with vertical displacement.

Sphincter disturbance

Sphincter disturbance also occurs following pelvic fractures (Henderson, 1989). Other papers reporting instances of at least one-third neurological disturbances are Semba et al. (1983) and Huittinen and Slatis (1972). Semba et al. (1983) reported two patients with faecal incontinence from a series of 30 vertically unstable fractures.

Walking ability/impairment of gait

Majeed (1989) describes walking aids, gait unaided and walking distance and grades level of activity within these parameters. Timed walking tests are often used in clinical practice to assess walking ability. These tests are usually self paced and require the patient to walk as far as possible in either 2, 6 or 12 minutes (Butland et al. 1982). However these protocols have no standardised pace or incremental facility, which limits their sensitivity. A standardised and externally paced shuttle walking-test has been developed and evaluated by Singh et al. (1992) to assess patients with chronic airways obstruction. It incorporates an incremental and progressive structure which requires the patient to walk for as long as possible, up and down a 10-m walkway, at a speed dictated by a tape cassette. The test has been shown to be a simple and reliable method of assessing walking capacity for patients with chronic low back pain and may be a useful outcome measure for other spinal and lower limb disabilities (Frost, 1993, unpublished data).

Outcome of visceral injuries (see also Chapter 6)

The vast majority of urological injuries associated with pelvic fractures occur in the male patient. The classical site of injury is at the membranous urethra, however direct injury to the bladder by bony fragments may also occur. Resultant complications include sexual dysfunction, stricture, impotence and incontinence. Classifications of these factors have been made by Colapinto and McCallum (1977) and by Colapinto (1980).

Sexual dysfunction

Sexual dysfunction may occur following pelvic fracture. In females there may be dyspareunia, particularly following tilt fractures (Kellam *et al.*, 1987). Male sexual dysfunction is common following pelvic fractures (Colapinto and McCallum, 1977). Majeed (1989) includes a reference of sexual dysfunction in his scoring system.

Leg-length discrepancy

Residual leg-length discrepancy is usually associated with vertical shear fractures. Tile (1988) describes a discrepancy greater than 25 mm as yielding an unsatisfactory result*.

Vascular injuries

Vascular injuries have been reported following pelvic fractures. Sember *et al.* (1983) reported an 8% instance. Outcome measures following vascular injuries are described in Chapter 14. There is a significant incidence of vascular injuries following pelvic fractures.

Infection

Infection is an important complication of open fractures. Eighteen percent of 71 patients treated surgically developed infection in a series from Sunnybrook (K. Willett, personal communication).

Scoring systems

The only reported scoring system specifically for pelvic fractures has been proposed by Majeed (1989) (Tables 16.1, 16.2). He stated his objectives in designing a numerical scoring system as;

*Note the comment in the group discussion.

Table 16.1 Functional assessment

Pain – 30 points		Standing – 36 points	
Intense, continuous at rest	0–5	*A Walking aids (12)*	
Intense with activity	10		
Tolerable, but limits activity	15	Bedridden or almost	0–2
With moderate activity, abolished by rest	20	Wheelchair	4
		Two crutches	6
Mild, intermittent, normal activity	25	Two sticks	8
Slight, occasional or no pain	30	One stick	10
		No sticks	12
Work – 20 points			
No regular work	0–4	*B Gait unaided (12)*	
Light work	8		
Change of job	12	Cannot walk or almost	0–2
Same job, reduced performance	16	Shuffling small steps	4
Same job, same performance	20	Gross limp	6
		Moderate limp	8
Sitting – 10 points		Slight limp	10
		Normal	12
Painful	0–4		
Painful if prolonged or awkward	6	*C Walking distance (12)*	
Uncomfortable	8		
Free	10	Bedridden or few metres	0–2
		Very limited time and distance	4
Sexual intercourse – 4 points		Limited with sticks, difficult without prolonged standing possible	6
Painful	0–1	One hour with a stick limited without	8
Painful if prolonged or awkward	2	One hour without sticks slight pain or limp	10
Uncomfortable	3		
Painfree	4	Normal for age and general condition	12

Table 16.2 Clinical grade

Working before injury	*Not working before injury*	*Grade*
≥ 85	≥70	Excellent
70–84	55–69	Good
55–69	45–54	Fair
≤ 55	≤ 45	Poor

- Ease of use.
- Comprehensive cover of clinical criteria and infrequently assessed functions such as sitting and sexual intercourse.
- Use of objective findings as far as possible.
- Functional ability of the whole patient as well as local specific findings.

Five criteria are included in the assessment: pain, standing, sitting, sexual intercourse and work. These are score weighted to give a maximum possible of 100 points. In this system, 44% of the maximum possible score is given over to either a direct or indirect measurement of pain.

Outcome following acetabular fractures

Acetabular fractures may occur as isolated injuries or in association with femoral head dislocation. Pennal and Massiah (1980) state that the prognosis is related to:

1. The type of fracture.
2. The presence of damage to the weight-bearing area of the acetabulum.
3. The persistence of displacement of the fracture.
4. Further pelvic ring damage.
5. The age of the patient.

There are two main measures describing outcome following acetabular fractures: clinical and radiological. These measures have been incorporated into scores to assess hip function. The scores have been successively refined with the results of arthroplasty in mind, but they may be justifiably applied to the results of treatment following acetabular fractures. The lack of uniformity of scoring systems in current practice often precludes comparison of different series. However, the majority of systems utilise indices of pain, hip mobility, level of activity and patient satisfaction. There are a number of systems described for the assessment of arthroplasty that may be particularly applied to the outcome of acetabular fractures.

Clinical evaluation

Gade (1947) attempted to quantify useful mobility around the hip by favourably weighting the important movements of the hip. He devised a single figure namely 'the mobility index', which he derived by measuring active movements of flexion, abduction, lateral rotation, adduction, medial rotation and extension. He specifically weighted the useful component of each movement. For example, abduction from 0–15 degrees was multiplied by 0.6; 15–30 degrees by 0.4 and 30–60 degrees by 0.1. By multiplying the different parts of different movements by varying weights and totalling them, a normal adult hip achieved a score of 100 (Figure 16.1). This attempts to measure impairment.

Sheperd (1954) used the moblity index in her assessment table. This assessment was derived for The British Orthopaedic Association to quantify outcome following arthroplasty. It was intended to obviate discrepancies in recording pre- and postoperative parameters by medical staff. In addition to the mobility index, ratings of pain, function by performance estimated by a comparison of activities before and after operation (Table 16.3) and the patient's own assessment were included. These parameters were graded to give an overall assessment of excellent, good, satisfactory or poor (Table 16.4). This scale tries to 'lump together' impairment, disability and handicap.

Epstein (1974) reported the use of both clinical and radiological criteria to assess the outcome following posterior fracture-dislocations of the hip. For each parameter an arbitrary overall grading of excellent, good, satisfactory or poor was assigned (Tables 16.5, 16.6). If the rating by the two

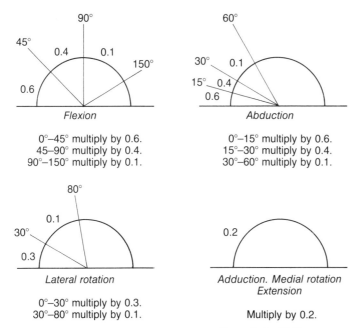

0°–45° multiply by 0.6.
45–90° multiply by 0.4.
90°–150° multiply by 0.1.

0°–15° multiply by 0.6.
15°–30° multiply by 0.4.
30°–60° multiply by 0.1.

0°–30° multiply by 0.3.
30°–80° multiply by 0.1.

Multiply by 0.2.

Figure 16.1 Gade's Mobility Index (from Gade, 1947)

methods differed the lower grading was assigned. This scale confuses impairment and handicap.

Merle d'Aubigne and Postel (1954) described a score based on pain (P), mobility (M) and ability to walk (W) (Table 16.7). Each parameter is scored from 0 to 6:

where M = 5 or 6, and
where P + W = 11 or 12   the result is very good
where P + W = 10   the result is good
where P + W = 9   the result is medium
where P + W = 8   the result is fair
where P + W = 7 or less   the result is poor

If M is 4, the result is scored one grade lower. If M is 3, it is scored two grades lower. This summates measures of impairment, handicap and disability.

A similar system assessing pain, mobility and walking ability with gradings from 1 to 6 was proposed by the Judet and Judet (1952), and Charnley (1972) modified the Merle d'Aubigne and Postel score by adding the annotations A, B and C to describe unilateral, bilateral and other relevant pathology respectively.

Lazansky (1967), drawing on experience of these methods, reiterated the sentiments of Aufranc (1957) when he stated: 'One should hesitate to judge the effect of a surgical procedure, even in a large series of cases, when any attempt to compare accurately the patient's condition before the operation with that after the operation was actually impossible'. He specifically addressed his system for use in bilateral disease. Again, he

Table 16.3 Assessment of functional activity (from Shepherd, 1954)

Activity	Black marks
Limp	
Yes	1
No	0
Trendelenburg test	
Positive	2
Negative	0
Walking outside	
Unaided	0
Requires one stick	1
Requires two sticks	3
Requires two crutches	4
Distance walked	
Not at all	4
100 yards	3
$\frac{1}{4}$ mile	2
Over a mile	0
Completely bedridden	10
Putting on own shoe and sock	
Yes	0
With difficulty	1
No	2
Stair climbing	
Yes	0
With difficulty	1
No	3
Toilet	
Yes	0
With difficulty	1
No	3
Bathing	
Yes	0
With difficulty	1
No	3
Work and activities	
Heavy physical	0
Moderate	1
Light	2
Slight	3
None	4

used the parameters of pain, functional capacity of the patient and mobility of the hips (Tables 16.8–16.10). These were assigned individual values for 16 specifically named parameters and summated to give a total score. The total scores in each category were divided by an appropriate integer to give a best possible score of 6 points in each category. For instance, the maximum possible score in the pain category is 12, so this is divided by two to give a maximum total of 6. Similarly, the maximum functional score is 23; this is divided by four to give a maximum subtotal close to 6.

Table 16.4 Assessment table (from Shepherd, 1954)

	Pain index	Mobility	Function by performance	Patient's assessment
Excellent	'None' or 'ignores'	$\geqslant 50$	5 or under and decreased post operatively by 3 or more or 6–10 and decreased by 5 or more	Enthusiastic 'yes' or 'Yes, but …'
Good	'None' or 'ignores' or 'less than before operation'	49–20	3 or under and decreased or 4–13 and decreased by 3 or more	Enthusiastic 'yes' or 'Yes, but …'
Fair	Less than, or the same as before operation, but not 'disabling' or 'gripping'	49–40	4 or over and decreased only by 2 or 1 or as preoperatively or increased by 1	Doubtful
Poor	'Makes concessions' and worse than before operation or 'disabling' or 'gripping'	< 40	Increased by 2 or more	Not worth while

Table 16.5 Roentgenographic criteria for evaluating results (from Epstein, 1974)

Excellent (normal)
All of the following: normal relationship between the femoral head and the acetabulum; normal articular cartilage space; normal density of the head of the femur; no spur formation; no calcification in the capsule

Good (minimum changes)
Normal relationship between the femoral head and the acetabulum; minimum narrowing of the cartilage space; minimum deossification; minimum spur formation; minimum capsular calcification

Fair (moderate changes)
Normal relationship between the femoral head and the acetabulum. Any one or more of the following: moderate narrowing of the cartilage space; mottling of the head, areas of sclerosis, and decreased density; moderate spur formation; moderate to severe capsular calcification; depression of the subchondral cortex of the femoral head

Poor (severe changes)
Almost complete obliteration of the cartilage space; relative increase in density of the femoral head; subchondral cyst formation; formation of sequestra; gross deformity of the femoral head; severe spur formation; acetabular sclerosis

---

Table 16.6 Clinical criteria for evaluating results (from Epstein, 1974)

Excellent
All of the following: no pain; full range of hip motion; no roentgenographic evidence of progressive changes

Good
No pain: free motion (75% of normal hip motion); no more than a slight limp; minimum roentgenographic changes

Fair
Any one or more of the following: pain, but not disabling; limited motion of the hip; no adduction deformity; moderate limp; moderately severe roentgenographic changes

Poor
Any one or more of the following: disabling pain; marked limitation of motion or adduction deformity; redislocation; progressive roentgenographic changes

---

Mobility is assessed using a modification of Gade's mobility index (Figure 16.2) which measures *passive* as opposed to *active* movements and specifically measures active abduction and straight-leg raising; the total is divided by 12 to give a maximum score of 6. When the mean of the subtotals has been calculated, it is arbitrarily assigned a description graded from very poor to excellent (Figure 16.3). This system is too complex. It attempts to summate ordinal data, and tries to assess impairment, disability and handicap in one scale.

The Toronto Hip Rating has been used by Pennal *et al.* (1980). This awards a maximum of 6 points each for pain, ability to walk and range of motion. Less than 12 points equates with poor function; 13–15 fair function; 16–18 good or excellent function. It is felt that assessment made 1 year postoperatively will give a reliable indication of final outcome. This attempts to measure impairment and disability.

Harris (1969) devised a hip score for the assessment of total hip-joint replacement; this comprises assessments of pain, function, range of motion and absence of deformity. These parameters are weighted in such a fashion as to give a maximum possible score of 100. Pain is allocated a maximum of 44 points in a six-category scale. Function carries a maximum of 47 points and is further divided into categories of gait (maximum 33) and an activity rating (maximum 14). Deformity is allocated 4 points

Table 16.7 Merle d'Aubigne and Postel hip score

Score	Pain	Mobility	Ability to walk
0	Pain is intense and permanent.	Anklylosis with bad position of the hip	None
1	Pain is severe even at night.	No movement; pain or slight deformity	Only with crutches
2	Pain is severe when walking: prevents any activity.	Flexion under 40 degrees.	Only with canes
3	Pain is tolerable with limited activity.	Flexion between 40 and 60 degrees	With one cane, less then 1 hour: very difficult without a cane
4	Pain is mild when walking; and disappears with rest	Flexion between 60 and 80 degrees: patient can reach his foot.	A long time with a cane: short time without cane and with limp
5	Pain is mild and inconstant: normal activity	Flexion between 80 and 90 degrees: abduction of at least 15 degrees.	Without cane but with slight limp
6	No pain	Flexion of more than 90 degrees: abduction to 30 degrees	Normal

Table 16.8 Allocation of points for pain (from Lazansky, 1967)

Severe, spontaneous	1
Severe on attempting to walk, prevents all activity	2
Tolerable, permitting limited activity	3
Only after some activity, disappears quickly with rest	4
Slight or intermittent: pain on starting to walk but getting less with normal activity	5
No pain	6

Table 16.9 Allocation of points for function (from Lazansky, 1967)

Use of walking aids	
Bedridden	1
Chair life	2
Two crutches	3
Two sticks	4
One stick always	5
One stick outdoors	6
No sticks	7
Walking ability	
Bedridden or a few yards	1
Time and distance very limited, with or without sticks	2
Limited with one stick (less than 1 hour). Difficult without stick. Able to stand long periods	3
Long distances with one stick, limited without a stick	4
No stick but a limp, little or no limitation of distance	5
Normal (for age and general condition of health)	6
Gait without aids	
Cannot walk	1
Shuffles with small steps or 'scissors'	2
Walks with gross limp	3
Walks with moderate limp	4
Slight limp	5
Normal gait	6
Shoes and stockings	
With help or aids	1
Without help or aids	2
Cuts toenails	
No	1
Yes	2

and range of motion 5 points. A score between 90 and 100 is considered to denote an excellent result, between 80 and 90, a good result, 70 and 80, a fair result and less than 70, a poor result (Table 16.11). This is widely used, but again suffers through the addition of ordinal data, and attempting to measure impairment, disability and handicap at once. This score has been widely used in a number of applications. Detailed discussions of it can be found by Murray (1993). This scoring method has been used by Heeg *et al.* (1990) to assess outcome in acetabular fractures. The Iowa Hip Score (Larson, 1963) also utilises a points allocation to a maximum of 100. This method has many similarities to the Harris score but employs different weightings for the individual parameters. The Iowa Hip Score is not known to have been applied to acetabular fractures.

Table 16.10 Allocation of points for mobility (from Lazansky, 1967)

Gade's index (passive)					
Index	*Right*	*Left*	*Index*	*Right*	*Left*
1–10	1	1	51–60	6	6
11–20	2	2	61–70	7	7
21–30	3	3	71–80	8	8
31–40	4	4	81–90	9	9
41–50	5	5	$\geqslant 91$	10	10
Abduction against gravity					
Range (degrees)	*Right*	*Left*	*Range (degrees)*	*Right*	*Left*
Unable	1	1	15–30	3	3
Neutral to 15	2	2	> 30	4	4
Straight-leg raising					
Range (degrees)	*Right*	*Left*	*Range (degrees)*	*Right*	*Left*
Unable	1	1	30–60	3	3
< 30	2	2	> 60	4	4
Shortening					
Amount (in)			*Right or left*		
> 1			1		
< 1			2		
0 or $< \frac{1}{4}$			3		
Separation of feet (intermalleolar distance)					
Range (in)			*Range (in)*		
$\leqslant 10$	1		21–25	4	
11–15	2		26–30	5	
16–20	3		> 30	6	
Contracture					
Range (degrees)			*Right*	*Left*	
Any adduction or flexion over 30			1	1	
Flexion contracture less than 30			2	2	
None or flexion less than 5			3	3	

Matta *et al.* (1986a) devised their own modification of the Merle d'Aubigne scoring system (Table 16.12).

Radiological evaluation

The outcome of fractures particularly affecting the weight-bearing portion of the acetabulum will be closely related to the anatomical reduction and hence radiological appearance (Letournel, 1980; Matta and Merrit, 1988).

Epstein's (1974) radiological grading was designed for use in conjunction with a clinical grading following posterior fracture-dislocations of the hip. Four grades are recognised, excellent, good, fair and poor. An excellent result denotes a normal hip with a normal anatomical relationship between the femoral head and acetabulum, normal joint space, normal head density and no capsular calcification. By contrast a poor radiological result was consistent with severe changes; obliteration of the joint space, an increase in femoral head density, deformity of the head, osteophyte formation and subchondral cysts (Tables 16.5, 16.6).

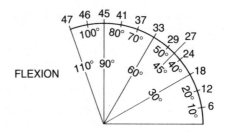

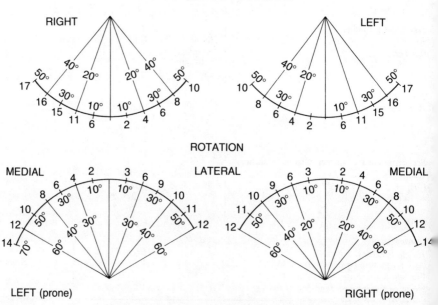

Figure 16.2 Mobility Index (from Lazansky)

Radiographs can be classified by the amount of degenerative change observed in the hip at follow-up. This is graded as nil, mild, moderate or severe by Pennal *et al.* (1980), but unfortunately the paper does not give a detailed description of their method. Matta (1986b) may have used Judet views to measure displacement of the acetabulum at follow-up, although this is unclear in the paper. They graded displacement from excellent to poor.

Matta and Merit (1988) described an assessment related to the amount of displacement on standard radiological views. Displacement of 1 mm or less was regarded as anatomical reduction. Displacement of 3 mm or less was graded satisfactory and greater than 3 mm was graded unsatisfactory.

The timing of the postinjury assessment is clearly of vital importance. Lowell recommended a 1-year follow-up. At this stage 94% of patients rated excellent or good are likely to remain so. Ninety-one per cent of patients ultimately developing significant osteoarthritis or avascular

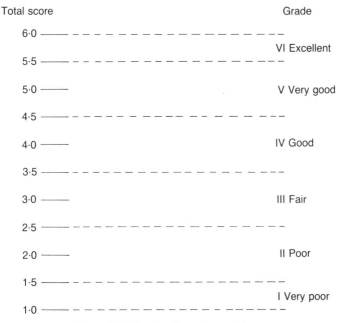

Figure 16.3 Grading (from Lazansky)

necrosis will show at least early changes at this stage. All will have failed to achieve good or excellent function. This work was originally published by Rowe and Lowell (1961). This view was also supported by Lansinger (1977).

Letournel (1980) described his own system for assessing X-rays at follow-up. He reported a 6% incidence of osteoarthrosis in 244 fractured acetabula that he had operated on. In addition, a separate category of 90 out of 244 with isolated osteophytosis was reported as another radio-logical group. A further group of 302 fractures had avascular necrosis of the bone in either the femoral head or the acetabular margin (6.6%), together with articular cartilage necrosis in 0.4% of the group.

The long-term results of traumatic posterior dislocation of the hip have been assessed by Upadhyay and Moulton (1981). Unfortunately, these authors have chosen to mix the radiological and clinical outcomes into four groups which makes it impossible to separate radiological osteo-arthritis from clinical symptoms. Epstein (1980) reported over 500 cases reviewed by his radiological system.

Pipkin fractures may also be assessed by Epstein's method, he reported 46 cases reviewed by his radiological system (Epstein *et al.*, 1985).

Complications

Heterotopic ossification

Most authors use the Brooker *et al.* (1973) grading. A good review paper using this system is that by Bosse *et al.* (1988). Up to 70% of patients may

Table 16.11 Harris hip score: synopsis of The Evaluation System

I. Pain (44 possible)
  A. None or ignores it   44
  B. Slight, occasional, no compromise in activities   40
  C. Mild pain, no effect on average activities, rarely moderate pain with unusual
      activity, may take aspirin   30
  D. Moderate pain, tolerable but makes concessions to pain. Some limitation of ordinary
      activity or work. May require occasional pain medicine stronger than aspirin   20
  E. Marked pain, serious limitation of activities   10
  F. Totally disabled, crippled, pain in bed, bedridden   0

II. Function (47 possible)
  A. Gait (33 possible)
      1. Limp
         a. None   11
         b. Slight   3
         c. Moderate   5
         d. Severe   0
      2. Support
         a. None   11
         b. Cane for long walks   7
         c. Cane most of the time   5
         d. One crutch   3
         e. Two canes   2
         f. Two crutches   0
         g. Not able to walk (specify reason)   0
  B. Activities (14 possible)
      1. Stairs
         a. Normally without using a railing   4
         b. Normally using a railing   2
         c. In any manner   1
         d. Unable to do stairs   0
      2. Shoes and socks
         a. With ease   4
         b. With difficulty   2
         c. Unable   0
      3. Sitting
         a. Comfortably in ordinary chair 1 hour   5
         b. On a high chair for half an hour   2
         c. Unable to sit comfortably in any chair   0
      4. Enter public transportation   1

III. Absence of deformity points (4) are given if the patient demonstrates:
  A. Less than 80° fixed flexion contracture
  B. Less than 10° fixed adduction
  C. Less than 10° fixed internal rotation in extension
  D. Limb-length discrepancy less than 3.2 cm

IV. Range of motion (index values are determined by multiplying the degrees of motion
    possible in each area by the appropriate index)
  A. Flexion 0–45 degrees × 40   C. External rotation in ext. 0–15 × 0.4
      45–90 degrees × 0.6   over 15 degrees × 0
      90–110 degrees × 0.3   D. Internal rotation in extension any × 0
  B. Abduction 0–45 degrees × 0.8   E. Adduction 0–45 degrees × 0.2
      15–20 degrees × 0.3
      over 20 degrees × 0

To determine the overall rating for range of motion, multiply the sum of the index values × 0.05. Record Trendelenburg
test as positive, level or neutral.

Table 16.12 Clinical grading criteria (from Mata *et al.*, 1986)

Pain		Ambulation		ROM	
No pain	6	Normal	6	100–95%	6
Slight or intermittent	5	No cane but slight limp	5	80–94%	5
Pain after ambulation but disappears	4	Long distances with cane/crutch	4	60–79%	4
Moderately severe permits ambulation	3	Limited even with support	3	40–59%	3
Severe with ambulation	2	Very limited	2		
Severe, prevents ambulation	1	Bedridden	1	0–39%	1
Clinical grade: (total points)		Excellent		18	
		Good		15–17	
		Fair		12–14	
		Poor		3–11	

develop this complication, which is almost universal when there is a head injury in combination with an acetabular fracture.

Neurological complications

Sciatic nerve palsy is a common complication following posterior disloca-tions and acetabular fractures. This may be either traumatic or iatrogenic in origin. Most authors seem to have used a clinical assessment of this, relying on foot-drop and sensory changes. EMG studies may also be used (Letournel, 1980). The incidence of sciatic nerve palsy in a conservatively treated series was 10% (Wilson, 1982).

Other complications

Infection following surgery is common; assessment of infection is dis-cussed in Chapter 12. Death following internal fixation of acetabular fractures is a recognised complication. The incidence of this may be as high as 10% in patients over 60 years (Letournel, 1980).

Children's fractures of the acetabulum

This is a rare injury. The main risk associated with this is damage to the triradiate cartilage which can produce severe incongruance between the acetabulum and the femoral head. This injury has been investigated by Heeg *et al.* (1989) who reviewed 23 patients below the age of 17 years; no formal outcome studies have been performed. There is a potential for differential growth of the three bones comprising the acetabulum, and this remains a difficult structure to measure.

Group discussion

Many of the discussion group's comments have been incorporated into the text of the chapter. Some of the more general comments are included here.

The group felt that for individual patients, and possibly for audit, inability to return to work, time to return to work and performance at work were appropriate measures but are surrounded by considerable difficulties when used in research.

It was the opinion of the group that the pain measurement methods described in Chapter 2 might be usefully applied to pelvic fractures. It might also be worth considering using disability indices, such as the Oswestry Disability Scale (Fairbank et al., 1980), as an outcome measure for these injuries.

When assessing walking ability and impairment of gait, the group suggested that the outcome measures could include energy consumption (Roberts and Carnes, 1990). Frost (unpublished data) also reported a technique involving a 10-m walking test which the group felt might well be applied to this group of patients.

The group could see little of value in the Majeed (1989) scoring system. The Epstein system has been quite widely used (mainly by Epstein), however, no reliability or repeatability studies have been done on this method and clearly these are needed if this radiological outcome measure is to be used in clinical research papers. Once again, it is important to emphasise that radiological outcome measures should be distinguished from other outcome measures.

The question of whether MRI offered a useful outcome measure following these injuries was debated At present, there are no reliable data available. There is evidence that MRI is probably the most sensitive measure for primary avascular necrosis of the femoral head, however this is a completely different condition from avascular necrosis seen following injury to the hip.

The group felt that if a hip score was going to be used, then the Charnley (1972) modification of the Merle d'Aubigne Score is probably the most appropriate. It was considered that the Epstein Classification was probably the best classification system to use. However, no validation of this classification was known This would be a valuable contribution to proving the reliability of this method of assessing radiological osteo-arthritis.

The incidence of total hip replacement following acetabular fracture may be used as an outcome measure. The group are not aware of any publication where this has been used formally as an outcome measure following this injury, but it can be seen that it would be an appropriate endpoint for survival analysis following acetabular fractures. One review of hip replacements following acetabular fractures is by Romnes and Lewallen (1990). Eighty-nine per cent of these were done for osteo-arthritis and 11% for avascular necrosis.

With regard to leg-length discrepancy, the discussion group pointed out that it is very difficult to measure following pelvic injuries. Scanograms probably offer the best available method. An alternative is to use wooden blocks. To our knowledge no reliability studies have been done in this area.

References

Aufranc OE (1957) Constructive hip surgery with the vitallium mould. *J. Bone Joint Surg.*; **39A**: 237

Bosse MJ, Poka A., Reinert CM, Ellwanger F, Slawson R, McDevitt ER (1988) Heterotopic ossification as a complication of acetabular fractures. *J. Bone Joint Surg.*; **70A**: 1231–1237

Brooker AF, Bowerman JW, Robinson RA, Riley LH Jr (1973) Ectopic ossification following total hip replacements. Incidence and a method of classification. *J. Bone Joint Surg.*; **55A**: 1629–1632

Burgess AR, Eastridge BJ, Young JWR, Ellison TS, Ellison PS, Poka A, Bathon GH, Brumback RJ (1990) Pelvic ring disruptions: effective classification system and protocols. *J. Trauma*; **30**: 848–856

Butland RJA, Gross ER, Pang J, Woodcock AA, Geddes DM. (1982) Two, six and twelve minute walking tests in respiratory diseases. *Br. Med. J.*; **284**: 1604–1608

Charnley J (1972) Long term results of low friction arthroplasty of the hip performed as a primary intervention. *J. Bone Joint Surg.*; **54B**: 61–76

Colapinto V (1980) Trauma to the pelvis: urethral injury. *Clin. Orthop. Rel. Res.*; **151**: 46–55

Colapinto V, McCallum RW (1977) Injury to the male posterior urethra in the fractured pelvis. A new classification. *J. Urol.*; **118**: 575

Epstein HC (1974) Posterior fracture dislocations of the hip. Long term follow up. *J. Bone Joint Surg.*; **56A**: 1103–1134

Epstein HC (1980) Traumatic Dislocations of the Hip. Williams and Williams, Baltimore

Epstein HC (1985) *Traumatic Dislocations of the Hip*. Williams & Wilkins: Baltimore, p. 3.

Epstein HC, Wiss DA, Cozen L (1985) Posterior fracture dislocation of the hip with fractures of the femora head. *Clin. Orthop.*; **201**: 9–17

Fairbank JCT, Davies J, Couper J, O'Brian JP (1980) Oswestry disability questionnaire. *Physiotherapy*; **66**: 271–273

Gade HG (1947) A contibution to the surgical management of osteoarthritis of the hip joint. A clinical study *Acta Chir. Scand.*; **120S**: 37–45

Goldstein A, Phillips T, Scafani SJA (1986) Early open reduction and internal fixation of the disrupted pelvic ring. *J. Trauma.*; **26**: 325–333

Harris WH (1969) Traumatic arthritis of the hip after dislocation in acetabular fractures: treatment by mould arthroplasty. *J. Bone Joint Surg.*; **51A**: 737–755

Henderson RC (1989) The long-term results of non-operatively treated major pelvic disruptions. *J. Orthop. Trauma*; **3**: 41–47

Heeg M, Klasen HJ, Vissa JD (1989) Acetabular fractures in children and adolescents. *J. Bone Joint Surg.*; **71B**: 418–421

Heeg M, Klasen HJ, Vissa JD (1990) Operative treatment for acetabular fractures. *J. Bone Joint Surg.*; **72B**: 383–386

Holdsworth FW (1948) Dislocations and fracture-dislocation of the pelvis. *J. Bone Joint Surg.*; **30B**: 461–466

Huittinen VM, Slatis P (1972) Nerve injury in double vertical pelvic fractures. *Acta Chir. Scand.*; **138**: 571–575

Judet R, Judet J (1952) Technique and results with the acrylic femoral head prosthesis. *J. Bone Joint Surg.*; **34B**: 1973–1980

Kellam JF, McMurtrie RY, Paley D, Tile M (1987) The unstable pelvic fracture: operative treatment. *Orthop. Clin. North Am.*; **18**: 25–41

Lansinger O (1977) Fractures of the acetabulum. *Acta Orthop. Scand. Suppl.*; 165

Larson CB (1963) Rating scale for hip disabilities. *Clin. Orthop. Rel. Res.*; **31**: 85–93

Lazansky MG (1967) A method for grading hips. *J. Bone Joint Surg.*; **49B**: 644–651

Letournel E (1980) Acetabular fractures: classification and management. *Clin. Orthop. Rel Res.*; **151**: 81–106

Majeed SA (1989) Grading the outcome of pelvic fractures. *J. Bone Joint Surg.*; **71B** 304–306

Matta J, Merrit PO (1988) Displaced acetabular fractures. *Clin. Orthop. Rel. Res.*; **230** 83–97

Matta JM, Anderson LM, Epstein HC, Hendricks P (1986a) Fractures of the acetabulum: a retrospective analysis. *Clin. Orthop. Rel. Res.*; **205**: 230–240

Matta JM, Mehne DK, Roffi R (1986b) Fractures of the acetabulum: early results of a prospective study. *Clin. Orthop. Rel. Res.*; **205**: 241–250

McMurtry R, Walton D, Dickinson D, Kellam J, Tile M (1980). Pelvic disruption in the polytraumatised patient: a management protocol. *Clin. Orthop. Rel. Res.*; **151**: 22–30

Merle D'Aubigne R, Postel M (1954) Functional results of hip arthroplasty with acrylic prosthesis. *J. Bone Joint Surg.*; **36A**: 451–475

Monahan PRW, Taylor RG (1974) Dislocation and fracture-dislocation of the pelvis. *Injury* **6**: 325–333

Murray D (1993) The hip. In Pynsent PB, Fairbank JCT, Carr A (eds) *Outcome Measures in Orthopaedics.* Oxford: Butterworth-Heinemann, chap. 10, p. 198

Neer CS II, Grantham SA, Shelton ML (1967) Supracondylar fracture of the adult femur: a study of one hundred and ten cases. *J. Bone Joint Surg.*; **49A**: 591–613

Pennal GF, Massiah KA (1980) Non-union and delayed union in fractures of the pelvis *Clin. Orthop. Rel. Res.*; **151**: 124–129

Pennal GF, Tile M, Waddell JP, Garside H (1980) Pelvic disruption; assessment and classification. *Clin. Orthop. Rel. Res.*; **151**: 12–21

Raf L (1966) Double vertical fractures of the pelvis. *Acta Chir. Scand.*; **131**: 298–305

Richardson JD, Harty J, Amin M, Flint LM (1982) Open pelvic fractures. *J. Trauma*; **22** 533–538

Roberts P, Carnes S (1990) The Orthopaedic Scooter: an energy-saving aid for assisted ambulation. *J. Bone Joint Surg.*; **72B**: 620–621

Romnes DW, Lewallen DG (1990) Total hip arthroplasty after fracture of the acetabulum long term results. *J. Bone Joint Surg.*; **73B**: 761–764

Rothenberger DA, Fischer RP, Strate RG, Velasco R, Pery JF (1978) The mortality associated with pelvic fractures. *Surgery*; **84**: 356–361

Rowe CR, Lawell JD (1961) Prognosis of fractures of the acetabulum. *J. Bone Joint Surg.* **43A**: 30–59

Semba RT, Yasukawa K, Gustilo RB (1983) Critical analysis of results of 53 Malgaigne fractures of the pelvis. *J. Trauma*; **23**: 535–537

Sheperd MM (1954) Assessment of function after arthroplasty of the hip. *J. Bone Join Surg.*; **36B**: 354–363

Singh SJ, Morgan MDL, Scott S, Walters D, Hardman AE (1992) Development of a shuttle walking test of disability in patients with chronic airways obstruction. *Thorax*; **47** 1019–1024

Slatis P, Karaaharju EO (1980) External fixation of unstable pelvic fractures: experience in 22 patients treated with trapezoid compression frame. *Clin. Orthop.*; **151**: 73–80

Tile M. (1984) *Fractures of the Pelvis and Acetabulum.* Baltimore: Williams and Wilkins

Tile M (1988) Pelvic ring fractures: should they be fixed? *J. Bone Joint Surg.*; **70B**: 1–12

Upadhyay SS, Moulton A (1981) The long term results of traumatic posterior dislocation of the hip. *J. Bone Joint Surg.*; **63B**: 548–551

Chapter 17

The shoulder and humerus

C. A. Pailthorpe

Introduction

The objective measurement of the results of treatment is often fraught with difficulties. A patient's expectation of outcome may be different to that defined by the doctor and may depend on the specific reason for treatment. Waddell has shown that in the treatment of low back pain, assessment of outcome appears to depend upon the final postoperative state rather than any change produced by surgery (Waddell *et al.*, 1988). Pain assessment is inevitably subjective and, as a result of pain, formal objective assessment may be affected. This is very relevant in the functional assessment of the shoulder, so outcome measures should include both subjective and objective indices.

The shoulder exhibits remarkable mobility which allows many of the normal activities of daily living (ADLs). This is particularly relevant in the assessment of patients with arthritic disorders and there have been several outcome scales proposed for such patients (Fries *et al.*, 1980; Jette, 1980; Boström *et al.*, 1991). There are a number of existing outcome measures available for the assessment of disorders of the shoulder. Some are specific to a disorder, e.g. the acromioclavicular joint (Imatani *et al.*, 1975) or fractures of the proximal humerus (Neer, 1970), whereas others, such as that described by Constant and Murley (1987), can be used for any condition of the shoulder.

The Constant assessment combines individual parameter assessments with a 100-point scoring system (Appendix 17.1). It was designed to be used in the clinical setting and does not use expensive equipment. This system has been accepted by the European Shoulder and Elbow Society. Future papers presented to the Society will have to use this system in their functional assessment.

As the shoulder is a complex joint, with varying traumatic disorders, outcome assessment will be considered in the following sections:

1. The acromioclavicular joint.
2. The rotator cuff.
3. Shoulder instability.
4. Proximal humeral fractures.
5. Humeral shaft fractures.

The acromioclavicular joint

The management of acromioclavicular injuries has been controversial for many years. Perhaps this is because there has been disagreement over both the classification of the injury and also the outcome assessment. For example, should the complete dislocation be treated operatively or conservatively?

In 1946 Urist reported on 41 cases of complete dislocation of the acromioclavicular joint (AC joint) and recognised that classification of the injury was important in comparing different types of treatment. He stated that there had been several papers in the literature reporting highly successful results but they were treating only minor injuries to the AC joint and not complete dislocations. His assessment of outcome was a return to military duty, usually within 2–3 months of injury. There were no long-term reviews.

In 1957 Arner et al., in Sweden, reported on 56 cases comparing conservative against surgical treatment. They distinguished between subluxation and dislocation and assessed the outcome using a simple scheme (Table 17.1). Lazcano et al., in 1961, reported on 43 patients with complete dislocation of the AC joint and used a different functional analysis. Urist, in a follow-up article in 1963, concluded that the functional results in conservatively managed cases were frequently equal or better than those of operated cases. However, there is no description of a formal functional assessment scheme applied to either group.

Some progress was made by Jacobs and Wade in 1966, who assessed their results on the basis of residual pain, deformity and shoulder motion. A year later, Weitzman (1967) reported his results of surgical treatment using both clinical and radiological criteria. Yet another variation on clinical outcome was used by Weaver and Dunn in their description of the surgical technique that is now known by their name (Weaver and Dunn, 1972). The first point scale for clinical evaluation of the outcome of treatment for complete dislocation of the AC joint was proposed by Imatani et al. in 1975 (Table 17.2). The scale is based on three categories, pain, function and motion. This outcome scale has not been universally accepted and it is surprising that in a 'current concepts' review article by Post in 1985, no mention of the score is made. Indeed, in this article there is little mention of any outcome evaluation of the different treatment methods.

In 1985, Walsh et al. evaluated the strength of shoulders following acromioclavicular injury using an isokinetic dynamometer in combination with a patient questionnaire. The latter included questions on pain, function, deformity and the patient's overall assessment of outcome of treatment. To each of these categories a score was allocated (Table 17.3).

Table 17.1 Assessment scheme as described by Arner et al. (1957)

Excellent	Normal mobility and power, asymptomatic
Good	Very slight restriction of movement or insignificant discomfort on unaccustomed exertion
Poor	More marked restriction of movement or discomfort at work or at rest

Table 17.2 Clinical evaluation system for acromiocla-vicular separation

Distribution	Points
Pain (40 points)	
None	40
Slight, occasional	25
Moderate, tolerable, limits activities	10
Severe, constant, disabling	0
Function (30 points)	
Weaknesses (percentage of preinjury)	20
Use of shoulder	5
Vocational change	5
Motion (30 points)	
Abduction	10
Flexion	10
Adduction	10

Reproduced from Imatani *et al.*, 1975.

Table 17.3 Study questionnaire

1. How would you describe any pain you are now experiencing with your injured shoulder?
No pain	4
Pain occasionally with heavy lifting	3
Pain after usual daily activities	2
Pain at all times	1

2. How would you describe any limitation of use you have in your injured shoulder?
No stiffness	4
Occasional stiffness after heavy activity	3
Stiffness after normal daily activity	2
Stiffness at all times	1

3. How would you describe any limitation of use you now have in your injured shoulder?
No limitation	4
Some heavy activities are limited	3
Some daily activities are limited	2
All activities are limited	1

4. When you look at youself, as in a mirror, do you now notice any deformities in your injured shoulder?
No deformity	4
Mild deformity	3
Moderate deformity	2
Severe deformity	1

5. Overall, how would you describe the outcome of your injury?
Excellent	4
Good	3
Satisfactory	2
Poor	1

Maximum score: 4 points in each category.

Reproduced from Walsh *et al.*, 1985 with permission.

It is interesting to note that patient satisfaction was lower in the operated group than in the non-operated group for complete dislocations. Also, there was no significant weakness in the latter group compared to the former. MacDonald *et al.*, in 1988, further refined Walsh's objective testing using a different isokinetic dynamometer and introduced a flexometer and grip strength. They modified the patient questionnaire to include two more sections, the assessor's own rating of pain and his own rating of the overall result. The use of isokinetic dynamometers is not feasible in everyday practice but they are a useful research tool.

Taft *et al.* in 1987 reviewed 127 patients with dislocation of the AC joint and used a rating system incorporating subjective (pain and stiffness), objective (strength and range of motion) and radiological criteria. A recent paper by Sunderam *et al.* reports on 31 patients with AC joint dislocation treated by a modified Bosworth technique (Sunderam *et al.*, 1992) and assesses the results using a modified Imatani score. A fourth section on clinical deformity has been introduced, maintaining an overall 100-point score but reducing the rating points of both function and motion.

A universally accepted system for reviewing the outcome of treatment would have many advantages. Taft comments in his paper that the authors were fully aware that assigning arbitrary values to measurements and subjective symptoms, which by their nature are imprecise, can give spurious impressions of scientific accuracy. Though the Constant assessment has been adopted as the 'shoulder outcome measurement', it has yet to be used in the assessment of treatment of AC joint injury.

Rotator cuff injury

Evaluation of the treatment of rotator cuff injuries has been bedevilled over the years by the difficulty in accurate diagnosis and classification. Originally, trauma was thought to be the principle aetiology of a cuff tear (Codman, 1934), but Neer has shown that impingement and hypovascularity are also important factors in the pathogenesis (Neer, 1983). Tears of the rotator cuff can be classified as incomplete or complete (communication with the glenohumeral joint). Cofield (1985) in a 'current concepts' review remarked that, though there had been many reports on the results of surgical treatment of cuff tears, there was a 'strange tendency' in those reports not to carefully analyse the extent of the tear seen at the time of operation and depict the results in relation to the anatomical position of the cuff lesion.

Various assessment schemes have been suggested (McLaughlin, 1962; Heikel, 1968; Godsil and Linscheid, 1970), with a more complex numerical scoring system described by Wolfgang (1974) (Table 17.4). Wolfgang's assessment scheme has been used recently by Itoi and Tabata (1992) to assess the conservative management of rotator cuff tears. As they found it difficult to classify patients into a satisfied or dissatisfied group, they omitted the section on patient satisfaction. They reviewed the literature on outcome of rotator cuff injury and concluded that the vari-

Table 17.4 Criteria for rating results

Pain
4 Absent regardless of activity
3 Mild with vigorous activity
2 Moderate, restricting some activity
1 Moderate, restricting most activity
0 Severe, constant, disabling

Motion (abduction)
4 More than 150 degrees
3 120 to 119 degrees
2 90 to 119 degrees
1 10 to 89 degrees
0 Less than 10 degrees

Strength
4 Normal
3 Mild weakness (against resistance)
2 Moderate weakness (against gravity)
1 Severe weakness (gravity eliminated)
0 Absent

Function
4 No impairment
3 Restricts strenuous working
2 Restricts all working
1 Prevents most common usage
0 No functional value

Satisfaction
1 Pleased
1 Not pleased*

Total points	*Overall rating:*
14–17	Excellent
11–13	Good
8–10	Fair
9–7	Poor

*1 implies that one point will be subtracted from the overall point total in computing the overall rating.
Reproduced from Wolfgang, 1974.

ations in the success rates reported can be explained by the differences in indications for conservative or operative treatment.

Post and Singh (1983) introduced a different assessment scheme based on pain and function (Table 17.5). Post measured the strength of the external rotators and the deltoid muscle subjectively using a simple grading system. A more accurate method of assessing muscle strength is to use force gauges (Gore *et al.*, 1986) or an isokinetic dynamometer (Walker *et al.*, 1987) but this is impractical in the outpatient setting and Constant's simplified system is more appropriate. Hawkins *et al.* (1985) reviewed 100 patients who were operated on for tears of the rotator cuff and utilised a assessment system based also on pain, function (use of the arm above and below shoulder height), strength, range of motion (both passive and active) and a subjective assessment by the patient of the outcome. They comment that it is difficult to distinguish true weakness from pain-related weakness.

Table 17.5 Assessment scheme as described by Post and Singh

Pain

Preoperation	75	No pain or discomfort with any activity
	30–74	Generally non-disabling pain
	0–29	Severe disabling pain that restricts activity
Postoperation	70–75	Excellent pain relief
	60–69	Good
	50–59	Fair
	< 50	Poor

Function

Preoperation	25	Active, full combined glenohumeral and scapulothoracic overhead motion and internal rotation (hand placed fully behind back)
	15–24	Forward flexion and abduction to 135 degrees
	11–14	Forward flexion and abduction to 90 degrees
	8–10	Forward flexion and abduction to 45 degrees
	0–7	Forward flexion and abduction to 30 degrees
Postoperation	Excellent	Active overhead motion more than 160 degrees
	Good	Active overhead motion more than 125 degrees
	Fair	Active overhead motion more than 75 degrees
	Poor	Active overhead motion less than 75 degrees

In addition the patient must have attained at least the same level of preoperative passive motion with no loss of significant motion

Reproduced from Post and Singh, 1983, with permission.

The outcome measures described are based mainly on pain, function and patient satisfaction. The Constant system does not take into consideration precise pathology.

Shoulder instability

The management of shoulder instability has remained controversial for many years. What is the outcome following the first dislocation? Is it simply a stable shoulder with no impairment of function? Simonet and Cofield in 1984 reviewed 116 patients following a first anterior dislocation of the shoulder using recurrence of dislocation as the main outcome measure, but did look at residual instability or pain. However, Hovelius in 1987, with an often quoted 5-year prospective study of anterior dislocation in teenagers and young adults, studied the recurrence rate and not function.

The usual yardstick of outcome following operation has been the recurrence of dislocation often with little reference to shoulder function. The only comment on outcome in Bankart's classic paper (Bankart, 1938) is in the summary and conclusions, where he states that the operation usually restores normal anatomy and invariably prevents recurrence. There must be over a hundred different procedures described for the surgical management of recurrent anterior dislocation of the glenohumeral joint. Many of these procedures are successful in the prevention of recurrent dislocation but it is often unclear if there is a functional penalty to be paid.

Rowe's classic paper in 1956 on the prognosis in dislocations of the shoulder introduced a functional evaluation (Table 17.6). Rowe has dominated the literature in promoting the Bankart procedure and, in 1978, produced a long-term end-result study. In this paper Rowe *et al.* describes a considerably more detailed rating system for the Bankart repair (Appendix 17.2).

There are many papers reporting the results of the different operations for stabilisation of the shoulder; some have evolved their own clinical and functional evaluation (e.g. Hovelius *et al.*, 1979; Sillár *et al.*, 1983; Symeonides, 1989; Varmarken and Jensen, 1989), whereas others have used the Rowe rating system (e.g. Weber *et al.*, 1984; Tsai *et al.*, 1991). Tsai also used an isokinetic dynamometer to assess strength.

It is inevitable that confusion reigns as to the ideal operation, when the outcome measures used are so inconsistent between papers. If the recurrence rate is the 'best' outcome measure, then there would appear to be little difference between the various operations. This is detailed by Rockwood *et al.* (1991) in a review of 53 studies with 3187 cases, finding recurrence rates of 3.2% for a Bankart, 3.0% for a Putti-Platt, 4.1% for a Magnusson-Stack and 1.7% for a Bristow. He comments that the problem at review was not the rate of recurrence but often poor function. The loss of external rotation, a complication of several of the procedures that involve shortening or tightening of subscapularis, is undesirable for those patients participating in sports using the upper arm. Regan *et al.* (1989) studied the dynamic outcome following three operative procedures, Putti-Platt, Magnusson-Stack and Bristow. They assessed the patient's return to throwing sports, the comparative loss of movement and objective measurement of strength using a dynamometer. They found a statistically significant weakness in external rotation following all three procedures. There was significant functional disability resulting in termination of all throwing activity in three of eight Magnusson-Stack, two of nine Bristow and four of the eight Putti-Platt patients who were all preoperatively recreational overhand or throwing athletes. In these days of competitive sport, a patient's expectation of return to that sport is an important part of outcome evaluation. It is possible for a patient to have an excellent result as determined by an assessment scheme, such as the Constant, and yet be bitterly disappointed in the outcome because of an inability to return to the high level of preinjury sporting activity. Clearly, it is important for the patient's expectation of outcome to coincide with the surgeon's operative goal of attaining stability!

Proximal humeral fractures

A classification system must be comprehensive enough to encompass all factors, yet specific enough to allow accurate diagnosis and treatment. Also, it must be flexible enough to accommodate variations and allow logical deductions for treatment. The classification of fractures of the proximal humerus remained controversial until 1970 when Neer proposed

Table 17.6 Evaluation of function following Bankart procedures

Poor	Fair	Good	Excellent
Marked limitation in all motions	50% limitation in external rotation 30% limitation of elevation	25% limitation in shoulder motion	Essentially normal motion
Limited in many activities and all sports	Limited in certain overhead work and sports	Moderate limitation in sport Useful shoulder for work	Very slight limitation in sports No limitation in work
Patients not satisfied	Patients satisfied	Patients satisfied	Patients very satisfied

Reproduced from Rowe, 1956.

a scheme (Neer, 1970) based upon Codman's earlier observation that fractures of the proximal humerus separate into four segments (Codman, 1934). This classification has stood the test of time and has been widely used (Clifford, 1980; Stableforth, 1984; Leyshon, 1984; Mills and Horne, 1985; Kristiansen and Christensen, 1987). It is likely to be superseded by the recent classification system proposed by Müller (Müller, 1990). Neer has described objective evaluation criteria to produce a numerical rating of function (Appendix 17.3), which has gained popularity and has been used by a number of authors (e.g. Svend-Hansen, 1974; Hägg and Lundberg, 1984; Kocialkowski and Wallace, 1990; Jakob et al., 1991).

Hägg compared the functional evaluation of three and four-part fractures of the proximal humerus using both the Neer rating and one originally proposed by Santee (Santee, 1924). The latter is based entirely on functional criteria and does not include radiological evaluation. This is an important point as, in Neer's rating, the presence of avascular necrosis incurs an automatic loss of 8–10 points and the overall result will always be worse than other cases with the same functional result but no radiological evaluation. Radiological criteria are not included in the Constant assessment and its presence may not be necessary. Hägg and Lundberg (1984) concluded that avascular necrosis results in 'failure', because of restricted motion and a low X-ray score. However, pain is often insignificant and the patients studied were fairly satisfied with the overall outcome. The Constant system should be used for the evaluation of these fractures.

Humeral shaft fractures

The management of humeral shaft fractures is generally conservative, with techniques varying from the hanging cast to functional bracing. Internal fixation techniques are indicated in certain circumstances, such as the multiply injured patient, and they have gained in popularity recently. In assessing their results many reports use the rates of union and non-union as the criteria of success (Winfield et al., 1942; Stewart and Hundley, 1955; Christiansen, 1967; Holm, 1970), others include greater functional assessment such as range of motion, weakness and recovery of activities (Mast et al., 1975; Sarmiento et al., 1977; Foster et al., 1985). The incidence of complications such as refracture, infection, nerve injury, flexion contractures, heterotopic bone formation and adhesive capsulitis have been described (Stern et al., 1984; Henley et al., 1992). Recent papers discussing both conservative and operative techniques such as intramedullary locking-nails continue to use much the same criteria (Camden and Nade, 1992; Jensen et al., 1992; Dabezies et al., 1992; Peter et al., 1992).

What is the correct outcome measure to use following a fracture of the shaft of the humerus? Clearly, when there is a risk of non-union, the rate of union and incidence of non-union are important factors. The incidence of complications associated with the particular technique used is also relevant. Some studies have investigated the functional outcome in more detail. Indeed Caldwell (1940), who is credited with the introduction of the hanging cast, reported that three of his 59 patients ultimately had poor motion of the shoulder and that some patients had restriction of elbow movement which took 3 months to recover. The advocates of functional bracing (Sarmiento *et al.*, 1977; Balfour *et al.*, 1982) have looked at function more thoroughly and recorded details of the range of elbow and shoulder motion.

Brumback *et al.* (1986) reviewed multiply injured patients with fractures of the humeral shaft treated by internal fixation using intra-medullary stabilisation with Rush rods and Enders nails. They specifically looked at the range of shoulder and elbow motion comparing the injured to the uninjured side at review. They describe a simple assessment scheme (Table 17.7).

Discussion

The assessment of shoulder function for traumatic disorders remains controversial. It is surprising that in his book on the shoulder, Rowe has a chapter on evaluation but hardly refers to it at all in the preceding chapters (Rowe, 1988). He clearly states the requirement for a standard method of assessing shoulder function and hopes that a single method will eventually become accepted.

None of the assessment systems introduces a score for age, a factor surely critical in the recovery of shoulder function. Lundgren-Lindquist and Sperling (1983) highlight the fact that the proportion of persons with limited functions in ADLs increases with age and that ageing per se results in a loss of mobility, muscle strength and coordination. Constant notes that power diminishes with age but does not discuss this factor further. Magnusson *et al.* (1990) have shown that there is a measurement error in normal healthy subjects of 19% in testing isokinetic shoulder abduction and 11% in hand-held dynamometer shoulder abduction. There is a normal day-to-day variation in motion in symptomatic patients and also variation in intra-rater and inter-rater assessment of some aspects of shoulder movement (Boström *et al.*, 1991). Thus, there is potential for substantial variability in the functional assessment if these factors are not taken into consideration. There is no comment on these factors by Constant, however his system appears to be the only one where observer error has been measured – three observers assessed 100 patients independently with only an interobserver error of 3% (range 0–8%).

Table 17.7 Assessment scheme for humeral shaft fractures

Excellent	Shoulder motion within 10 degrees of the normal side in all planes with the total decrease in elbow flexion and extension 10 degrees or less
Good	Painless shoulder motion of at least 120 degrees abduction or a loss of no more than 20 degrees elbow flexion and extension
Poor	A painful arc of either, or both, shoulder or elbow movement or does not meet the above criteria

Reproduced from Brumback *et al.*, 1986.

Their test group was a random selection of patients with abnormal shoulders but there is no breakdown of the patients' shoulder disorders. This may not be as relevant in the degenerative diseases where pain is often the most critical factor, but could assume more relevance in the variety of traumatic disorders described above.

Conclusions

The shoulder is a complex joint affected by many traumatic disorders. Outcome measures have been presented for selected traumatic categories. There is a clear requirement for accurate classification of injuries and subsequent evaluation of the available outcome measures. Extensive research is required to determine if a single outcome assessment scheme is suitable for all conditions of the shoulder.

References

Arner O, Sandahl U, Öhrling H (1957) Dislocation of the acromio-clavicular joint. *Acta Chir. Scand.*; **113**; 140–152

Balfour GW, Mooney V, Ashby ME (1982) Diaphyseal fractures of the humerus treated with a ready made brace. *J. Bone Joint Surg.*; **64A**: 11–13

Bankart ASB (1938) The pathology and treatment of recurrent dislocation of the shoulder joint. *Br. J. Surg.*; **26**: 23–29

Boström C, Harms-Ringdahl K, Nordemar R (1991) Clinical reliability of shoulder function assessment in patients with rheumatoid arthritis. *Scand. J. Rheumatol.*; **20**: 36–48

Brumback RJ, Bosse MJ, Poka A, Burgess AR (1986) Intramedullary stabilization of humeral shaft fractures in patients with multiple trauma. *J. Bone Joint Surg.*; **68A**: 960–970

Caldwell JA (1940) Treatment of fractures of the shaft of the humerus by hanging cast. *Surg. Gynecol. Obstet.*; **70**: 421–425

Camden P, Nade S (1992) Fracture bracing of the humerus. *Injury*; **23**: 245–248

Christensen S (1967) Humeral shaft fractures: operative and conservative treatment. *Acta Chir. Scand.*; **133**: 455–460

Clifford PC (1980) Fractures of the neck of the humerus: a review of the late results. *Injury*; **12**: 91–95

Codman EA (1934) *The Shoulder. Rupture of the Supraspinatus Tendon and Other Lesions about the Subacromial Bursa.* Boston: Thomas Todd

Cofield RH (1985) Current concepts review: rotator cuff disease of the shoulder. *J. Bone Joint Surg.*; **67A**: 974–979

Constant CR, Murley AHG (1987) A clinical method of functional assessment of the shoulder. *Clin. Orthop. Rel. Res.*; **214**: 160–164

Dabezies EJ, Banta CJ II, Murphy CP, d'Ambrosia RD (1992) Plate fixation of the humeral shaft with and without radial nerve injuries. *J. Orthop. Trauma*; **6**: 10–13

Foster RJ, Dixon GL, Bach AW, Appleyard RW, Green TM (1985) Internal fixation of fractures and non-unions of the humeral shaft. *J. Bone Joint Surg.*; **67A**: 857–864

Fries JF, Spitz P, Kraines RG, Holman HR (1980) Measurement of patient outcome in arthritis. *Arthritis Rheum.*; **23**: 137–145

Godsil RD Jr, Linscheid RL (1970) Intratendinous defects of the rotator cuff. *Clin. Orthop. Rel. Res.*; **69**: 181–188

Gore DR, Murray MP, Sepic SB, Gardner GM (1986) Shoulder muscle strength and range of motion following surgical repair of full thickness-rotator cuff tears. *J. Bone Joint Surg.*; **68A**: 266–272

Hägg O, Lundberg B (1984) Aspects of prognostic factors in comminuted and dislocated proximal humeral fractures. In Bateman JE, Welsh RP (eds) *Surgery of the Shoulder* Philadelphia: BC Decker, pp. 51–59

Hawkins RJ, Misamore GW, Habieka PE (1985) Surgery for full thickness rotator cuff tears. *J. Bone Joint Surg.*; **67A**: 1349–1355

Heikel HVA (1968) Rupture of the rotator cuff of the shoulder. *Acta Orthop. Scand.*; **39**: 477–492

Henley MB, Chapman JR, Claudi BF (1992) Closed retrograde Hackethal nail stabilization of humeral shaft fractures. *J. Orthop Trauma*; **6**: 18–24

Holm CL (1970) Management of humeral shaft fractures. *Clin. Orthop. Rel. Res.*; **71**: 132–139

Hovelius L (1987) Anterior dislocation of the shoulder in teen-agers and young adults. *J. Bone Joint Surg.*; **69A**: 393–399

Hovelius L, Thorling J, Fredin H (1979) Recurrent anterior dislocation of the shoulder. *J. Bone Joint Surg.*; **61A**: 566–569

Imatani RJ, Hanlon JJ, Cady GW (1975) Acute, complete acromioclavicular separation. *J. Bone Joint Surg.*; **57A**: 328–332

Itoi E, Tabata S (1992) Conservative treatment of rotator cuff tears. *Clin. Orthop. Rel. Res.*; **275**: 165–173

Jacobs B, Wade PA (1966) Acromioclavicular joint injury. *J. Bone Joint Surg.*; **48A**: 475–486

Jakob RP, Miniaci A, Anson PS, Jaberg H, Osterwalder A, Ganz R (1991) Four-part valgus impacted fractures of the proximal humerus. *J. Bone Joint Surg.*; **73B**: 295–298

Jensen CH, Hansen D, Jørgensen U (1992) Humeral shaft fractures treated by interlocking nailing: a preliminary report on 16 patients. *Injury*; **23**: 234–236

Jette AM (1980) Functional capacity evaluation: an empirical approach. *Arch. Phys. Med. Rehabil.*; **61**: 85–89

Kocialkowski A, Wallace WA (1990) Closed percutaneous K-wire stabilization for displaced fractures of the surgical neck of the humerus. *Injury*; **21**: 209–212

Kristiansen B, Christensen SW (1987) Proximal humeral fractures. Late results in relation to classification and treatment. *Acta Orthop. Scand.*; **58**: 124

Lazcano MA, Anzel SH, Kelly PJ (1961) Complete dislocation and subluxation of the acromioclavicular joint. *J. Bone Joint Surg.*; **43A**: 379–391

Leyshon RL (1984) Closed treatment of fractures of the proximal humerus. *Acta Orthop. Scand.*; **55**: 48–51

Lundgren-Lindquist B, Sperling L (1983) Functional studies in 79 year olds. *Scand. J. Rehabil. Med.*; **15**: 117–123

MacDonald PB, Alexander MJ, Frejuk J, Johnson GE (1988) Comprehensive functional analysis of shoulders following complete acromioclavicular separation. *Am. J. Sports Med.*; **16**: 475–480

Magnusson SP, Gleim GW, Nicholas JA (1990) Subject variability of shoulder abduction strength testing. *Am. J. Sports Med.*; **18**: 349–353

Mast JW, Spiegel PG, Harvey JP, Harrison C (1975) Fractures of the humeral shaft. *Clin. Orthop. Rel. Res.*; **112**: 254–262

McLaughlin HL (1962) Rupture of the rotator cuff. *J. Bone Joint Surg.*; **44A**: 979–983

Mills HJ, Horne G (1985) Fractures of the proximal humerus in adults. *J. Trauma*; **25**: 801–805

Müller ME (1990) *The Comprehensive Classification of Fractures of Long Bones*. Berlin: Springer-Verlag

Neer CS (1970) Displaced proximal humeral fractures. Part I. Classification and evaluation. *J. Bone Joint Surg.*; **52A**: 1077–1089

Neer CS (1983) Impingement lesions. *Clin. Orthop. Rel. Res.*; **173**: 70–77

Peter RE, Hoffmeyer P, Henley MB (1992) Treatment of humeral diaphyseal fractures with

Hackethal stacked nailing: a report of 33 cases. *J. Orthop. Trauma*; **6**: 14–17

Post M (1985) Current concepts in the diagnosis and management of acromioclavicular dislocation. *Clin. Orthop. Rel. Res.*; **200**: 234–247

Post M, Singh M (1983) Rotator cuff tear. *Clin. Orthop. Rel. Res.*; **173**: 78–91

Regan WD, Webster-Bogaert S, Hawkins RJ, Fowler PJ (1989) Comparative functional analysis of the Bristow, Magnusson-Stack, and Putti-Platt procedures for recurrent dislocation of the shoulder. *Am. J. Sports Med.*; **17**: 42–48

Rockwood CA, Green DP, Bucholz RW (1991) *Fractures in Adults*, 3rd edn. Philadelphia: Lippincott, pp. 1110–1111

Rowe CR (1956) Prognosis in dislocations of the shoulder. *J. Bone Joint Surg.*; **38A**: 957–977

Rowe CR (1988) *The Shoulder*. New York: Churchill Livingstone.

Rowe CR, Patel D, Southmayd WW (1978) The Bankart procedure. A long-term end-result study. *J. Bone Joint Surg.*; **60A**: 1–16

Santee HE (1924) Fractures about the upper end of the humerus. *Ann. Surg.*; **80**: 103–114

Sarmiento A, Kinman PB, Calvin EG, Schmitt RH, Phillips JG (1977) Functional bracing of fractures of the shaft of the humerus. *J. Bone Joint Surg.*; **59A**: 596–601

Sillár P, Cser I, Kéry L (1983) Results of the Putti-Platt operation for recurrent anterior dislocation of the shoulder. *Acta Chir. Hung.*; **24**: 31–35

Simonet WT, Cofield RH (1984) Prognosis in anterior shoulder dislocation. *Am. J. Sports Med.*; **12**: 19–24

Stableforth PG (1984) Four-part fractures of the neck of the humerus. *J. Bone Joint Surg.*; **66B**: 104–108

Stern PJ, Mattingly DA, Pomeroy DL, Zenni EJ, Kreig JK (1984) Intramedullary fixation of humeral shaft fractures. *J. Bone Joint Surg.*; **66A**: 639–646

Stewart MJ, Hundley JM (1955) Fractures of the humerus: a comparative study in methods of treatment. *J. Bone Joint Surg.*; **37A**: 681–692

Sunderam N, Patel DV, Porter DS (1992) Stabilization of acute acromio-clavicular dislocation by a modified Bosworth technique: a long-term follow-up study. *Injury*; **23**: 189–193

Svend-Hansen H (1974) Displaced proximal humeral fractures. A review of 49 patients. *Acta Orthop. Scand.*; **45**: 359–364

Symeonides PP (1989) Reconsideration of the Putti-Platt procedure and its mode of action in recurrent traumatic anterior dislocation of the shoulder. *Clin. Orthop. Rel. Res.*; **246**: 8–15

Taft TN, Wilson FC, Ogleby JW (1987) Dislocation of the acromioclavicular joint. *J. Bone Joint Surg.*; **69A**: 1045–1051

Tsai L, Wredmark T, Johansson C, Gibo K, Engström B, Törnqvist H (1991) Shoulder function in patients with unoperated anterior shoulder instability. *Am. J. Sports Med.*; **19**: 469–473

Urist MR (1946) Complete dislocations of the acromioclavicular joint. *J. Bone Joint Surg.*; **28A**: 813–837

Urist MR (1963) Follow-up notes on articles previously published in the Journal. Complete dislocation of the acromioclavicular joint. *J. Bone Joint Surg.*; **45A**: 1750–1753

Varmaken JE, Jensen CH (1989) Recurrent anterior dislocation of the shoulder. *Orthopaedics*; **12**: 453–455

Waddell G, Reilly S, Torsney B, Allan DB, Morris EW, Di Paola MP, Bircher M, Finlayson D (1988) Assessment of the outcome of low back surgery. *J. Bone Joint Surg.*; **70B**: 723–727

Walker SW, Couch WH, Boester GA, Sprowl DW (1987) Isokinetic strength of the shoulder after repair of a torn rotator cuff. *J. Bone Joint Surg.*; **69A**: 1041–1044

Walsh WM, Peterson DA, Shelton G, Neumann RD (1985) Shoulder strength following acromioclavicular injury. *Am. J. Sports Med.*; **13**: 153–158

Weaver JK, Dunn HK (1972) Treatment of acromioclavicular injuries, especially complete acromioclavicular separation. *J. Bone Joint Surg.*; **54A**: 1187–1194

Weber BG, Simpson LA, Hardegger F (1984) Rotational humeral osteotomy for recurrent anterior dislocation of the shoulder associated with a large Hill–Sachs lesion. *J. Bone Joint Surg.*; **66A**: 1443–1450

Weitzman G (1967) Treatment of acute acromioclavicular joint dislocation by a modified Bosworth method. *J. Bone Joint Surg.*; **49A**: 1167–1178

Winfield JM, Miller H, LaFerte AD (1942) Evaluation of the 'Hanging Cast' as a method of treating fractures of the humerus. *Am. J. Surg.*; **55**: 228–249

Wolfgang GL (1974) Surgical repair of tears of the rotator cuff of the shoulder. *J. Bone Joint Surg.*; **56A**: 14–26

Appendix 17.1 Functional assessment of the shoulder.

Scoring for individual parameters

Pain	15
Activities of daily living	20
Range of motion	40
Power	25
Total	100

Scoring for pain

None	15
Mild	10
Moderate	5
Severe	0

Scoring for activities of daily living

Activity level	
Full work	4
Full recreation/sport	4
Unaffected sleep	2
Positioning	
Up to joint	2
Up to xiphoid	4
Up to neck	6
Up to top of head	8
Above head	10
Total for ADLs	20

Points for forward and lateral elevation

Elevation (degrees)	Points
0–30	0
31–60	2
61–90	4
91–120	6
121–150	9
152–180	10

External rotation scoring

Position	Points
Hand behind head with elbow held forward	2
Hand behind head with elbow held back	2
Hand on top of head with elbow held forward	2
Hand on top of head with elbow held back	2
Full elevation from top of head	2
Total	10

Internal rotation scoring

Position	Points
Dorsum of hand to lateral thigh	0
Dorsum of hand to buttock	2
Dorsum of hand to lumbosacral junction	4
Dorsum of hand to waist (3rd lumbar vertebra)	6
Dorsum of hand to 12th dorsal vertebra	8
Dorsum of hand to interscapular region (DV 7)	10

Appendix 17.2 Rating sheet for Bankart Repair

Scoring system	Units	Excellent (100–90)	Good (89–75)	Fair (74–51)	Poor (50 or less)
Stability					
No recurrence, subluxation, or apprehension	50	No recurrences	No recurrences	No recurrences	Recurrence of dislocation
Apprehension when placing arm in certain positions	30	No apprehension when placing arm in complete elevation and external rotation	Mild apprehension when placing arm in elevation and external rotation	Moderate apprehension during elevation and external rotation	Marked apprehension during elevation or extension
Subluxation (not requiring reduction)	10	No subluxations	No subluxations	No subluxations	
Recurrent dislocation	0				
Motion					
100% of normal external rotation, internal rotation, and elevation	20	100% of normal external rotation; complete elevation and internal rotation	75% of normal external rotation; complete elevation and internal rotation	50% of normal external rotation; 75% of elevation and internal rotation	No external rotation; 50% of elevation (can get hand only to face) and 50% of internal rotation
75% of normal external rotation, and normal elevation and internal rotation	15				
50% of normal external rotation and 75% of normal elevation and internal rotation	5				
50% of normal elevation and internal rotation; no external rotation	0				

Function

Function	Units	Description
No limitation in work or sports; little or no discomfort	50	Performs all work and sports; no limitation, in overhead activities; shoulder strong in lifting, swimming, tennis, throwing; no discomfort
Mild limitation and minimum discomfort	25	Mild limitation in work and sports: shoulder strong; minimum discomfort
Moderate limitation and discomfort	10	Moderate limitation doing overhead work and heavy lifting; unable to throw, serve hard in tennis, or swim; moderate disabling pain
Marked limitation and pain	0	Marked limitation; unable to perform overhead work and lifting; cannot throw, play tennis, or swim; chronic discomfort
Total units possible	100	

Reproduced from Rowe *et al.*, 1978.

Appendix 17.3 Neer's criteria for evaluation of the results of treatment of fractures of the proximal humerus

1. *Pain (35 units)*
   a. None/ignores — 35
   b. Slight, occasional, no compromise in activity — 30
   c. Mild, no effect on ordinary activity — 25
   d. Moderate, tolerable, makes concessions, uses aspirin — 15
   e. Marked, serious limitations — 5
   f. Totally disabled — 0

2. *Function (30 units)*
   a. Strength
      Normal — 10
      Good — 8
      Fair — 6
      Poor — 4
      Trace — 2
      Zero — 0
   b. Reaching
      Top of head — 2
      Mouth — 2
      Belt buckle — 2
      Opposite axilla — 2
      Brassiere hook — 2
   c. Stability
      Lifting — 2
      Throwing — 2
      Pounding — 2
      Pushing — 2
      Hold overhead — 2

Extension
   45° — 3
   30° — 2
   15° — 1
   <15° — 0

Abduction (coronal plane)
   180° — 6
   170° — 5
   140° — 4
   100° — 2
   80° — 1
   <80° — 0

External rotation (from anatomical position with elbow bent)
   60° — 5
   30° — 3
   10° — 1
   <10° — 0

Internal rotation (from anatomical position with elbow bent)
   90° (T6) — 5
   70° (T12) — 4
   50° (L5) — 3
   30° (gluteal) — 2
   <30° — 0

3. *Range of motion (25 units)*
   Flexion (sagittal plane)

180°	6
170°	5
130°	4
100°	2
80°	1
<80°	0

4. *Anatomy (10 units)* (rotation, angulation, joint incongruity, retracted tuberosities, failure metal, myositis, non-union, avascular necrosis)

None	10
Mild	8
Moderate	1
Marked	0–2

Total points   100 units

Excellent, above 89 units; satisfactory, 80 units; unsatisfactory, 70 units; failure, below 70 units.

Chapter 18

The elbow and forearm

D. M. Williamson

Introduction

Outcome measures in trauma are unsophisticated when compared with the scoring systems that have been developed for assessing the results of orthopaedic procedures and in particular those of joint replacement surgery. Elbow replacement is in its infancy relative to knee or hip arthroplasty and this is reflected in the paucity of reliable and validated scoring systems for the elbow. Similarly there is a dearth of tried and tested methods of measuring outcome following injury of the elbow or forearm in comparison to those for trauma to the hip or knee. The few comprehensive scoring systems for elbow arthroplasty have not been applied to the trauma setting.

Papers describing results of particular injuries commonly implement scoring schemes that have been utilised by a 'landmark' historical series. For example the criteria of Boyd and Boals (1969) for assessing Monteggia fracture-dislocations in adults are used by the authors of several subsequent series on the Monteggia injury. Although different treatment regimens are compared in this way, the only factor measured by this method is the range of elbow movement which in an arbitrary fashion is categorised as 'excellent', 'good', 'fair' or 'poor' without inclusion of any other measures which influence overall outcome such as pain score, parameters of function of the arm, radiographic criteria and subjective assessment.

The concept of retesting to determine the reliability of a grading system or measurement of interobserver error is rarely noted in the trauma literature. Validation of outcome measures is also uncommon.

Factors contributing to overall outcome

In simple terms the overall outcome after a particular type of injury relates to a great extent to the severity of that injury. Hence accurate description of an injury is mandatory to ensure that like is compared with like. Analysis of these systems is beyond the scope of this chapter but there are classifications such as that produced by the AO for fractures (Müller *et al.*, 1990) which are sufficiently detailed and reproducible to meet this objective. For research purposes it is essential that the range of

severity of injury is recorded using such a classification to allow meaningful comparison between different series. For audit and quality assurance a
broad diagnosis may commonly be used but one must be aware that
failure to subclassify the fracture or dislocation may introduce significant
error into the results by omitting an important variable.

The interval between injury and the assessment of outcome is of critical
importance. In the early phase after an injury there is likely to be marked
disability while a fracture is uniting or a soft tissue injury is healing. It is
not always easy to determine the length of the recovery phase for a
particular injury but caution in interpretation of results should be exer-
cised if assessment is made within 1–2 years of a significant injury. Indeed
for injuries to the major nerves at the elbow the recovery period may be
as long as 6 years.

After the recovery stage there is usually a plateau when the condition is
static. There may then be a final period where the outcome deteriorates,
for example due to the development of post-traumatic arthritis after
intra-articular fracture. The timing of this phase is not known for many
injuries but it is often assumed that a follow-up study at 15–25 years
postinjury will determine this aspect (Josefsson et al., 1984).

When considering injuries to children the timing of assessment is even
more critical. It is well known that extensive remodelling of children's
fractures may occur, and this will affect the outcome. For example, in a
study of forearm fractures in children the incidence of 'unsatisfactory'
results at 3 months was 23%, but at 4 years was only 2.9% (Thomas et
al., 1975). The age of the child at the time of injury is also important.
Thus gross malunion of the midshaft of the forearm bones will spontaneously correct in an infant but little useful correction of deformity can be
anticipated when the child is more than 8–10 years of age at the time of
injury (Fuller and McCullough, 1982).

Injuries which affect the epiphyseal plate of a growing child may give
rise to progressive deformity. This can take 3–4 years to become clinically
apparent and therefore early reviews may be falsely optimistic.

The length of follow-up is also important when assessing the results
after open fractures or after open reduction and internal fixation since
overt manifestation of bone infection may be delayed for a considerable
time.

The vast majority of published series reporting the outcome of specific
injuries to the elbow or forearm give arbitrary grades of 'excellent',
'good', 'fair' or 'poor' depending on a combination of measures of the
following; range of motion at the elbow and radioulnar joints, pain,
function, strength and deformity (the latter includes anatomical, cosmetic
and radiographic criteria).

Range of motion

This is included in all papers reporting outcome. There is considerable
variation however in the criteria used for 'good' versus 'poor' results.
Thus Steindler (1949) states that the most useful range of flexion and
extension of the elbow is between 60 and 120 degrees, and of the forearm
pronation to 80 degrees and supination to 45 degrees. Therefore a combined loss of 130 degrees (that is 60 degrees extension, 15 degrees flexion,

10 degrees pronation and 45 degrees supination) may still be considered to be within the useful range of movement of the elbow. Similarly Evans (1953) reporting the results of supracondylar-Y fractures of the humerus described a good result as one that included 60 degrees movement at the elbow. On the other hand Radin and Riseborough (1966) describing the outcome after radial head fracture state that loss of 30 degrees of movement in any direction constitutes a poor result and Flynn et al. (1974), whose grading system for supracondylar fractures in children is very widely used, only allows loss of 20 degrees from the arc of flexion and extension before allocating a poor outcome. The clinical and functional significance of reduced forearm rotation has not been clearly established and grading of the range of movement remains arbitrary.

All systems measure the extent of passive range of motion rather than active movement, whereas the latter correlates better with subjective and functional outcome.

Pain

Pain, when it is included in the grading system, tends to be categorised into three or four grades such as 'none', 'mild', 'moderate' and 'severe' without adequate definitions of each grade. In some papers (e.g. Coleman et al., 1987) the degree of pain is subdivided into the pain experienced at rest and with use. This is further refined in the system used by Inglis and Pellicci (1980) for outcome of elbow joint replacement but, in the latter, points are allocated to each severity of pain either at rest or when bending the elbow up to a maximum of 30 points for no pain at any time. Bruce et al. (1974) have five categories of pain measurement, namely no pain (15 points), annoying pain with no compromise of activity (13), pain interfering with activity (10), pain preventing some activity (5) and pain causing outcries and preventing activities (0). These definitions are rather loose and open to interpretation. The pain score, however, contributes only 15% of the total in that scoring system which is a sufficiently low proportion given the known difficulties of scoring pain*.

Strength

This variable is rarely measured in trauma reviews. In reviewing the results of tension band fixation of olecranon fractures, Holdsworth and Mossad (1984) assessed strength of flexion and extension of the elbow using a Cybex II dynamometer. They allocated 4 points for 75% or more of peak strength of the normal side, 3 points for 50–75%, 2 points for 25–50% and 1 point for 0–25%. Its value as an outcome measure is questionable since only one of the several patients scoring a subnormal strength rating was actually concerned about weakness of the elbow.

Deformity

Residual deformity can cause functional impairment. For instance, malunion of the shafts of the forearm bones may result in significant reduc-

* This may contribute to the reliability of the measure but is likely to reduce the validity.

tion of forearm rotation. More commonly however, deformity affects outcome by the cosmetic appearance of the upper limb. In a review of the results of supracondylar fractures of the humerus in children, Smith (1960) noted a 30% incidence of cubitus varus, acknowledged as the unsightly 'gunstock' deformity. There is rarely any functional deficit from this deformity however. According to the Flynn (1974) grading of outcome of supracondylar fractures any degree of cubitus varus automatically yields a 'poor' result, yet 40% of the parents of children with cubitus varus to measurement are unaware of a cosmetic deformity (Williamson and Cole, 1993). The validity of this grading system is therefore questionable when a poor result is allocated to a child who has no functional or obvious cosmetic deficit. Deformity remains highly subjective.

Other anatomical considerations include the radiographic appearance, particularly following intraarticular fractures. It is accepted that a significant malunion in this situation is likely to prejudice the long-term outcome due to development of post-traumatic osteoarthritis. Thus accuracy of reduction is included in some scoring systems. For instance, Holdsworth and Mossad (1984) allocate 4 points out a total of 16 points for the appearance of the immediate postreduction radiograph. The grading gives 4 points for a fracture which is barely visible, 3 points for an obvious fracture but no step, 2 points for a step up to 2 mm and 1 point for a step greater than 2 mm. The literature has failed to confirm that post-traumatic osteoarthritis and its functional consequences is related so simply to this type of grading.

Function

Simple scoring systems may judge whether the elbow is 'satisfactory' or 'not satisfactory' for activities of daily living (ADLs) (Goldberg et al., 1986). ADLs and work status are allotted a maximum of 20 points out of a total score of 100 points by Bruce et al. (1974). Work handicaps are defined as decreases in salary, in working hours, in physical demands of the job, or in decreased work volume due to the injured arm. Twenty points is scored if function is equal to the opposite arm; 15 points for independent ADLs and no more than two work handicaps; 10 points for inability to do up to three ADLs or three or more work handicaps, or necessity for change of occupation; and 5 points for inability to do four or more ADLs or occupational disability.

Since the function of the arm depends on a combination of strength, range of movement, level of pain and possibly deformity, assessment of function should provide a measure of the validity of the other aspects of a scoring system. Unfortunately this is lacking in the literature.

Elbow scoring systems

Several authors have derived scoring systems which contain some or all of the above factors that affect outcome. These will be discussed in more detail.

Bruce *et al.* 1974 (Table 18.1)

This paper assesses the results of Monteggia fracture-dislocations in adults and children. The maximum score is 100, comprising range of motion (60), ADL and work status (20), pain (15) and anatomy (5). The score for range of motion is calculated from the *Guides to the Evaluation of Permanent Impairment* published by the American Medical Association Committee on Rating of Mental and Physical Impairment (1971). The Committee developed the 'Guides' after study of the literature and taking the views of 'recognised authorities'. Loss of passive range of motion measured with a goniometer is awarded a percentage impairment value from a table. Separate percentages are given for loss of flexion, extension, pronation and supination and are added to give a total impairment. Flexion/extension contribute 60% and pronation/supination 40%. Further tables give impairment percentages for ankylosis either of radio-ulnar or humeroulnar movement at different positions of their respective arcs of movement. This is a very detailed analysis of range of movement with close scales of grading but it lacks validation against function.

The scoring for ADL and pain have been described already. There is an unusual section allocating up to 5 points for anatomy. One point is given for each of: acceptable cosmetic appearance, no clinical angulation, no clinical displacement, clinical change of carrying angle less than 10 degrees and radiographic union.

Table 18.1 The assessment of Monteggia fractures

Range of motion (60 points)
Number of points of ROM = 60 − (per cent impairment of upper extremity × 0.6)

Activities of daily living and work status (20 points)
20 – Function equal to opposite arm
15 – Independent ADL; no more than two work handicaps
10 – Unable to do more than three ADL; three or more work handicaps; occupational change required
 5 – Unable to do four or more ADL; occupational disability

Pain (15 points)
15 – No pain
13 – Annoying pain with no compromise of activity
10 – Pain interfering with activity
 5 – Pain preventing some activity
 0 – Pain causing outcries and preventing activities

Anatomy (5 points)
 1 – Acceptable cosmetic appearance
 1 – No clinical angulation
 1 – No clinical displacement
 1 – Clinical change of carrying angle less than 10 degrees
 1 – Roentgenographic union

Results (total points – 100)
Excellent – 96–100
Good – 91–95
Fair – 81–90
Poor – < 80

Reproduced from Bruce *et al.*, 1974.

Hospital for Special Surgery Assessment System (Table 18.2)

This system was developed to assess the outcome of total elbow arthroplasty and allocates points to pain (30), function (20), strength (10) and

Table 18.2 The scoring sytem of the hospital for special surgery

I Pain – 30 points	
1 No pain at any time	30
2 No pain when bending	15
3 Mild pain when bending	10
4 Moderate pain when bending	5
5 Severe pain when bending	0
6 No pain at rest	15
7 Mild pain at rest	10
8 Moderate pain at rest	5
9 Severe pain at rest	0
II Function – 20 points	
A 1 Bending activities for 30 min	8
2 Bending activities for 15 min	6
3 Bending activities for 5 min	4
4 Cannot use elbow	0
B 1 Unlimited use of elbow	12
2 Limited only for recreation	10
3 Household and employment	8
4 Independent self-care	6
5 Invalid	0
III Sagittal arc – 20 points	
One point for each 7 degree arc of motion	
IV Muscle strength – 10 points	
1 Can lift 5 lb (2.3 kg) to 90 degrees	10
2 Can lift 2 lb (0.9 kg) to 90 degrees	8
3 Move through arc of motion against gravity	5
4 Cannot move through arc of motion	0
V Flexion contracture – 6 points	
1 Less than 15 degrees	6
2 Between 15 and 45 degrees	4
3 Between 45 and 90 degrees	2
4 Greater than 90 degrees	0
VI Extension contracture – 6 points	
1 Within 15 degrees of 135 degrees	6
2 Less than 125 degrees	4
3 Less than 100 degrees	0
4 Less than 80 degrees	0
VII Pronation – 4 points	
1 Greater than 60 degrees	4
2 Greater than 30 to 60 degrees	3
3 Greater than 0 degrees	0
4 Less than 0 degrees	0
VIII Supination – 4 points	
1 Greater than 60 degrees	4
2 Greater than 45–90 degrees	3
3 Greater than 15–45 degrees	2
2 Less than 0 degrees	0

Reproduced from Inglis and Pellici, 1980.

range of movement (40). The pain score suffers in requiring interpretation of mild, moderate and severe pain. Part of the function section is specific to use of the elbow for bending activities and the remainder to its use in recreation, work and ADL. There is a surprisingly small (25%) proportion of the range of movement score allocated to pronation/supination. Thus a total lack of pronation, which will cause significant disability, only results in the loss of 4 points from the total score.

There seems no reason why this scoring system would not be suitable for assessing the outcome of trauma to the elbow, perhaps with the addition of a section allocating points for deformity.

Holdsworth and Mossad, 1984 (Table 18.3)

This scoring system, which was used to assess olecranon fractures, has sections for symptoms (4 points), range of movement (4), strength (4) and accuracy of reduction of the fracture (4). The symptoms section relates mainly to pain, but there are some odd features such as, downgrading from 4 points (maximum) to 2 points for 'occasional spontaneous pain' or 'clicking' of the elbow. In the range of movement category a point is lost for the loss of 10 degrees of movement, which for the majority of patients would probably not be noticed, and 3 points are lost for more than 30 degrees loss of movement. As this system is to assess function after olecranon fracture, only flexion/extension is described. As discussed pre-

Table 18.3 The assessment of elbow function following tension band fixation of displaced fractures of the olecranon

Symptoms	
No symptoms	4
Pain only if knocked	3
Occasional, spontaneous pain or clicking	2
Frequent or constant pain	1
ROM	
Normal	4
Excellent – up to 10 degrees loss	3
Good – up to 30 degrees loss	2
Poor – > 30 degrees loss	1
Strength (flexion/extension with Cybex II dynamoneter)	
Normal 75% or more of peak strength on normal side	4
Satisfactory 50–75%	3
Poor 25–50%	2
Very weak 0–25%	1
Accuracy of reduction	
Excellent – barely visible	4
Satisfactory – obvious but no step	3
Fair – up to 2 mm step	2
Poor – > 2 mm step	1
Total	
Poor	< 11
Good	12–13
Excellent	14–16

Reproduced from Holdsworth and Mossad, 1984.

viously the strength section and accuracy of reduction section have not been validated.

Broberg and Morrey, 1986 (Table 18.4)

In assessing the outcome after radial head excision following trauma, these authors used their 'functional rating index'. There are sections for range of motion (40), pain (35), strength (20) and stability (5). The range of motion score is calculated by adding 0.2 times the flexion arc to 0.2 times the rotation arc. Thus there is a maximum score of 27 for the flexion arc, 6 for pronation and 7 for supination. Grip strength is measured with a torque dynamometer but there is no assessment of elbow strength. Stability is a subjective statement by the patient of mild loss (perceived but no limitation), moderate loss (limits some activity) or severe loss (limits everyday tasks). Stability, of course, is of great interest following radial head excision but is probably not of particular relevance to most post-traumatic situations. Pain scoring in this system is essentially a subdivision into mild, moderate and severe.

Group discussion

The elbow instruments outlined in the chapter were discussed and all were considered to have shortcomings. Many sections on pain, range of movement and ADLs were deficient in some respect. None had any evidence of attempts to validate or perform repeatability studies. The group felt that evidence of ischaemic contracture and myositis ossificans were important complications and these should be recorded. Radiological

Table 18.4 The functional rating index

Motion	
Degree of flexion (0.2 × arc)	27
Degree of pronation (0.1 × arc)	6
Degree of supination (0.1 × arc)	7
Strength	
Normal	20
Mild loss (appreciated but not limiting, 80% of opposite side)	13
Moderate loss (limits some activity, 50% of opposite side)	5
Severe loss (limits everyday tasks, disabling)	0
Stability	
Normal	5
Mild loss (perceived by patients, no limitation)	4
Moderate loss (limits some activity)	2
Severe loss (limits everyday tasks)	0
Pain	
None	35
Mild (with activity, no medication)	25
Moderate (with or after activity)	15
Severe (at rest, constant medication, disabling)	0

Reproduced from Broberg and Morrey, 1986.

measurement of cubitus varus using Baumann's angle (Baumann, 1929) is a useful measure of deformity and has a place in assessing outcome after fractures of the distal humerus. The group was not able to suggest a best buy for outcome instruments in this anatomical region.

References

American Medical Association Committee on Rating of Mental and Physical Impairment (1971) *Guides to the Evaluation of Permanent Impairment*. Chicago: AMA

Baumann E (1929) Beiträge zur Kenntnis der Frakturen an Ellbogengelenk. Unter besonderer Berücksichtigung der Spätfolgen. 1. Allgemeines und Fractura supra condylica. *Beitr. Klin. Chir.*; **146**: 1–50

Boyd HB, Boals JC (1969) The Monteggia lesion. *Clin. Orthop. Rel. Res.*; **66**: 94–100

Broberg MA, Morrey BF (1986) Results of delayed excision of the radial head after fracture. *J. Bone Joint Surg.*; **684**: 669–674

Bruce HE, Harvey JP, Wilson JC (1974) Monteggia fractures. *J. Bone Joint Surg.*; **56A**: 1563–1576

Coleman DA, Blair WF, Churr D (1987) Resection of the radial head for fracture of the radial head. Long-term follow-up of 17 cases. *J. Bone Joint Surg.*; **69A**: 385–392

Evans EM (1953) Supracondylar-Y fractures of the humerus. *J. Bone Joint Surg.*; **35B**: 381–385

Flynn JC, Matthews JG, Benoit RL (1974) Blind pinning of displaced supracondylar fractures of the humerus in children. *J. Bone Joint Surg.*; **56A**: 263–272

Fuller DJ, McCullough CJ (1982) Malunited fracture of the forearm in children. *J. Bone Joint Surg.*; **64B**: 364–367

Goldberg I, Peylan J. Yosipovitch Z (1986) Late results of excision of the radial head for an isolated closed fracture. *J. Bone Joint Surg.*; **68A**: 675–679

Holdsworth BJ, Mossad MM (1984) Elbow function following tension band fixation of displaced fractures of the olecranon. *Injury*; **16**: 182–187

Inglis AE, Pellici PM (1980) Total elbow replacement. *J. Bone Joint Surg.*; **62A**: 1252–1258

Müller ME, Nazarin S, Koch P, Schatzker J (1990) *The Comprehensive Classification of Fractures of the Long Bones*. Berlin: Springer-Verlag

Josefsson PO, Johnell O, Gentz CF (1984) Long-term sequelae of simple dislocation of the elbow. *J. Bone Joint Surg.*; **66A**: 927–930

Radin EL, Riseborough EJ (1966) Fractures of the radial head. *J. Bone Joint Surg.*; **48A**: 1055–1064

Smith L (1960) Deformity following supracondylar fractures of the humerus. *J. Bone Joint Surg.*; **42A**: 235–252

Steindler A (1949) The reconstitution of the upper extremity in spinal cerebral paralysis. In *Instructional Course Lectures, The American Academy of Orthopaedic Surgeons*, vol. 6. Ann Arbor: JW Edwards, pp. 120–133

Thomas EM, Tuson KWR, Browne PSH (1975) Fractures of the radius and ulna in children. *Injury*; **7**: 120–124

Williamson DM, Cole WG (1993) Treatment of selected extension supracondylar fractures of the humerus by manipulation and strapping in flexion. *Injury*; **24**: 249–252

Chapter 19

The wrist

J. J. Dias

Introduction

The wrist joint is the most complex joint in the body including, as it does, 10 bones, many intrinsic and extrinsic ligaments with five primary motors for the wrist joint and four for forearm rotation. Its main function is to provide stability so that the hand can be precisely positioned to perform a task efficiently. The wrist and forearm work essentially as a single unit in most tasks and it is probably artificial to separate the two.

Assessment of wrist function, therefore, is always a composite assessment with the consequent difficulty in attributing impairment to a single anatomical structure. Indirect measures, such as grip strength, are required to provide a 'rough' guide on outcome.

Most studies which assess outcome of wrist injury and disease have concentrated on movement and strength. Very few include a functional assessment or even an accurate document of the patient's problems.

Treatment aims

The aim of treatment of any wrist injury is to resolve the patient's problems completely with the least cost in terms of impairment, additional disability, handicap and especially distress. The steps involved, therefore, are:

1. To clearly define the problem(s) and expectations.
2. To establish the cause(s).
3. To weigh the potential gains with the potential losses if intervention is considered and to select, given the patient's expectations, functional requirements and overall state the most appropriate intervention for that individual.
4. To anticipate and prevent complications.
5. To assess the outcome.

Assessment of outcome should be (a) appropriate to the goals established prior to intervention and (b) appropriately timed.

An assessment of the wrist is a snapshot of the condition of the wrist at that time. Outcome assessment should answer two questions; first, has the treatment goal been achieved and second, is further change, for the better or worse, expected.

An illustrative example is a patient with an acute scaphoid fracture. The patient expects to have a pain free mobile and strong wrist. The orthopaedic goal is union of the fracture, as well as the patient's goal. Immobilisation of the injured wrist in a plaster cast for 8 weeks without union may, after an interval, meet the patient's expectation but not the surgeons. The surgeon would expect change for the worse because of the onset of degenerative arthritis. The short-term impairment of wrist motion is a direct consequence of intervention, that is immobilisation in a plaster cast.

Anatomy

The wrist joint includes the distal radius and ulna and the joint between these bones, the radiocarpal joint between the proximal carpal row and the radius and the midcarpal joint between the proximal carpal row and the distal carpal row.

The distal radius has two articular surfaces, one for the proximal carpal row and the other for the ulna. The articular surface for the ulna, the sigmoid notch, is concave and at a slight (approximately 20 degrees) forward inclination. Its radius of curvature is 4–7 mm greater than that of the corresponding surface of the ulna (af-Ekemstam, 1992). Dorsally it extends more distal and thereby accounts for the effective shortening of the radius in pronation when the radius lies obliquely over the ulna.

The distal ulna behaves like the convex side of a condylar joint. Its radius of curvature is smaller than the corresponding articular surface of the radius.

The distal radioulnar joint has two main 'ligaments': the triangular fibrocartilage which arises from the styloid fossa and is inserted into the ulnar rim of the distal radius, and the interosseus membrane. The configuration of the triangular fibrocartilage is similar to the collateral ligaments of the other condylar joints of the hand. It is triangular, the apex is inserted near the axis of rotation on the condylar side and its base is inserted into the concave side. The joint capsule is a less important structure. The volar capsule becomes tight in supination and the dorsal capsule becomes tight in pronation.

The main movement is forearm rotation with an effective arc of almost 180 degrees. In pronation the radius slides forwards and proximally in addition to rotation. Most tasks are performed with the radius in slight pronation.

The radiocarpal joint is a complex joint. The distal end of the radius has an articular surface that is inclined volar-wards (11 degrees average) and ulnar-wards (26 degrees average). The articular surface is divided by a ridge into a lateral styloid fossa for articulation with the scaphoid and an ulnar fossa which articulates with the lunate. The distal articular surface of the radius along with the triangular fibrocartilage articulates with the proximal carpal row.

The proximal carpal row is formed by the scaphoid, the lunate and the triquetrium. These three bones are connected by strong interosseous attachments along their proximal contiguous margins. This row demonstrates a twisting motion. The twist increases on radial deviation and decreases in ulnar deviation of the wrist. This complex movement is essential to provide circumduction of the wrist as the twisting motion flexes the scaphoid to allow radial deviation of the wrist.

The distal carpal row is formed by the capitate and the hamate. The centre of wrist motion lies within the head of the capitate (Youm et al., 1978). The trapezium and the trapezoid provide the offset base for thumb motion.

There are numerous named extrinsic ligaments in the wrist. The volar ligaments are stronger than the dorsal ligaments. Like all condylar joints these are fan shaped and the apex lies close to the centre of wrist motion on the head and neck of the capitate. They are arranged in an inverted 'V' manner and are well described by Taliesnik (1976).

All tendons crossing the wrist can move it. The primary motors of the wrist are the flexors carpi radialis and ulnaris and the extensors carpi radialis (longus and brevis) and ulnaris. The extensor carpi ulnaris with its sheath is an important contributor to the stability of the distal ulna.

The posterior interosseous nerve and the terminal branches of the anterior interosseous nerve provide proprioception and sensation to the radiocarpal joint. Articular branches of the ulnar nerve provide sensation to the distal radioulnar joint.

Outcome assessment

Outcome assessment is the documentation of change.

From the patient's point of view the principal positive outcome is the resolution of symptoms. It is therefore of primary importance to carefully document the patient's problem so that comparison may be made after intervention.

Pain

The most common presenting problem in the wrist is pain. Injury, inflammation, abnormal movement, impingement, tension and occasionally pressure on a nerve account for most causes of wrist pain. A careful assessment of the type, site, severity, aggravating, relieving and associated factors of the pain before and after treatment is, therefore, a fundamental requirement in assessing outcome. Severe unremitting pain in the wrist is uncommon. A careful assessment of function before treatment is therefore required. Such an assessment must take into account the patient's level of activities and dominance in addition to assessing the patient's own reaction to the pain. The single most difficult aspect in assessing pain is the assessment of its severity, which has been dealt with in Chapter 2.

The primary goal in most wrist conditions is to abolish pain. Therefore the outcome of most wrist conditions can be assessed in terms of pain relief. Intervention can of course make the pain worse or may leave the pain unchanged. Slight relief is such that the patient experiences less pain but there is no improvement in function. Significant relief of pain is such that patients can undertake those activities which prior to intervention were either not possible or were difficult. The best outcome, however, is complete pain relief.

Appearance of the wrist and hand

Swelling

Assessing outcome of treatment of a discrete swelling around the wrist is usually not difficult. The possible outcomes are that the swelling has increased, there has been no change, there is incomplete resolution, there is complete resolution or that there is recurrence. Recurrence can be quantified in terms of the period to recurrence. A common example is a wrist ganglion. Surgical excision which includes a capsulotomy has a recurrence rate of around 5%. The outcome in such a case is only satisfactory if the swelling is completely abolished and does not recur.

Deformity

Assessing outcome for correction of deformity is unambiguous. Measurement of the deformity before and after intervention provides a reasonable assessment of the degree of correction achieved. The measurement may be clinical or radiographic. Provided the measurement is carried out by a single observer and is reproducible, it provides an accurate assessment of correction of the deformity.

Loss of movement

This can be the result of an abnormality of the motor function (division or neuromuscular abnormality) or stiffness or pain. In the former the passive movement of the wrist is possible but active movement is either incomplete or impossible. Assessing the outcome of treatment is relatively straightforward and is detailed below.

Instability

Patients can present with abnormality of movement. This usually accompanies wrist pain and presents as an associated click or clunk in the distal radioulnar joint or the proximal carpal row. Standard clinical tests are used to establish the presence or absence of instability. Quantifying the degree of instability is difficult and arbitrary – the simplest way is to designate the instability as probable (if only just different from the opposite side) or definite.

Abnormal movement should be distinguished from joint laxity. A routine assessment for joint laxity should be carried out and a comparison made to the contralateral side if it is normal. This is usually not possible in the presence of disease such as rheumatoid arthritis which can involve both wrists.

Strength

Almost all conditions affecting the wrist alter the grip strength. Hence careful assessment of this is essential in establishing whether any intervention has been beneficial. Assessment of strength is an indirect assessment and is dependent on many factors, ranging from motivation, intact neuromuscular structure and anatomical and functional integrity of the forearm, wrist and hand. In assessing the outcome of wrist conditions it is only of value if the wrist is considered to be the predominant, if not the only, cause of weakness.

Function

Like abolishing pain, improving function is a primary aim of most intervention for the wrist. It is therefore surprising that very few assessments of outcome include an assessment of function before and after intervention.

Assessing change

Assessment of outcome for wrist conditions involves assessment of change in subjective, objective and investigative parameters before and after intervention in order to establish whether the goal of intervention has been attained. There is a fundamental requirement therefore that a clear goal is established prior to treatment and that parameters are assessed prior to intervention and that the timing of postintervention assessment is adequate.

Wrist movement

Range of wrist movement

Wrist movement is complex. It allows circumduction of the hand and involves movement of the wrist and forearm.

Clinical assessment of wrist movement is done by measuring the range of wrist movement using an ordinary goniometer. The range of dorsiflexion, palmar flexion, radial and ulnar deviation is measured. Forearm rotation is assessed by measuring supination and pronation.

Wrist movement is usually measured with the wrist in full pronation and the fingers extended so that the middle finger is in line with the third metacarpal. The neutral position is one in which the third metacarpal is in line with the radius. For practical purposes it is easier to measure dorsiflexion and palmar flexion from the ulnar side. One limb of the goniometer is placed along the ulna and the centre of rotation over the tip of the ulnar styloid. The hand is then moved into maximum dorsiflexion and the distal limb of the goniometer is brought to lie in line with the third metacarpal. The change in angle from the neutral position is then noted as the angle of active/passive dorsiflexion. Similarly the range of palmar flexion is assessed by moving the hand into maximum palmar flexion (American Academy of Orthopaedic Surgeons, 1965).

Radioulnar deviation is measured with the elbow flexed and the forearm pronated. The forearm and hand lie on the table with the palm facing downwards. The neutral position is one in which the third metacarpal is in line with the radius. One limb of the goniometer is placed parallel to the axis of the radius while the centre of rotation is placed over the head of the capitate. The distal limb of the goniometer is placed along the third metacarpal. The hand is then moved into maximum radial deviation and the angle measured. Ulnar deviation is similarly measured by moving the hand into maximum ulnar deviation (Moore, 1949).

Forearm rotation is measured with the elbow flexed and the forearm placed in the midprone position. In this position the plane of the palm should lie in the parasagittal plane. The forearm is then rotated into maximum supination and the angle of the plane of the palm to the neutral is measured as the angle of supination. Similarly the angle of pronation can also be measured (American Academy of Orthopaedic Surgeons, 1965).

Impairment assessment

Based on these measurements it is possible to assess the percentage of impairment of wrist movement which can be related to the loss of the whole arm and impairment to the whole body. This method of assessment is well documented and standardised by the International Federation of Societies for surgery of the hand in 1980. Each part of the upper limb is assigned a percentage value in terms of impairment to the whole limb. The wrist is assigned 60%; dorsal and palmar flexion movement is given 70% value of the total range of wrist motion while radioulnar deviation is given 30%. The usual range of wrist motion is taken from 60 degrees of dorsiflexion to 60 degrees of palmar flexion, and from 20 degrees of radial deviation to 30 degrees of ulnar deviation. The impairment is assessed by adding that of dorsopalmar flexion and radioulnar deviation (Swanson et al., 1990).

Wrist circumduction

Recently the introduction of biaxial flexible goniometers has made it possible to assess both planar motions simultaneously. This is done by fixing the two end blocks of the electrogoniometer at the neck of the third metacarpal and at the forearm and then performing a circumduction motion of the wrist with or without constraint of forearm rotation. When connected to the appropriate software the system can generate figures of wrist circumduction, known as Lissajous's figures. These describe the arc of wrist movement and in the normal wrist are oval with the long axis inclined from dorsal and radial to palmar and ulnar. The figure gives a more functional assessment of wrist movement.

Comparison of these figures assist in determining the deviation from normal and establishing any change with time especially after intervention (Ojima et al., 1991).

Comparison

In the assessment of movement of the wrist the contralateral unaffected wrist usually serves as a frame of reference. However the difference between the dominant and non-dominant sides must be considered. This varies for each individual and is not available when the opposite wrist is affected. The range of movement may itself vary during the course of the day depending on the presence of stiffness or pain. This may confound any single measurement.

In assessing outcome, however, the magnitude of change is of greater value than an absolute measurement.

Finally the method of measurement itself is not accurate and the possibility of inter- and intraobserver error must be borne in mind (Moore, 1949).

Strength

The next commonly assessed parameter for wrist disorders is grip strength.

This can be measured crudely by getting the patient to squeeze two fingers of the examiner's hand while the examiner tries to pull his fingers out of the patient's grip. The strength can be simply recorded as equal of good, weak or absent. This method has not been validated.

When the grip is weak it can be assessed using a sphygmomanometer. The cuff is rolled into a 5-cm diameter roll and then inflated to 50 mmHg. The patient squeezes the cuff and any change in the height of the mercury column in millimetres is recorded as the power of grip.

The most commonly recommended device to assess grip strength is the hand dynamometer. The handles of such a device are set apart at 6 cm. The two handles are squeezed together and the strength assessed using a strain gauge. In men grip strength varies between 30.4 and 70.4 kg while in females it ranges from 14 to 38.6 kg. It can vary with age, time of day and dominance. The grip strength can vary between the dominant and non-dominant hand by 5–10% (Bechtol, 1954). On average grip strength is weak in the non-dominant hand in 5.4% of men and 8.9% of women. The position of the wrist has a significant impact on grip strength (O'Driscoll *et al.*, 1992). There is a variation in strength of around 20% over a 2-week period (Young *et al.*, 1989).

The method of assessing grip strength using a hydraulic dynamometer with adjustable handle settings is well established and has been shown to be reliable (Mathiowetz *et al.*, 1984). There are published norms for children and adults (Mathiowetz *et al.*, 1985, 1986).

Assessment of fatigue and endurance is now possible by linking a dynamometer to a computer with the appropriate software. Such a system assists in identifying malingerers.

Functional assessment

The simplest form of functional assessment for the wrist is to ask the patient to list those tasks that cannot be performed and those that are difficult. Assessment of outcome could then include assessing whether the difficulty of these tasks has changed and whether tasks that could not be performed can now be done. This system assesses each individual's disability and is independent of the dominance of the hand but it does not allow comparison between patients.

A standard assessment of daily activities should be used. These activities should ideally be independent of dominance or sex and should include household, work-related and leisure tasks. There are many such tests for the hand and some can be used for the wrist. These have been examined in detail by Macey and Kelly (1993). The form shown in Table 19.1 has been used in assessing outcome for various wrist conditions in the Leicester Group of Hospitals. In order to avoid ambiguity only three categories are recognised for each task: (1) cannot perform; (2) has difficulty and (3) can perform normally.

While Predetermined Motion Time Systems (PMTS) is widely used in industry to improve, analyse and time industrial work it is difficult to use it in the clinical environment. The availability of the BTE work simulator has helped analyse motor performance and perform motion time measurements in order to quantify the physical aspects of disability. It allows the evaluation of manual dexterity and helps predict skills (Curtis and Engalitcheff, 1981).

This system is not, however, universally available. For the wrist it is possible to assess certain tasks in an occupational therapy setting, similar to the functional timed assessment for rheumatoid hands. One such assessment validated and used in the Leicester Group of Hospitals is outlined in Table 19.2. Tasks such as lifting a full kettle with the forearm supinated and pronated assess the function of the wrist in the parasagittal plane, while lifting a full saucepan assesses wrist function in the radio-ulnar plane. These tasks can be timed to provide a methods time measurement (MTM) system for the wrist.

Performance of these tasks provides a global assessment of the wrist

---

Table 19.1 Functional wrist assessment: tasks

A. Home	B. DIY
1. Washing clothes	1. Painting/decorating
2. Hoovering	2. Screwdriver use
3. Dusting	3. Hammer use
4. Washing/drying up	4. Saw use
5. Ironing	
6. Opening jars	C. Hobbies/leisure
7. Lifting heavy saucepans	1. Playing sports
8. Picking up heavy items	2. Gardening
9. Cutting bread/cheese/vegetables	3. Sewing/knitting
10. Cleaning windows	
D. Personal	E. Work difficulties
1. Getting into/out of the bath	
2. Eating	
3. Dressing/undressing	
4. Driving	

For each task, if applicable, ability is graded as: unable to perform, has difficulty, can perform without any difficulty.

Table 19.2 Functional wrist assessment: objective

---

1. Flexion/extension
   a. In sitting position, forearm resting on a box file, pick up 4 oz weight from table with forearm prone; 5 times each hand (time in seconds)
   b. In sitting position, forearm resting on a box file, lift 4 oz weight from table with forearm supine; 5 times each hand (time in seconds)
   c. As above in neutral forearm rotation

2. Forearm rotation
   a. Lift and pour 1 pint of water from saucepan to another and back again each hand
   b. In sitting position pick up a heavy book and turn over to each side; 10 times in 20 seconds each hand

3. Power grip
   Pick up hammer and strike block of wood; 5 times each hand in 10 seconds

4. Hook grip
   Pick up suitcase holding 1 brick from chair and hold for 30 seconds, each hand

5. Cylinder grip
   Hold jug of water containing 1 pint of water for 30 seconds, each hand

---

and provides insight into the actual disability that an individual may have as a result of a multitude of underlying factors including motivation and pain. Such an assessment also helps highlight the various trick manoeuvres a patient may develop to overcome an impairment.

Radiographic assessment

Radiographic views

Radiographs provide a picture of the anatomical abnormality within the wrist (Wilson *et al.*, 1990). Comparison of radiographs obtained before intervention and at a reasonable time after the intervention for wrist conditions provides a further objective assessment of outcome for several conditions of the wrist which involve the bones and joints.

Radiographs provide us with information regarding the integrity of the individual bones making up the wrist, the alignment of these bones and the state of the joints. It is usual to obtain at least two views of the wrist, the posteroanterior and the lateral. It is essential to obtain standard views if radiographs are to be used for measurement.

Any radiograph of the wrist must include at least the distal third of the radius and ulna and the whole of the third metacarpal in the image. The third metacarpal must always (if possible) lie in line with the radius. The distance of the radiographic plate must be standard at 1 m and the thumb placed in maximum abduction.

The posteroanterior view must be taken with the shoulder abducted at 90 degrees and the elbow flexed to 90 degrees. In this position the forearm is in the anatomical midprone position and not in the usual full prone position.

The position of forearm rotation when obtaining wrist radiographs is important, as in full pronation the radius lies across the ulna and hence is effectively shortened. The assessment of ulnar variance (Palmer *et al.*, 1982) which assesses the proximal-distal distance of the articular surface of the ulna from that of the radius depends on accurate radiographs obtained in a midprone anatomical position (Epner *et al.*, 1982). Measurements taken in full pronation will overestimate the ulnar plus variance when the distal ulna articular surface lies distal to that of the radius.

Standardising the position of the wrist in these radiographs contributes greatly to comparison with future radiographs and hence assists in the accuracy of measurements.

Radiographic anatomy

The distal radius is inclined volar-wards by 11 degrees and ulnar-wards by 26 degrees. The distal ulna is usually level with the distal radius or within 2 mm proximal to it. The gap between the distal radius and ulna is usually less than 4 mm.

Parameters

When viewing the radiographs of the wrist four parameters are assessed:

1. LINES

The proximal articular surfaces of the scaphoid, lunate and triquetrium form a uniform curve, as do the distal articular surfaces of these bones and the articular surface of the capitate and hamate. Any abnormality of these lines should suggest an abnormality of the carpal bones or in their alignment (Gilula, 1979).

2. SHAPE, SIZE AND ORIENTATION OF CARPAL BONES

Deviation from normal should be noted. The scaphoid and lunate in particular deserve attention.

The lunate is quadrilateral in a posteroanterior view when its axis is in line with the long axis of the radius. When it tilts forward or backward it assumes a more triangular shape. Similarly a foreshortened scaphoid with the tuberosity superimposed on it like a ring suggests abnormal forward tilting of the scaphoid in neutral radiographs. Abnormal increase in size usually indicates a dislocation of part of the carpus, usually around the lunate.

The orientation of the carpal bones is best seen on the lateral view. The axis of the capitate, lunate and radius are in the same line. The scaphoid is tilted forward by 56 degrees. A deviation of more than 5 degrees from similar measurements on the opposite unaffected wrist suggests an abnormality. The method of assessment of the axis is established and found to be reliable on standard radiographs (Larsen *et al.*, 1991a, 1991b).

3. JOINT SPACE

A solitary joint narrowing usually suggests a dislocation. Diffuse narrowing in the presence of cysts, sclerosis and osteophytes indicates arthritis. It is important to document the precise location and severity of joint space narrowing and include information regarding cysts, sclerosis and osteophytes. The joint space may be either normal, reduced in comparison to other joints or the opposite unaffected side, or absent. Sclerosis, cyst formation and osteophytes are usually documented as present or absent. The size of the cyst need only be noted if it is large and especially if it is solitary. The usual site for an osteophyte, apart from the radioulnar joint, is the radial styloid.

It is important to compare initial radiographs with subsequent ones if any comment regarding the onset of osteoarthritis is to be made. This is of particular importance when assessing outcome, as the professed goal of several wrist procedures is to delay the onset of osteoarthritis even when there is no good information on the natural history of the condition. For example, in the treatment of scaphoid fracture non-union the goal is to prevent osteoarthritis. There is now good evidence in literature that this goal is achieved following operations to promote union.

4. GAPS

The possibility of ligamentous disruption should be considered if the gap between two carpal bones is greater than 4 mm and especially when this appearance is unilateral.

Assessment of radiographs before and after intervention when bone union is intended depends on establishing that no gap exists. It must be appreciated that unless the X-ray beam is perpendicular to the gap none will be recorded on the radiograph. A spurious impression of bone union may be formed. When doubt exists tomograms, MRI or ultrasonographic assessment for movement at that site should be carried out.

There are several scoring systems to document the degree of arthritis. These are used especially with regard to rheumatoid arthritis. The commonest one is the Larsen scoring system, although the Steinbrocker staging system is more comprehensive. Both suffer from the drawbacks of most scoring methods in that the scores are arbitrary as is the final categorisation. Recent studies (Kaye et al., 1990; O'Sullivan et al., 1990) cast doubts on their value in assessing both progression of disease and outcome. Kaye (1991) has presented a good overview of the scoring systems used for rheumatoid arthritis.

Conclusions

Assessment of outcome for wrist conditions, like the outcome assessment for virtually every other site, is limited, even if an accurate and reproducible protocol could be defined, by the fact that each assessment is merely a snapshot of the wrist at that moment in time. If the assessment is done when the wrist is at its worst any subsequent assessment even in the absence of intervention would demonstrate improvement. Conversely assessment before intervention with the wrist at its best compared with an assessment following treatment with the wrist at its worst may indicate little change. This is particularly true when assessing change in pain and stiffness. Some parameters can be established with confidence, such as union of a fracture. Most parameters such as range of movement, strength, function and pain vary with different factors in any one patient, thereby making the task of assessing outcome difficult.

There is no doubt that the principal aim in assessing outcome of wrist conditions is to establish whether for each individual the goals set before intervention have been met.

Group discussion

The discussion group felt the most important aspects of outcome were grip strength, appearance of the hand, pain and return to work. The group considered the radiographic features of the wrist and agreed that the goals in treatment were restoration of anatomy, especially in relation to joint injuries. There was discussion concerning the appropriateness of the use of ultrasound, CT, MRI and fluoroscopy. The author of the chapter felt that CT for him offered no more than well-controlled X-rays. The development of MRI was useful in defining avascular necrosis in relation to trauma. It was decided that wrist arthroscopy did not deserve mention in this outcome chapter.

Radiographic measurement was discussed and it was agreed that the disturbed measurements of carpal height, carpal dissociation and instability could affect outcome. Growth abnormality in these variables also affected outcome. It was felt that classifications of arthritis and fractures, such as the Frickman or the Larsen classifications, were of limited use and validity.

The group agreed that appearance was an important aspect of outcome assessment and could be divided into three groups, namely deformity, scars and swellings. Deformity could be subdivided into soft tissue and bony deformity, scars into contracture scars, hypertrophic scars, etc. Swellings might also be subdivided into diffuse and local. The concept of contour deformity was considered but it was felt this was not, in general, understood by the group.

The author's section on 'Measurement of Change' and the strong emphasis on the three so-called objective measurements of outcome were discussed. These measures are wrist movement, strength and radiographic measurement. With regard to wrist movement, it was noted that goniometric observations in the wrist had figures for validity and reproducibility and circumduction, as a relatively new method of assessing wrist movement deserves mention as it appears to be accurate and reproducible. The point was emphasised that this is an instrument that is only in its developmental infancy.

Under the section on strength, the group emphasised the very subjective nature of the finger squeezing test mentioned at the start of the section. Bulb and sphygmomanometer dynamometers are commonly used and deserve mention. They are most useful on the lower end of the spectrum with weak grips, especially in diseases such as rheumatoid arthritis, as they do not match the validity and reproducibility of the more scientific Jaymar dynamometer. There is a lack of information on the bulb and sphygmomanometer as opposed to the wealth of publications on the Jaymar dynamometer. The group felt it was worth mentioning the tests of submaximal effort, such as the rapid exchange test and also the Mathiowetz flat-curve test.

Functional assessment in the hand was then considered. The Leicester functional assessments (Tables 19.1, 19.2) met with approval but these are subjective and similar instruments exist in most hand units. The reader's attention is drawn to the functional assessments outlined in the ASHT assessment of 1990 (King and Walsh, 1990), which is discussed in the previous volume (Macey and Kelly, 1993). The point was made that these so-called American tests are not in common use in the UK.

References

af-Ekemstam F (1992) Anatomy of the distal radioulnar joint. *Clin. Orthop. Rel. Res.*; **275**: 14–18

American Academy of Orthopaedic Surgeons (1965) *Joint Motion: method of measuring and recording*. Chicago: American Academy of Orthopaedic Surgeons

Bechtol C (1954) Grip test: the use of a dynamometer with adjustable handle spacings. *J. Bone Joint Surg.*; **36A**: 820–832

Curtis RM and Engalitcheff J Jr (1981) A work simulator for rehabilitating the upper extremity – preliminary report. *J. Hand Surg.*; **6**: 499

Epner RA, Bowers WH, Guilford WB (1982) Ulnar variance – the effect of wrist positioning and roentgen filming technique. *J. Hand Surg.*; **7A**: 298–305

Gilula LA (1979) Carpal injuries: analytic approach and case excercises. *AJR*; **133**: 503

Larsen CF, Stigsby B, Lindquist S, Bellstrom T, Mathiesen FK, Ipsen T (1991a) Observer variability in measurements of the carpal bones angles on lateral wrist radiographs. *J. Hand Surg.*; **16A**: 893–898

Larsen CF, Mathiesen FK, Lindquist S (1991b) Measurements of carpal bone angles on lateral wrist radiographs. *J. Hand Surg.*; **16A**: 888–893

Kaye JJ (1991) Radiographic methods of assessment (scoring) of rheumatic disease. *Rheum. Dis. Clin. North Am.*; **17**: 457–470

Kaye JJ, Fuchs HA, Moseley JW, Nance EP, Callahan LF, Pincus T (1990) Problems with the Steinbrocker staging system for radiographic assessment of the rheumatoid hand and wrist. *Invest. Radiol.*; **25**: 536–544

King TI, Walsh WW (1990) Computers in hand therapy practice. *J. Hand Ther.*; **3**: 157–159

Macey A, Kelly CP (1993) The Hand. In Pynsent PB, Fairbank JCT, Carr AJ (eds) *Outcome Assessment in Orthopaedics*. Oxford: Butterworth-Heinemann, pp. 174–197

Mathiowetz V, Weber K, Volland G, Kasnman N (1984) Reliability and validity of grip and pinch strength evaluations. *J. Hand Surg.*; **9A**: 222–226

Mathiowetz V, Kasnman N, Volland G, Weber K, Dowe M, Rogers S (1985) Grip and pinch strength: normative data for adults. *Arch. Phys. Med. Rehabil.*; **66**: 69–74

Mathiowetz V, Wiemer DM, Federman SM (1986) Grip and pinch strengths: norms for 6 to 19 year olds. *Am. J. Occup. Ther.*; **40**: 705–711

Moore ML (1949) The measurement of joint motion. Part II. The technic of goniometry. *Phys. Ther. Rev.*; **29**: 256

O'Driscoll SW, Horii E, Ness R, Calahan TD, Richards RR, Au KN (1992) The relationship between wrist position, grasp size, and grip strength. *J. Hand Surg.*; **17**: 169–177

Ojima H, Miyake S, Kumashiro M, Togami H, Suzuki K (1991) Dynamic analysis of wrist circumduction: a new application of the biaxial flexible electrogoniometer. *Clin. Biomech.*; **6**: 221–229

O'Sullivan HH, Lewis PA, Newcombe RG, Broderick NJ, Robinson DA, Coles EC, Jessop JD (1990) Precision of Larsen grading of radiographs in assessing progression of rheumatoid arthritis in individual patients. *Ann. Rheum. Dis.*; **49**: 286–289

Palmer AK, Glisson RR, Werner FW (1982) Ulnar variance determination. *J. Hand Surg.*; **7A**: 376–379

Swanson AB, Swanson G, Goran-Hagert C (1990) Evaluation of impairment of hand function In Hunter JM, Schneider LJ, Mackin EJ, Callahan AD (eds) *Rehabilitation of the Hand: surgery and therapy*, 3rd edn. St Louis: CV Mosby

Taleisnik J (1976) The ligaments of the wrist. *J. Hand Surg.*; **1**: 110

Wilson AJ, Mann FA, Gilula LA (1990) Imaging the hand and wrist. *J. Hand Surg.*; **15B**: 153–167

Youm Y, McMurty RY, Flatt AE, Gillespie TE (1978) Kinematics of the wrist: I. an experimental study of radial-ulnar deviation and flexion-extension. *J. Bone Joint Surg.*; **60A**: 423–431

Young VL, Pin P, Kraemer BA, Gould RB, Nemergut L, Pellowski M (1989) Fluctuations in grip and pinch strength among normal subjects. *J. Hand Surg.*; **14A**: 125–129

Chapter 20

Hand and flexor tendon injury

C. Kelly and A. Macey

> . . . what is more remarkable than this hand of ours with the intricate design, marvellous mechanism and exquisite sensibility (Boyes, 1975)

Introduction

The variable quality of assessment and the lack of standard outcome methods for common hand trauma has made comparison of results difficult. Variables that influence outcome include the severity of injury, the ability of the surgeon, the quality of postoperative splinting and last, but by no means least, the rehabilitation programme. The hand is a complex organ of sensation and manipulation and relies heavily on these factors after injury. No universal system has evolved for the evaluation of hand trauma. Without standardised assessment, the results of surgery or therapy in hand injuries will be confused by 'splinter' publications using various 'home-brewed' instruments. Patient treatment, education and growth of the hand surgery speciality is dependent on the policing of papers and publications on hand trauma by individuals and hand societies who are expert in the field of outcome assessment (Fess, 1990). The national and international hand societies continue to set standards for outcome measures. It is the responsibility of authors of prospective and retrospective studies to use those instruments that are well established, recognising and, as much as possible, compensating for their weaknesses. In this chapter, the instruments that have evolved for the assessment of hand trauma are examined, with special reference to flexor tendon injuries. Good results after flexor tendon injury reflect a standard of care and rehabilitation that is desirable.

In assessing outcome we must consider the relationship between impairment, handicap and disability. This is not a constant, even in seemingly straightforward injury. Paul Brown's classic article 'Less than Ten' (Brown, 1982) describes 180 of 183 surgeons with finger amputations who all managed to pursue a surgical career. In other circumstances a digit amputation may mean permanent disability with loss of employment and even psychosocial disturbance. The common instruments used in assessment of the injured hand will now be considered.

Range of motion

Range of motion (ROM) is a valuable instrument for which 'norms' are available and accepted. The goniometer is a reliable tool providing it is used in a standard way (AAOS, 1965). Hamilton and Lachenbruch (1969) found that goniometer placement (i.e. either dorsal or lateral) was independent of the result and more reliant on consistency of technique by a single observer. Estimation of joint angles is commonly practised especially in the busy outpatient clinic, indeed Schneider (1986) claims reliability for his measurements using a straight edge. However, most would agree that the goniometer when used properly gives more reliable joint angle measurements (Low, 1976; Boone *et al.*, 1978). The recent introduction of electronic goniometers has increased ease of use and more rapid and accurate data acquisition. Greenleaf (1991) claims an accuracy of 1% with their electronic goniometer and a reduction in examination time by half for their system as a whole. In 1976 the Clinical Assessment Committee of the American Society for Surgery of the Hand (ASSH) suggested the use of Total Active Motion (TAM) and Total Passive Motion (TPM) as useful measures for assessing hand function. This system of measures has been extensively used in the assessment of flexor tendon surgery and will be discussed later in this chapter.

Volumetric assessment

Swelling in the hand, by reducing the passive range of digital motion, is a major cause of hand stiffness and is high priority in rehabilitation of the traumatised hand. It is, therefore, logical that it is an important instrument in hand evaluation. There are two methods of measuring swelling:

1. By a water displacement volumeter.
2. Circumferential measurements of digits.

The volumeter and its design have been attributed to Brand and Wood. It has been found to be accurate to within 10 ml when used in a standard way (Waylett and Sebley, 1981). Circumferential measurements are also useful in monitoring progress of treatment and depend for reliability on tape placement and tension (Seddon, 1975).

Nerve function

The goal of treatment in the nerve-injured hand is a pain-free hand with normal sensation. Disturbed feeling can have a devastating effect in areas of sensory priority. This can take the form of loss of feeling or altered sensibility with or without pain. Examples of altered sensibility include dysaesthesias, cold intolerance and algodystrophy.

Nerve function can be measured using one or more of the following modalities:

- Sensory testing.
- Motor testing.

- Electrophysiological testing.
- Integrated hand function, e.g. the Moberg Pick-up Test (Moberg, 1958).

Sensory testing can be subdivided into tests of spatial or threshold testing. In the former, the patient is asked to discriminate between one- and two-point application of a stimulus, e.g. the Weber two-point discrimination test. However, as in all hand-held tests, application force differs between tests and between observers.

In threshold testing variable force stimuli are applied, for example, Semmes–Weinstein monofilaments can produce a controlled reproducible force stimulus when used as recommended (Bell-Krotoski, 1990). Moberg (1958) described the functional value of sensibility in three ways using two point discrimination (2-PD):

1. Tactile gnosis – 2-PD < 6 mm.
2. Sensibility for gross grip – 2-PD 7–15 mm.
3. Protective sensibility.

At the lowest level of protective sensibility the ability to feel anything is regarded as positive. Both two-point discrimination and moving two-point discrimination, described by Dellon (1978), have been endorsed by the American Society for Surgery of the Hand Clinical Assessment Committee and are widely regarded as useful tests of nerve function. The tests must be applied rigorously to produce valid results (Moberg, 1990). Recent critical work by Marsh (1989) has questioned the validity of using 2-PD.

Ideally there should be a simple valid test of nerve function. None are available at present and the clinician in a busy outpatient clinic gets more value from documenting a Tinel sign, observing function and identifying pain syndromes. Quantitative nerve testing is time consuming and may only be appropriate in the study of specific injuries and in the field of research.

More detailed discussion of the injured peripheral nerve is found in Chapter 13.

Strength assessment

Estimation of strength in the hand is a useful outcome measure and commonly reported in the literature. Hand grip strength and key pinch are commonly measured, various dynamometers and pinch meters are commercially available. The hydraulic Jamar Dynamometer as designed by Bechtol (1954) has stood the test of time and has excellent figures for validity and reproducibility (Fess, 1990). Despite progress in the design of similar types of equipment, the Jamar dynamometer remains as the 'industry standard'. Recent technological advancements in this area include the BTE (Baltimore Therapeutic Equipment Company) work simulator and the EVAL Hand Evaluation Workstation (Greenleaf Medical). Both combine electronic grip meters with other elements in hand assessment to produce detailed and graphical reports.

Integrated hand function tests

Total hand function after injury is of more interest to the surgeon and the therapist than individual measurements of joint motion and strength. Historically, the Moberg Pick-up Test (Moberg, 1958) was the first attempt to test integrated hand function. Since then a multiplicity of tests have been designed, all claiming to closely evaluate hand function. A survey of members of the American Society of Hand Therapists in 1990 listed the use of the more popular tests among its members (King and Walsh, 1990) (Table 20.1). The Jebsen hand function test has been adopted as the preferred measure of hand dexterity by a number of special interest groups though it does not test bilateral hand function (Jebsen et al., 1969). However, all of these timed tests are only part of the picture and instruments that record and quantify movement and force generated by the hand are needed (Jones, 1989).

Imaging of the hand

Plain radiographs are helpful in determining the result of treatment of skeletal injury, particularly in relation to non-union, malunion and artic-ular incongruity. The key to X-rays in follow-up is the matching to previous investigations (Wilson et al., 1990). MRI can identify avascular necrosis before plain X-rays. However, the role of MRI and CT in the traumatised hand has yet to be defined.

Cosmesis

'My face is ugly I don't mind, I don't see it I'm behind' (ASSH, 1988). This quotation must be contrasted with the visual exposure the hand receives from the patient and the public. Often patients complain of the cosmetic aspects of hand deformity after injury. Swanson et al. (1990) emphasise the assessment of both the passive and active cosmesis in the hand. In this system the patient and examiner rate the cosmetic improve-ment after surgery on a three-point scale of 'minimum', 'moderate' and

Table 20.1 Integrated hand function tests – ASHT survey

	Percent of respondents using test
Purdue pegboard	70%
Activities of daily living	68%
BTE work simulator	66%
Moberg Pick-up Test	54%
Minnesota Rate of Manipulation	52%
Jebsen Hand Function Test	48%
O'Connor Dexterity Test	26%
Valpar Work Sample Series	26%
Other	21%

Reproduced from King and Walsh, 1990, with permission.

'marked'. Psychological factors must also be taken into account and Grunert *et al.* (1988) reported that 95% of patients with hand injuries experience nightmares after injury. If these injuries are sustained at work, there is an understandable reluctance to return to that same job. Quantifying the influence on outcome presents a problem. Patient satisfaction has a strong influence on the result of treatment. As in other specialties it is only recently that it has managed to deserve mention in the published work on hand trauma. It is inextricably linked to patients' expectations of surgery. General health assessment profiles such as the Nottingham Health Profile have not gained popular support in hand surgery as they are considered not sensitive or specific enough to document changes in outcome after hand surgery. Recently the concept of a 'Hand Health Profile' was discussed at an audit subcommittee meeting of the British Society for Surgery of the Hand and work is under way on its development (F. D. Burke, 1993, personal communication).

Instruments specific to flexor tendon injury

'One of the most baffling problems in surgery is to restore normal function to a finger in which the tendons have been injured' (Bunnell, 1956)

The principles of management of flexor tendon injuries are now well established. Outcome is determined by injury severity, the quality of surgery and rehabilitation. Probably the greatest challenge to the hand surgeon in dealing with trauma is to achieve good results in the severed flexor tendons in 'no man's land'. The major contribution of Doyle and Blythe (1975) in the description of the anatomy of the annular and cruciate pulleys of the flexor tendon in the digit and also the classification of flexor tendon injuries into individual zones (Table 20.2) has helped to accurately define the site of injury.

Assessment of results

Various factors directly influence the results of tendon repair. These include:

1. The mechanism and force of injury.
2. Patient factors such as age, occupation and motivation.
3. Associated injury to skin vessels and nerves.
4. The local response of tissues to trauma.

Boyes (1971) felt that the preoperative condition was probably the most important factor affecting flexor tendon grafting. His evaluation rated the finger from 'good', which is the ideal situation for considering grafting, to 'salvage', where the initial injury was devastating and involved many tissues (Table 20.3). Examples of other presurgical assessments are given in Tables 20.4 and 20.5.

In 1956 Bunnell, in a discussion of evaluation of the results of tendon repair, made the following statement: 'A rough conception based on estimation from experience is probably as accurate and as practically

Table 20.2 Flexor tendon zones in the fingers and thumb

In the finger	
Zone I	Distal to the superficialis insertion
Zone II	From A-1 pulley to insertion of superficialis
Zone III	From distal end of carpal tunnel to A-1 pulley
Zone IV	Within carpal tunnel
Zone V	Proximal to carpal tunnel
In the thumb	
Zone I	Distal to the interphalangeal joint
Zone II	From A-1 pulley to interphalangeal joint
Zone III	In the thenar eminence
Zone IV	In the carpal tunnel
Zone V	Proximal to the carpal tunnel

Reproduced from Kleinert and Verdan, 1983.

Table 20.3 Boyes' pre-tendon grafting evaluation

Good	Minimal scar, supple joints, no trophic changes
Scar	Cicatrix impairing exposure or gliding of graft (e.g. destroyed pulley)
Joint	Impaired passive motion of digit
Multiple	More than one digit with tendon injury
Salvage	Initial injury was devastating and required flaps or grafts and involved nerve or bone reconstruction

Reproduced from Boyes and Stark, 1971.

Table 20.4 Grading severity of tendon injury

Group 1	Isolated tendon (sublimis, profundus or both)
Group 2	Tendon injury with damage to one neurovascular bundle
Group 3	Tendon injury with skin damage or injury to the floor of the fibro-osseus canal, with or without associated neurovascular injury

Reproduced from Langlais *et al.*, 1989, with permission © Springer-Verlag.

useful'. This philosophy has been ignored over the past 30 years by those surgeons eager to formulate a standardised assessment in order to validate the results of their surgery and compare them with similar series. Many excellent papers and symposia publications have devoted attention to this critical problem (Boyes and Stark, 1971; Buck-Gramcko *et al.*, 1976; Kleinert and Verdan, 1983; Strickland, 1985; Tubiana, *et al.*, 1979). Despite this, it is estimated that there are no less than ten assessment systems used throughout the world, although a few have recently been favoured (Nielsen and Jensen, 1985; So *et al.*, 1990).

Boyes is credited with much of the original attempts at introducing a standard instrument of flexor tendon injury assessment. In Boyes' method the pulp to palm distance previously described was used so that for each finger with a tendon injury there was a single result. This is a simple method of evaluation and is readily understood. However, it is being criticised on two major points. First, there is the difficulty of consistent selection of reference points in the measurement of pulp to palm distance, secondly Boyes' method does not take into account any extension deficit.

Table 20.5 Tubiana and Pulvertaft's preoperative assessment for flexor tendon surgery

Degree	Type of injury/time	Early (within 12 hr)	Late (after 3 weeks)
I	Clean wound (skin + tendon)	Primary repair	1-stage tendon graft
II	Clean wounds with neurovascular lesion	One neurovascular bundle injured: primary repair of tendon and nerve. Two neurovascular bundles: primary repair of tendon, nerves and at least one artery	One neurovascular bundle: 1-stage tendon graft with nerve repair or nerve graft secondarily. Two neurovascular bundles: repair at time of tendon graft.
III	Tendon section associated with bone or joint lesion	Satisfactory stabilisation, primary repair. Unsatisfactory stabilisation, secondary tendon repair after bone healing	Any necessary bone or joint procedure to regain functional ROM before performing tendon grafting
IV	Tendon section associated with several aggravating factors	With skin loss: skin coverage primarily, tendon repair second. With many structures involved, a complex situation; repair depends on experience of surgeon, age and occupation of patient, state of entire hand	Scar tissue is present after extensive soft tissue damage, infection or previous surgery. Poor results expected. Either arthrodesis or amputation is considered as an alternative procedure

Reproduced from Kleinert and Verdan, 1983.

Furthermore, it fails to compensate for the functionally good result when the pulp touches the palm proximal to the distal flexor crease. Boyes and Stark (1971) reported on 1000 tendon grafts using this method and since then there have been many reports using this assessment alone or in combination with other assessments. Van't Hof and Heiple (1958) identified the shortcomings of the latter method and added a linear measurement of the extension lag to their scoring system (Figure 20.1). The latter does not allow for different sized fingers and angular measurement systems are preferred by some (So *et al.*, 1990). Lister *et al.* (1977) measured the extension lag in angular degrees and combined this with pulp to palm distance to score results (Table 20.6).

In 1976, Buck-Ggrameko reported on the results of tendon repair and recommended a method of flexor tendon evaluation (Table 20.7). This method of evaluation has been widely accepted especially by the German Speaking Society for Surgery of the Hand (Kleinert and Verdan, 1983). It is complex and considered generous in its assessment of excellent results compared to other methods (Nielsen and Jensen, 1985; So *et al.*, 1990). At the same time, the Clinical Assessment Committee of the American Society for Surgery of the Hand recommended the use of total active movement (TAM) and total passive motion (TPM) of the digit and extensor deficit (Kleinert and Verdan, 1983). This involved summation of the range of movement of the three joints, the metacarpophalangeal joint (MCP), the proximal interphalangeal joint (PIP) and the distal inter-

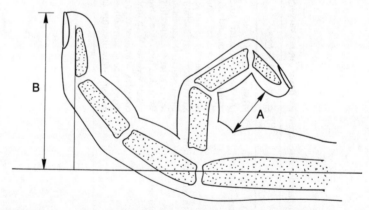

Figure 20.1 The Van't Hof and Heiple method. A = pulp to palm distance, B = extension deficit, A + B = index of excursion. Index of excursion: 0–1″ = good; 1–2″ = fair; 2–3″ = poor; >3″ = failure. (Reproduced from Van't Hof and Heiple, 1958.)

Table 20.6 Lister's Method

Result	Flexion deficit (cm)	Extension deficit (degrees)
Excellent	< 1	< 15
Good	1–1.5	15–30
Fair	1.6–3	31–50
Poor	> 3	> 50

Reproduced from Lister *et al.*, 1977.

Table 20.7 The Buck-Gramcko assessment of flexor tendon repair

		Points
A. Distance between finger tip and distal palmar crease, composite flexion		
0–2.5 cm	⩾ 200 degrees	6
2.5–4 cm	⩾ 180 degrees	4
4.0–6.0 cm	⩾ 150 degrees	2
> 6 cm	< 150 degrees	0
B. Extension deficit		
0–30 degrees		3
31–50 degrees		2
51–70 degrees		1
> 70 degrees		0
C. Composite flexion minus composite extension (total active movement)		
⩾ 160 degrees		6
⩾ 140 degrees		4
⩾ 120 degrees		2
< 120 degrees		0
Evaluation: A + B + C		
Excellent		14–15
Good		11–13
Fair		7–10
Poor		0–6

Reproduced from Buck-Gramcko *et al.*, 1976.

phangeal joint (DIP). Measurements were taken with a fisted hand and hyperextension was considered abnormal:

TPM = total flexion minus total extension lag

TAM is the sum of the angles formed by the MCP, PIP and DIP joints in maximum active flexion, minus the total active extension deficit for each joint. A percentage normal TAM can be got by comparing with the contralateral uninjured finger and a single figure result obtained by applying a further formula to rate the result from poor to excellent (Table 20.8). This system is widely used but is not applicable to bilateral injuries, especially as there are no universally accepted normal TAM values. This rating system was further developed by Tubiana *et al.* (1979) and their work culminated with a recommendation at the Congress of the International Federation of Societies for Surgery of the Hand that the system be adopted throughout the world as a standard assessment. Strickland (1989) makes the point that 30% of total digital motion is intrinsic muscle mediated and independent of extrinsic flexor tendon function. He believes that the range of movement of the MCP joint is rarely impaired after tendon surgery and feels the inclusion of this joint in

Table 20.8 TAM Codification System

Excellent	= normal
Good	= TAM greater than 75% normal side
Fair	= TAM greater than 50% normal side
Poor	= TAM worse than before surgery

Reproduced from Kleinert and Verdan, 1983.

the assessment has a falsifying influence on the assessment of digital function. This is generally true in finger injuries, however, in more proximal injury a deficit in MCP motion can result. He recommends the use of a formula which gives a figure for the percentage range of movement compared to the normal side for the PIP and DIP joints (Table 20.9). Strickland's system has been criticised because it fails to represent joint posture in the given range of motion (So *et al.*, 1990). For instance, 100 degrees of active motion may be functionally useless if the finger fails to touch the palm. The result is then rated from poor to excellent according to the recommendation of the International Federation for Hand Surgeons. Schneider (1986), in an excellent review of the subject, recommended the use of TAM, however, he felt that the usual presentation of data into poor to excellent ratings was too judgemental. He suggested four 'groups' instead.

One of the most important contributions on assessment of tendon injuries was made by The Federation for Surgery of the Hand and their subcommittee on tendon injuries (Kleinert and Verdan, 1983). A selected group of interested hand surgeons from around the globe examined the problem of the injured flexor tendon. They recommended that the TAM and Buck-Gramcko systems be more widely accepted and proposed further discussion on a single universal system.

Few papers have compared the different evaluation systems. So *et al.* (1990) looked at five systems of evaluation of flexor tendon injuries, namely:

1. The Buck-Gramcko system.
2. The Linear system or LMS (So *et al.*, 1990).
3. The Grossman system 11 (Grossman *et al.*, 1986).
4. The TAM system (ASSH).
5. The revised Strickland system (Strickland, 1985).

They found that the systems differed significantly in their evaluation of good and excellent results. They ranked the five systems in order of decreasing leniency, thus:

- Buck-Gramcko.
- Strickland.
- LMS.
- Grossman 11.
- TAM.

Table 20.9 The Strickland Formula

$$\frac{\text{PIP} + \text{DIP flexion} - \text{extension lag}}{175° \times 100} = \% \text{ of normal PIP plus DIP motion}$$

Group	PIP plus DIP (%) return	PIP plus DIP − (degrees) extension loss
Excellent	75–100	132+
Good	50–74	88–131
Fair	25–49	44–87
Poor	< 25	< 44

Reproduced from Strickland, 1985.

They concluded by favouring the Buck-Grameko system which gave the best results in their series but recommended modifications of the scoring of TAM which they felt was too lenient. Another system, introduced by Tsuge *et al.* (Table 20.10), has been compared, by Nielsen and Jensen (1985), with the systems of Buck-Gramcko and Kleinert. They examined 67 tendon injuries in Zone 2 and demonstrated obvious differences in grading of the functional results. They felt that the Buck-Gramcko system closely correlated with the overall function of the three finger joints.

Complications

Reporting of complications is an important feature of outcome assessment and clearly depends on the diligence of the researcher. In Gault's series (1987) 55% of patients suffered cold intolerance and 10% of these had no associated neurovascular injury. It is interesting that this problem gets little attention in most published series of flexor tendon repair. Common complications include:

• Rupture of the repair.
• Adhesions.
• Joint contracture.
• Cold intolerance.

These are not always easily identified. For instance, tendon rupture is a definite event in the patient with good movement but can be masked by joint stiffness. In the literature on outcome of flexor tendon surgery little is mentioned about return of strength or function, apart from the various assessments of digital motion. More recently authors have included return of grip strength in their assessment. Ejeskar (1982) looked at finger flexion force and grip strength after tendon repair. He found poor correlation between grip strength and hand function but that normal finger flexion force was associated with a good range of DIP motion. The patient's opinion of outcome is important but not commonly reported. Here the process of care and the results of medical intervention must be separated. Once again no standard method exists for recording this information.

Conclusions

Despite exhaustive efforts by the international societies no one universal system of hand evaluation has emerged. The essential instruments are

Table 20.10 Evaluation of repair using Tsuge method

	Excellent	Good	Fair	Poor
Finger tip to distal palmar crease (cm)	0–1	1–2	2–4	4+
Composite flexion (degrees)	> 200	180–200	150–180	< 150

Reproduced from Tsuge *et al.*, 1977.

well described and should be used. However, much work is still required in validation of established instruments and development of new ones. The variable results of flexor tendon repair probably reflect the variation in assessment criteria and pattern of injury seen in different hand units. Also, the quality of the surgical repair and rehabilitation is not amenable to standardised outcome measures and statistical analysis.

Group discussion

A single assessment system for tendon injury would be ideal. The present systems can be faulted on three points:

1. There is extra emphasis on range of motion and little on function.
2. There is no allowance made for the different movement requirements of different digits.
3. The commonly reported 'excellent to poor' divisions are too judgemental and difficulties arise in deciding where to draw the line between these groups.

When reporting results, the group recommend documentation of the 'raw data'. This should include:

1. The range of motion (passive and active) of all three finger joints.
2. Pulp to palm distance.

Acknowledgements

The authors would especially like to thank the Derby Hand unit for their inspiration, also Marie Carter and Ann Kelly in Oswestry for their help in the preparation of the text.

References

AAOS (1965) *Joint Motion: method of measuring and recording*. Chicago: American Academy of Orthopaedic Surgeons

ASSH (1988) Cosmetic aspects of hand surgery

Bechtol C (1954) Grip test: the use of a dynamometer with adjustable handle spacings. *J. Bone Joint Surg.*; **36A**: 820–824, 832

Bell-Krotoski JA (1990) Light touch-deep pressure testing using Semmes–Weinstein monofilaments. In Hunter JM, Schneider LH, Mackin EJ, Callahan AD (eds) *Rehabilitation of the Hand*, 3rd edn. St Louis: CV Mosby

Boone DC, Azen SP, Lin CM et al. (1978) Reliability of goniometric measurements. *Phys. Ther.*; **58**: 1355–1360

Boyes JH (1975) The philosophy of tendon surgery. In *AAOS: symposium on tendon surgery in the hand*. St Louis: CV Mosby

Boyes JH, Stark HH (1971) Flexor tendon grafts in the fingers and the thumb. *J. Bone Joint Surg.*; **53A**: 1332–1342

Brown PW (1982) Less than ten – surgeons with amputated fingers. *J. Hand Surg.*; **7**: 31–37

Buck-Gramcko D, Dietrich FE, Gogge S (1976) Bewertungskriterien bei Nachuntersuchungen von Beugesehnenwiederherstellungen. *Handchirurgie*; **8**: 65–69

Bunnell S (1956) *Surgery of the Hand*. London: Pitman Medical

Dellon AL (1978) The moving two-point discrimination test: clinical evaluation of the quickly adapting fiber/receptor system. *J. Hand Surg.*; **3**: 474–481

Doyle JR, Blythe WF (1975) The finger flexor tendon sheath and pulleys: anatomy and reconstruction. In *AAOS: Symposium on Tendon Surgery in the Hand*. St Louis: CV Mosby

Ejeskar A (1982) Finger flexor force and hand grip strength after tendon repair *J. Hand Surg.*; **7**: 61–65

Fess EE (1990) Documentation: essential elements of an upper extremity assessment battery. In: Hunter JM, Schneider LH, Mackin EJ, Callahan AD (eds) *Rehabilitation of the Hand* 3rd edn. St Louis: CV Mosby

Gault DT (1987) A review of repaired flexor tendons. *J. Hand Surg.*; **12B**: 321–325

Greenleaf W (1991) *EVAL Computer Workstation for the Clinical Evaluation of the Hand*. Palo Alto, CA: Greenleaf Medical

Grossman JAI, Wilkins L, Maurer G, Tubiana R (1986) An analysis of methods for evaluating the results of flexor tendon surgery and proposal of a universal system. Paper presentation at 3rd Congress of International Federation of Societies for Surgery of the Hand, Tokyo, pp. 12–13

Grunert BK, Devine CA, Matloub HS, Sanger Jr, Yousif NJ (1988) Flashbacks after traumatic hand injuries: prognostic indicators. *J. Hand Surg.*; **13A**: 125–127

Hamilton GF, Lachenbruch PA (1969) Reliability of goniometers in assessing finger joint angle. *Phys. Ther.*; **49**: 465–469

Jebsen RH, Taylor N, Trieschmann RB, Trotter MJ, Howard LA (1969) An objective and standardized test of hand function. *Arch. Phys. Med. Rehabil.*; **50**: 311–319

Jones LA (1989) The assessment of hand function: a critical review of techniques. *J. Hand Surg.*; **14A**: 221–228

King TI, Walsh WW (1990) Computers in hand therapy practice. *J. Hand Ther.*; **3**: 157–159

Kleinert HE, Verdan C (1983) Report of the Committee on Tendon Injuries. *J. Hand Surg.*; **8**: 794–798

Langlais F *et al.* (1989) Early mobilisation after primary flexor tendon repair in 152 fingers (excluding zone II) and in 60 thumbs. *Int. Orthop.*; **13**: 269–274

Lister GE, Kleinert HE, Kutz JE, Atasoy E (1977) Primary flexor tendon repair followed by immediate controlled immobilisation. *J. Hand Surg.*; **2**: 441–451

Low JL (1976) The reliability of joint measurement. *Physiotherapy*; **62**: 227–229

Marsh DR (1989) *The Measurement of Peripheral Nerve Function in the Upper Limb*. Thesis, University of Cambridge

Moberg E (1958) Objective methods for determining the functional value of sensibility in the hand. *J. Bone Joint Surg.*; **40B**: 454–476

Moberg E (1990) Two-point discrimination test. *Scand. J. Rehabil. Med.*; **22**: 127–134

Nielsen AB, Jensen PO (1985) Methods of evaluation of the functional results of flexor tendon repair of the fingers. *J. Hand Surg.*; **10B**: 60–61

Schneider LH (1986) Assessment of results in flexor tendon surgery In Hunter JM (ed) *Tendon Surgery in the Hand*. St Louis: CV Mosby

Seddon H (1975) *Surgical Disorders of the Peripheral Nerves*. New York: Churchill Livingstone

So YC, Chow SP, Pun WK, Luk KDK, Crosby C, Ng C (1990) Evaluation of results of flexor tendon repair: a critical analysis of five methods in ninety-five digits. *J. Hand Surg.*; **15B**: 258–264

Strickland JW (1985) Results of a flexor tendon surgery in zone 2. *Hand Clin.*; **1**: 167–179

Strickland JW (1989) Flexor tendon surgery Part 1: primary flexor tendon repair. *J. Hand Surg.*; **14B**: 261–272

Swanson AB, Swanson G, Göran-Hagert C (1990) Evaluation of impairment of hand function. In: Hunter JM, Schneider LH, Mackin EJ, Callahan AD (eds) *Rehabilitation of the Hand* 3rd edn. St Louis: CV Mosby

Tsuge K, Yoshikazu Y, Matsuishi Y (1977) Repair of flexor tendon by intratendinous tendon suture. *J. Hand Surg.*; **2**: 436–440

Tubiana R, McMenamin P, Gordon S (1979) Évaluation des résultats après réparation des tendons longs fléchisseurs des doigts. *Ann. Chir.*; **33**: 659–662

Van't Hof A, Heiple KG (1958) Flexor tendon injuries in the fingers and thumb. A comparative study. *J. Bone Joint Surg.*; **40A**: 256–261

Waylett J, Seibly D (1981) A study to determine the average deviation accuracy of a commercially available volumeter. *J. Hand Surg.*; **6**: 300

Wilson AJ, Mann FA, Gilula LA (1990) Imaging the hand and wrist. *J. Hand Surg.*; **15B**: 153–167

Chapter 21

Femoral head and neck fractures

D. A. Macdonald and S. J. Calder

Proximal femoral fracture is a potentially lethal injury and leads to high usage of hospital resources. Assessment of outcome in trauma to this region has focused on trying to identify patient and treatment variables which have an effect on both prognosis and also on the use of resources. Instruments used in such research must, therefore, be of a wider scope than merely evaluating the effectiveness of treatment of the fracture alone. There must be an adequate description of the population being studied and the setting in which treatment occurred. Assessment of the patient should include mental state, mobility, fracture type, presence of co-morbidity, age and social dependence.

A variety of outcome measures have been used in the assessment of hip fractures and these include:

1. Mortality.
2. Mobility score.
3. Cost–benefit analysis.

The incidence of femoral head and neck fracture appears to be increasing. It has been estimated that proximal femoral fractures account for 82% of all operative trauma cases in the elderly and 12% in the under-60 age group (Bannister, 1989). Controversies in treatment still exist despite the high frequency of these injuries and a large clinical experience of their management. Major controversies revolve around the timing and type of surgical intervention, methods of rehabilitation and the timing of discharge from hospital to some form of community or home-based care. This chapter will outline the commonly used outcome measures used in studies of fractures and describe in each section how these may be influenced by different patient populations and different methods of treatment.

Mortality

Mortality studies have been reported following hip fractures since the 1950s and they are usually quoted at 6 months from surgery. These mortality rates must take into account the underlying mortality of the population being studied. The mortality rates quoted in the literature vary from 14% to 41% at 6 months (Table 21.1). A number of factors need to be taken into consideration when mortality is expressed, as there may be explanatory variables which affect mortality.

These factors were first described by Evans *et al.* (1979). The majority of studies reported indicate that the most significant factor affecting mortality is mental ability. This factor also has the greatest effect on outcome. Ions and Stephens (1987) and Wood *et al.* (1992) describe the most significant predictors of 6-month mortality as being dementia, postoperative chest infection, malignant neoplasia, old age and deep wound infection, in that order. They found that a simple test of mental ability was the most significant prognostic indicator.

Studies of mortality are fundamental to the assessment of outcome in patients with proximal femoral fractures and it is from these types of studies that prognostic indicators can be determined. It is important to use standardised mortality figures.

Table 21.1 A summary of the mortality rates quoted in the literature

Reference	Patients (no.)	Time from operation	Mortality (%)
Addison, 1959	53	6 weeks	25*–30†
Garcia et al., 1961	205	6 months	18
Hinchey and Day, 1964	288	6 months	14
Frangakis, 1966	179	1 year	21
Burwell, 1967	131	1 month	14
		6 months	27
Davie, 1968	39	3 months	31
Hunter, 1969	94	1 month	16
		6 months	41
Riska, 1971	122	5 months	20
Wrighton and Woodyard, 1971	154	6 months	39
Lunt, 1971	98	6 months	31
Polyzoides, 1971	110	4 months	23
Beals, 1972	607	1 year	50
Salvati and Wilson, 1973		3 months	13
Raine, 1973–4	42*	6 months	12
	52†	6 months	33
Kavlie and Sundal, 1974	269	6 months	23
Hunter, 1974	200	6 months	18
Chan and Hoskinson, 1975	107	6 weeks	6.5
	136		20.6
Kavlie et al., 1975	300	6 months	21
D'Arcy and Devas, 1976	361	6 months	23
Barnes et al., 1976	1503	1 month	7.4
			13.3
		6 months	> 15
			> 23
Tillberg, 1976, 1977 (revisions)	163	6 weeks	9
	105	6 weeks	3
Sikorski and Barrington, 1981	57	6 months	20 (approx.)
	57		38 (approx.)

* Displaced subcapital fracture treated by internal fixations.
† Displaced subcapital fracture treated by hemiarthroplasty.

Functional analysis

Functional analyses are not commonly performed in assessing the out-come of a hip fracture. However, it may be relevant to use some of the standardised hip scores that are used in the assessment of total hip replacement. These hip scores have been discussed at some length in the previous volume of this series (Murray, 1993). The most commonly used of the hip scores are the Merle d'Aubigne–Charnley, the Harris Hip Score, the Iowa Hip Score and the Mayo Hip Score. The scores have been used to describe outcome after acetabular fractures in hip disloca-tions (Letournel, 1979, 1980; Matta et al., 1986a,b; Matta and Merritt, 1988). Some of these studies also included radiographic assessments (Epstein, 1974; Matta et al., 1986a,b). Hip scores have also been used after treatment of fractured neck of femur with hemiarthroplasties, reports in the literature include those by Langan (1979), Bartucci et al. (1985) and Yamagata et al. (1987). Studies of internally fixed subcapital fractures also include radiographic analysis of evidence of avascular necrosis of the femoral head (Stromquist et al., 1984; Madsen et al., 1987).

In addition to these standardised hips scores, mobility scores are also used in the assessment of outcome following hip fracture. These mobility scores have been described as having a predictive value in determining mortality after hip fracture (Parker and Pryor, 1992). The latter authors describe an assessment of mobility ranging between nought and 13 (Table 21.2).

The evaluation of outcome from treatment should also include an assessment of complications. Complications from fractures are discussed in more detail in Chapters 9 and 12 of this volume. The reader may also wish to refer to the classification of complications described by the BOA (1993).

Cost–benefit analysis

The relative costs of different forms of treatment are of increasing import-ance in the assessment of outcome from hip fracture. A number of methods of assessing cost can be used. The quality adjusted life years (QUALY) give an indication of benefit or utility of a particular treat-ment. The use of QUALYs is described in detail by Williams (1985, 1987). A number of relevant studies have been published (Parker and

Table 21.2 Assessment of mobility before the fracture

Mobility	No difficulty	With an aid	With help from another person	Not at all
Able to get about the house	3	2	1	0
Able to get out of the house	3	2	1	0
Able to go shopping	3	2	1	0

Score is the total, 0–9.
Reproduced from Parker and Pryor, 1992, with permission.

Pryor, 1992; Hollingworth *et al.*, 1993). Such studies demonstrated that about 40% of patients with fractured neck of femur are suitable for early discharge using a scheme such as 'hospital at home'. The use of these schemes can lead to significant reductions in costs of treatment. These analyses may also be used to determine differences in costs between different methods of treatment, either different forms of surgery or between surgery and conservative treatment. This is particularly true in the assessment of undisplaced subcapital fractures in which a non-surgical option can be demonstrated to be almost as cost effective as surgery (Parker and Pryor, 1992). However, non-surgical treatment of extra-capsular fractures results in a high likelihood of non-union and an esti-mated 1-year mortality of 60% (Hornby *et al.*, 1989; Parker and Pryor, 1992). The use of QUALYs has been questioned by some authors (Klein, 1989; La Puma and Lawlor, 1990) and they should be used with caution in the assessment of orthopaedic surgical procedures (Fitzpatrick, 1993).

Mental test score

Mental test score are commonly used in the assessment of outcome from hip fracture and a number of different scores have been used. Evans *et al.* (1979) describes a mental test score based on that proposed by Blessed *et al.* in 1969. This modified questionnaire has a score range of 0–13, standard errors for test, re-test and for observer variation are approxi-mately 1.0. An alternative mental test score has been described by Qureschi and Hodkinson (1974) (Table 21.3).

Classification

Although the purpose of this book is not to describe classifications of fractures, in the case of the femoral head and neck some account must be made of the type of fracture used as this has implications for outcome. The most significant distinction is between those fractures which occur within the capsule of the joint, so-called intracapsular fractures, and those outside the capsule. Intracapsular fractures have a high association with avascular necrosis of the femoral head, which can lead to permanent

Table 21.3 Abbreviated mental test: the score is the number of questions answered correctly (0–10)

State age
Give the current time to the nearest hour
Remember an address and repeat it at the end of the test
State the current year
Name the institution to which you have been admitted
Recognise two persons
State date of birth (day and month are sufficient)
Give the year of the start of the Second World War
Name the present monarch or head of state
Count backwards from 20 to 1

Reproduced from Qureschi and Hodkinson, 1974, by permission of Oxford University Press.

disability and secondary arthritic change. The second major group of fractures, occurring outside of the capsule between the trochanters of the femur, are called the intertrochanteric fractures. The most commonly used classification for fractures of the femoral head and femoral neck was described by Garden in 1961. DeLee (1991) has also described a classification based on patient characteristics, which is illustrated in Table 21.4. Other fractures that may occur in this vicinity involve the femoral head itself. These are termed Pipkin fractures and were first described by Pipkin in 1957. They have also been discussed by other authors (Lang-Stevenson and Getty, 1987; Swiontkowski, 1991). There does appear to be significant difficulty with assigning patients to particular classification groups described in studies by Frandsen *et al.* (1988) and Anderson *et al.* (1990). The AO group have also attempted a classification of fractures. This is described in their fracture classification manual (Gustillo, 1991). Some authors have used bone scintigraphy in assessing these fractures (Stromquist, 1983; Stromquist *et al.*, 1984; Alberts *et al.*, 1987; Alberts, 1990). This examination does not appear to have a great prognostic significance but can be used in the diagnosis of avascular necrosis. MRI can also be used in the diagnosis of avascular necrosis (Speer *et al.*, 1990).

Fractures in childhood

Childhood proximal femoral fractures differ from those in the adult. A number of different types of fracture have been identified and these were described by Ratliff in 1960. These are:

1. Transepiphyseal.
2. Transcervical.
3. Basal.
4. Trochanteric.

It appears that the transcervical is the most common. A number of complications can arise from these fractures of which avascular necrosis is the most catastrophic. Some studies have demonstrated an early satisfactory result following a fracture, but describe a deterioration with growth

Table 21.4 Classification based on patient characteristics

1. Femoral neck fracture in elderly patient
   a.   Impacted fractures
   b.   Displaced fractures
2. Fractures of the femoral back neck diagnosed late
3. Femoral neck fracture in the young adult less than 40 years of age
4. Stress fracture of the femoral neck
5. Ipsilateral fracture of the femoral neck and femoral shaft
6. Femoral neck fractures in patients with Paget's disease
7. Femoral neck fractures in patients with Parkinson's disease
8. Fractures of the femoral neck in patients with spastic hemiplegia
9. Postradiation fracture of the femoral neck
10. Pathological femoral neck fractures secondary to metastatic disease of the bone
11. Femoral neck fractures in patients with hyperparathyroidism

Reproduced from DeLee, 1991, with permission.

into adulthood (Leung and Lam, 1986). This deterioration is usually in the form of degenerative change within the joint.

Group discussion

Preinjury status

It was felt that preinjury status was of paramount importance in the assessment of femoral neck fractures as, in the vast majority of cases, this was not an isolated skeletal injury but the latest of a series of multisystem failures. A number of different forms of assessment were considered.

Mental test score

This is a dementia score, originally described correlating the histological findings of presenile dementia with a questionnaire. This questionnaire was modified and validated by Evans *et al.* (1979) to a 13-point scale. This group also demonstrated that it could predict mortality. Blakemore has reduced this to a single question, finding that if the patient is unable to give their age to within 5 years, the mortality rate is tripled (unpublished data).

Patients with femoral neck fractures are often admitted in a state of acute confusion, affecting the validity of their answer to the question. It was felt that the question should be posed when the patient had been resuscitated, a few hours before planned surgical intervention.

The group concluded that the mental test score should be abbreviated to two questions

1. How old are you?
2. Where do you live?

administered either by medical, physiotherapy or nursing staff after the conclusion of resuscitation, 2–3 hours before planned surgery.

Independence

Independence can be tested by history of acts of daily living, such as ability to bath, toilet, transfer, dress, feed and avoid incontinence. It was felt that the validation of this, while probably sound, could be flawed by the increasing practice of 'granny dumping'. This occurs when either residential home proprietors or relatives are finding the patient too demanding and, therefore, exaggerate their disabilities in order to have them placed in different residential accommodation.

Severity of injury

Intracapsular fractures should either be described as 'displaced' or 'undisplaced'. Undisplaced corresponding to Garden's categories 1 and 2 and displaced, 3 and 4.

Trochanteric fractures should be regarded as stable or unstable with particular emphasis being placed on an intact medial cortical buttress for stable cases.

Subtrochanteric fractures were best classified by Russell and Taylor's method (Taylor *et al.*, 1987) which identifies the problem of greater trochanteric fracture or insertion of intramedullary nail. The classification is based on whether or not the fracture lines extend to the piriform fossa or whether or not there is an intact medial cortical buttress.

Radiological outcome

Union appeared to be the most reliable radiological outcome, measured after 1 year in displaced intracapsular fractures and after 6 months in peritrochanteric injuries. Avascular necrosis could present late and as only 25% of such cases have pain, this seemed an insufficiently specific measure.

Preoperative assessment of femoral head vitality

Intraosseous, venography, pressure monitoring, isotope bone scan, laser Doppler, vital dyes and MRI scanning have not proven sufficiently reproducible to distinguish the living from the dead femoral head.

Management

It was considered that management had to be efficient and that undisplaced intracapsular fractures should be held with either two or three multiple pins on a single dynamic hip screw. Displaced intracapsular fractures should be either reduced within Garden's angles and undergo a stable fixation or replaced with an uncemented or cemented hemiarthroplasty or a total hip replacement.

Trochanteric fractures in younger patients should be treated by anatomical fixation, whereas in the elderly it was felt that a sliding device with a screw placed centrally or inferiorly in the head was the treatment of choice. The continuing use of fixed length devices in stable fractures was considered entirely justifiable. In subtrochanteric fractures a nail could be used which should be securely locked proximally and distally.

Timing of assessment of fixation

Displaced intracapsular fractures should be assessed for union after 1 year. Hemiarthroplasties should also be assessed for thigh pain and acetabular erosion after 5 years and total hip replacement for loosening also after 5 years. Peritrochanteric fractures should be assessed for union at 6 months.

Functional outcome

Pain

The Charnley scoring system appears reliable, validated and reproducible, and could be supplemented with analgesic requirement.

Mobility

This should be measured by functional satisfaction alone and correlated with preinjury status.

Independence

This should be correlated with preinjury housing status. Assessment should be made at 1 year.

Femoral head fractures

Few members of the group had a large personal experience of femoral head fractures and considered that the chapter should remain unchanged in this area.

Children's fractures

It was immediately apparent that the few series that were available were subject to sampling problems of sufficient magnitude that only vague conclusions could be drawn. Radiological assessment should be at skeletal maturity, assessing head congruity, this should be correlated with pain, limp and leg-length inequality.

References

Addison J (1959) Prosthetic replacement in primary treatment of fracture of femoral neck (abridged) *Proc. R. Soc. Med.*; **52**: 908–910

Alberts KA (1990) Prognostic accuracy of preoperative and postoperative scintimetry after femoral neck fracture. *Clin. Orthop. Rel. Res.*; **250**: 221–225

Alberts KA, Dahlborn M, Ringertz H (1987) Sequential scintimetry after femoral neck fracture. Methodologic aspects and prediction of healing. *Acta Orthop. Scand.*; **58**: 217–222

Anderson E, Jorgensen LG, Hededam LT (1990) Evans' classification of trochanteric fractures: an assessment of the interobserver and intraobserver reliability. *Injury*; **21**: 377–378

Bannister G (1989) In: Bunker TD, Colton LC, Webb JK (eds) *Frontiers in Fracture Management*. London: Martin Dunitz

Barnes R, Brown JT, Garden RS, Nicholl AE (1976) Subcapital fractures of the femur; a prospective review. *J. Bone Joint Surg.*; **58B**: 2–24

Bartucci EJ, Gonzales MH, Cooperman DR, Freedburg HI, Barmada R, Laros GS (1985) The effect of adjunctive methylmethacrylate on failures of fixation and function in patients with intertrochanteric fractures and osteoporosis. *J. Bone Joint Surg.*; **67A**: 1094–1107

Beals RK (1972) Survival following hip fracture: long follow-up of 607 patients. *J. Chron. Dis.*; **25**: 235–244

Blessed G, Tomlinson BE, Roth M (1968) The association between quantitative measures of demential and of senile change in the cerebral grey matter of elderly subjects. *Br. J. Psychiatr.*; **114**: 797–811

BOA (1993) *British Orthopaedic Association Trauma Lexicon*. London

Burwell HN (1967) Replacement of the femoral head by a prosthesis in subcapital fractures. *Br. J. Surg.*; **54**: 741–749

Chan RNW, Hoskinson J (1975) Thompson prosthesis for fractured neck of femur: a comparison of surgical approaches. *J. Bone Joint Surg.*; **57B**: 439–443

D'Arcy J, Devas M (1976) Treatment of fractures of the femoral neck by replacement with the Thompson prosthesis. *J. Bone Joint Surg.*; **58B**: 279–286

Davie B (1968) Experiences with the Austin Moore prosthesis with special reference to mortality from recent femoral neck fractures. *Med. J. Aust.*; **1**: 92–93

DeLee JC (1991) In Rockwood CA Jr, Green DP, Bucholz RW (eds) *Rockwood and Green's Fractures in Adults*, 3rd edn. 2 Philadelphia: JB Lippincott, pp. 1481–1651

Epstein HC (1974) Posterior fracture dislocations of the hip. Long term follow up. *J. Bone Joint Surg.*; **56B**: 1103–1134

Evans J Grimley, Prudham D, Wandless I (1979) A prospective study of fractured proximal femur – factors associated with survival. *Age Ageing*; **8**: 246–250

Fitzpatrick R (1993) Patient satisfaction and quality of life measures. In Pynsent PB, Fairbank JCT, Carr AJ (eds) *Outcome Measures in Orthopaedics*. Oxford: Butterworth-Heinemann

Frandsen PA, Anderson E, Madsen F, Skjodt T (1988) Gardens classification of femoral neck fractures. An assessment of inter-observer variation. *J. Bone Joint Surg.*; **70B**: 588–590

Frangakis EK (1966) Intracapsular fractures of the neck of the femur: factors influencing non-union and ischaemic necrosis. *J. Bone Joint Surg.*; **48B**: 17–30

Garcia A Jr, Neer CS II, Ambrose GB (1961) Displaced intracapsular fractures of the neck of the femur: 1. Mortality and morbidity. *J. Trauma*; **1**: 128–132

Garden RS (1961) Low-angle fixation of the femoral neck. *J. Bone Joint Surg.*; **43B**: 647–663

Garden W, Newman RJ, Hamblen DL, Williams BO (1988) Prospective randomised study of an orthopaedic geriatric in-patient service. *Br. Med. J.*; **297**: 1116–1118

Gustillo RB (1991) *The Fracture Classification Manual*. St Louis: Mosby Year Book

Hinchey JJ, Day PL (1964) Primary prosthetic replacement in fresh femoral neck fractures: a review of 294 consecutive cases. *J. Bone Joint Surg.*; **46A**: 223–240

Hollingworth W, Todd C, Parker M, Roberts JA, Williams R (1993) Cost analysis of early discharge after hip fracture. *Br. Med. J.*; **307**: 903–906

Hornby R, Grimley Evans J, Vardon V (1989) Operative or conservative treatment for trochanteric fractures of the femur: a randomised epidemiological trial in elderly patients. *J. Bone Joint Surg.*; **71B**: 619–623

Hunter GA (1969) A comparison of the use of internal fixation and prosthetic replacement for fresh fractures of the neck of the femur. *Br. J. Surg.*; **56**: 229–232

Hunter GA (1974) A further comparison of the use of internal fixation and prosthetic replacement for fresh fractures of the neck of the femur. *Br. J. Surg.*; **61**: 382–384

Ions GK, Stevens J (1987) Prediction of survival in patients with femoral neck fractures. *J. Bone Joint Surg.*; **69B**: 384–387

Kavlie H, Sundal B (1974) Primary arthroplasty on femoral neck fractures: a review of 269 consecutive cases treated with the Christiansen endoprothesis. *Acta Orthop. Scand.*; **45**: 579–590

Kavlie H, Norderval Y, Sundal B (1975) Femoral head replacement with the Christiansen endoprosthesis; a follow-up study, and a report on 175 arthroplasties with the present model of the prosthesis with acrylic cement fixation. *Acta Chir. Scand.*; **141**: 96–103

Klein KR (1989) The role of health economics. *Br. Med. J.*; **299**: 275–276

Kyle RF, Gustillo RB, Premer RF (1979) Analysis of six hundred and twenty-two inter-trochanteric hip fractures – a retrospective and prospective study. *J. Bone Joint Surg.*; **61A**: 216–221

Langan P (1979) The Giliberty Bipolar Prosthesis – A clinical and radiographic review. *Clin. Orthop. Rel. Res.*; **141**: 169–175

Lang-Stevenson A, Getty CJM (1987) The Pipkin fracture – dislocation of the hip. *Injury*; **18**: 264–269

La Puma J, Lawlor EF (1990) Quality-adjusted life-years: ethical implications for physicians and policy makers. *JAMA*; **263**: 2917–2921

Leung PC, Lam SF (1986) Long term follow-up of children with femoral neck fractures. *J. Bone Joint Surg.*; **68B**: 537–540

Letournel E (1979) The results of acetabular fractures treated surgically: twenty-one years experience in the hip. *Proceedings of 7th Open Scientific Meeting of the Hip Society*. St Louis: CV Mosby

Letournel E (1980) Acetabular fractures: classification of management. *Clin. Orthop. Rel. Res.*; **151**: 81–106

Lunt HRW (1971) The role of prosthetic replacement of the head of the femur as primary treatment for subcapital fractures. *Injury*; **3**: 107–113

Madsen F, Linde F, Andersen E, Birke H, Hvass L, Poulsen TD (1987) Fixation of displaced femoral fractures – comparison between sliding screw, plate and four cancellous bones screws. *Acta Orthop. Scand.*; **58**: 212–216

Matta JM, Merritt PO (1988) Displaced acetabular fractures. *Clin. Orthop. Rel. Res.*; **230**: 83–97

Matta JM, Anderson LM, Epstein HC, Hendrick P (1986a) Fractures of the acetabulum: a retrospective analysis. *Clin. Orthop. Rel. Res.*; **205**: 230–240

Matta JM, Mehne DK, Roffi R (1986b) Fractures of the acetabulum: early results of a prospective study. *Clin. Orthop. Rel. Res.*; **205**: 241–250

Murray D (1993) The hip. In Pynsent PB, Fairbank JCT, Carr AJ (eds) *Outcome Measures in Orthopaedics*. Oxford: Butterworth-Heineman

Parker MJ, Pryor GA (1992) The timing of surgery for proximal femoral fractures. *J. Bone Joint Surg.*; **74B**: 203–205

Pipkin G (1957) Treatment of grade IV fracture-dislocation of the hip. *J. Bone Joint Surg.*; **39A**: 1027–1042

Polyzoides AJ (1971) Prosthetic replacement after femoral neck fractures (short- and long-term follow-up). *Injury*; **2**: 283–286

Qureschi KN, Hodkinson HM (1974) Evaluation of a ten-question mental test in the institutionalized elderly. *Age Ageing*; **3**: 152–157

Raine GET (1973–4) A comparison of internal fixation and prosthetic replacement for recent displaced subacpital fractures of the neck of the femur. *Injury*; **5**: 25–30

Ratliff AHC (1960) Fractures of the neck of the femur in children. *J. Bone Joint Surg.*; **44B**: 528–542

Riska EB (1971) Prosthetic replacement in the treatment of subcapital fractures of the femur. *Acta Orthop. Scand.*; **42**: 281–290

Salvati EA, Wilson PD Jr (1973) Long-term results of femoral head replacement. *J. Bone Joint Surg.*; **55A**: 516–524

Sikorski JM, Barrington R (1981) Internal fixation versus hemiarthroplasty for the displaced subcapital fracture of the femur: a prospective study. *J. Bone Joint Surg.*; **63B**: 357–361

Speer KP, Spritzer CE, Harrelson JM, Nunley JA (1990) Magnetic resonance imaging of the femoral head after acute intracapsular fracture of the femoral neck. *J. Bone Joint Surg.*; **72A**: 98–103

Stromquist B (1983) Femoral head vitality after intracapsular hip fracture. *Acta Orthop. Scand.*; **54**: suppl. 200

Stromquist B, Brismar J, Hansson L, Palmer J (1984) Technetium-99m-methylene-diphosphonate scintimetry after femoral neck fracture; a three year follow-up study. *Clin. Orthop. Rel. Res.*; **182**: 177–189

Swiontkowski MR (1991) Femoral head fractures. *Curr. Orthop.*; **5**: 99–105

Taylor JC, Russell TA, LaVelle DG, Callandruccio RA (1987) *Clinical Results of 100 Femoral Shaft Fractures Treated with Russel–Taylor Interlocking Nail System*. San Francisco: American Academy of Orthopaedic Surgery

Tillberg B (1976) Treatment of fractures of the femoral neck by primary arthroplasty. *Acta Orthop. Scand.*; **47**: 209–213

Tillberg B (1977) Endoprosthesis as treatment for necrosis and pseudarthrosis after transcervical femoral fractures: a clinical review. *Acta Orthop. Scand.*; **48**: 296–300

Williams A (1985) Economics of coronary artery by pass grafting. *Br. Med. J.*; **291**: 326–329

Williams A (1987) How should NHS priorities be determined? *Hosp. Updated*; **13**: 261–263, 341

Wood DJ, Ions GK, Quinby JM, Gale DW, Steven J (1992) Factors which influence mortality after hip fracture. *J. Bone Joint Surg.*; **74B**: 199–202

Wrighton JD, Woodyard JE (1971) Prosthetic replacement for subcapital fractures of the femur: a comparative surgery. *Injury*; **2**: 287–293

Yamagata M, Chao EY, Ilstrup DM, Melton LJ, Coventry MB, Stauffer RN (1987) Fixed head and bipolar universal hip endoprostheses – a retrospective clinical and radiographic study. *J. Arthroplasty*; **2**: 327–341

Chapter 22

Femoral and tibial shaft fractures

E. F. Wheelwright

Fractures of the femoral and tibial shafts make a significant contribution to the workload of most orthopaedic units. Tibial shaft fractures are relatively more common than those of the femoral shaft, but it is estimated that such injuries together account for approximately 1 in 10 admissions to those orthopaedic wards dealing with trauma (Edinburgh Royal Infirmary Trauma Unit admissions data, 1991).

The literature abounds with studies to ascertain the best treatment for these fractures. Unfortunately, the majority of articles are based on retrospective series, usually considering a single method of treatment or of operative fixation. The choice of treatment for diaphyseal fractures of the femur has always been less contentious than that for tibial fractures, and there is currently a virtual consensus of opinion that early surgical intervention is justified in most cases of femoral fracture. For the tibia, however, there is considerable divergence of opinion as to whether conservative or surgical intervention is justified. Frequently, authors have adopted individualised classifications to describe the fractures being dealt with, and have employed essentially subjective and non-standardised criteria to report their findings.

This chapter relates to outcome following femoral and tibial shaft fractures. Because of the greater incidence of tibial shaft fractures and the controversy surrounding their treatment, much of this chapter concentrates upon issues raised in relation to fractures of the tibia. However, many of the points made are equally pertinent to similar fractures of the femoral shaft.

Clinical measures of outcome

Most reports in the literature concentrate on three main clinical measures of outcome, namely: the speed of healing, complication rates, and the incidence of joint stiffness and deformity. There is little doubt that these three areas of interest are primarily affected by the severity of the injury, but only rarely in the literature is injury severity used for stratifying patients in reports of a given treatment. It is therefore difficult to use published data to compare different forms of treatment. Although the purpose of this chapter is to discuss measurement of ultimate outcome, it is of relevance to briefly list the various systems of classification which have been used to grade injury severity. The major difficulty with these systems is that there is no universally agreed classification, various researchers tending to adopt their own systems which range from simple ratings to more complex multivariate classifications.

Ellis (1958) grouped tibial fractures into three classes according to whether he considered them to be of minor, moderate or major severity. Nicoll (1964) devised a more systematic classification, to control for the effects of displacement, fracture comminution, and the presence or absence of an open wound. Bauer et al. (1962) and Edwards (1965) noted that the type of trauma had a significant effect on outcome and as a result, related outcome to the extent of soft tissue damage. The contrast between direct or high energy injury versus indirect or low energy trauma has been extended by the work of Gustilo and others (Gustilo and Anderson, 1976; Gustilo et al., 1984), with reference to open fractures, and by Tscherne (Oestern and Tscherne, 1984), primarily for closed injuries.

Fracture morphology has also been studied in relation to the degree of soft tissue injury. Winquist et al. (1984) graded the extent of fracture comminution, initially for femoral fractures, but more recently this system has been applied to tibial fractures (Henley, 1989). Johner and Wruhs (1983) also used this approach, and this classification has been recently adopted by the AO/ASIF group in their comprehensive classification of long bone fractures (Muller et al., 1990).

Classification systems have also been used in an attempt to provide the surgeon with objective criteria for reliably predicting which limbs can be salvaged rather than amputated in lower extremity trauma with associated vascular compromise (Hutchins, 1981; Gregory et al., 1985; Lange et al., 1985; Hansen, 1987; Bondurant et al., 1988; Court-Brown et al., 1990). The most recent of these, the Mangled Extremity Severity Score (MESS – Helfet et al., 1990), attempts to relate limb salvage decision-making variables (Table 22.1) at the time of presentation to eventual outcome. A MESS (Table 22.2) of 6 or less is said to be likely to result in a viable limb, for which limb salvage procedures are recommended. In contrast, a score in excess of 7 is said to occur in limbs where there is a greatly increased morbidity and mortality if attempts are made at limb salvage, thereby guiding the attending surgeon towards primary amputation for such severe injuries. In their prospective evaluation of the MESS score, Helfet et al. (1990) reported that a score greater than 7 had 100% predictable value for amputation.

Unfortunately, all these classifications have disadvantages. The ideal fracture classification system should predict results and guide treatment. Because injuries respond differently to varying treatments, the choice of treatment itself may effect the validity of the grading system chosen. Another important limitation of these classification systems is that they have been validated with end-points such as average time to union, risk of non-union or risk of infection rather than ultimate function, risk of deformity and response to a given treatment. For further details, the reader is referred to the individual reports of the classification systems listed above.

Table 22.1 Limb salvage decision-making variables

Patient
  Age
  Underlying chronic disease (diabetes)
  Occupational considerations
  Patient and family desires

Extremity
  Mechanism of injury
  Fracture pattern
  Arterial/venous injury (location)
  Neurological (anatomical status)
  Injury status of ipsilateral foot
  Intercalary ischaemia zone after revascularisation

Associated
  Magnitude of associated injury
  Severity and duration of shock
  Warm ischaemia time

Reproduced from Helfet *et al.*, 1990, with permission.

Union (see also Chapter 9)

The time for healing for femoral or tibial shaft fractures has been the main focus of most studies on the management of these injuries. A numerical value assigned to the time to union would, on first impressions, appear to be unequivocal. In reality, however, this figure is, at best, based on clinical and radiological judgement made at outpatient visits occurring at intervals of at least several weeks. This instrument is clearly, therefore, insensitive. There are also considerable doubts regarding the reliability of such data, since fracture healing is an on-going process, the end-point of which is differently interpreted by different observers. In addition, healing is not uniform throughout a given fracture site, and since the process is continuous, it is not possible to pin down healing as a discrete event to a particular date. Despite this observation, accepted norms for femoral and tibial fracture healing are regularly stated, some authors suggesting that union takes 3–4 months (e.g. Crawford-Adams, 1983) or up to 6 months by others (e.g. Nicoll, 1964).

Although it is therefore meaningless to refer to an average period for union, mean time to union is frequently used as the basis for comparison between different series of patients and for different treatment modalities. An alternative suggestion was proposed by Austin (1977) who demonstrated the value of plotting cumulative percentage curves to represent healing time (Figure 22.1). Using this method, Austin analysed six different studies, suggesting that only 50% of fractures had healed 16 weeks after injury, while 80% had healed by 26 weeks. The other main advantage of using cumulative percentage curves is that they can be used to show end-points other than fracture healing (e.g. time to return to work – Rokkanen *et al.*, 1969; and see below).

The implication of this work is that there is good reason for compiling a database on the natural history of tibial and femoral fracture healing, based upon information from a large number of fractures. Some authors

Table 22.2 The Mangled Extremity Severity Score (MESS)

Type	Characteristics	Injuries	Points
Skeletal/soft tissue			
1	Low energy	Stab wounds, simple closed fractures, small-calibre gunshot wounds	1
2	Medium energy	Open or multiple level fractures, dislocations, moderate crush injuries	2
3	High energy	Shotgun blast (close range), high velocity gunshot wounds	3
4	Massive crush	Logging, railroad, oil rig accidents	4
Shock			
1	Normotensives haemodynamics	BP stable in field and in OR	0
2	Transiently hypotensive	BP unstable in field but responsive to intravenous fluids	1
3	Prolonged hypotension	Systolic BP less than 90 mmHg in field and responsive to intravenous fluid only in OR	2
Ischaemia			
1	None	A pulsatile limb without signs of ischaemia	0*
2	Mild	Diminished pulses without signs of ischaemia	1*
3	Moderate	No pulses by Doppler, sluggish capillary refill paraesthesia, diminished motor activity	2*
4	Advanced	Pulseless, cool, paralysed and numb without capillary refill	3*
Age group			
1	≤ 30 years		0
2	31–49 years		1
3	≥ 50 years		2

* Points ×2 if ischaemic time exceeds six hours
OR = operating room; BP = blood pressure.
Reproduced from Helfet *et al.*, 1990, with permission.

have pursued this approach (Oni *et al.*, 1988). From these data, it would then be possible to gain a more accurate assessment of different types of recovery curve under various different conditions.

Delayed union

It follows that since there is at present no agreed concept of 'average' time to union, there cannot be an absolute time beyond which fractures are said to be in a state of 'delayed' union. Not surprisingly, therefore, reports of the incidence of delayed union fluctuate considerably. In Keller's substantial review of published data, reported delayed union rates ranged from 0% to 83% (Keller, 1983). Usually the median value is taken as the dividing point between what is defined as normal, and what is defined as delayed, but it would seem to be more reasonable to revise the

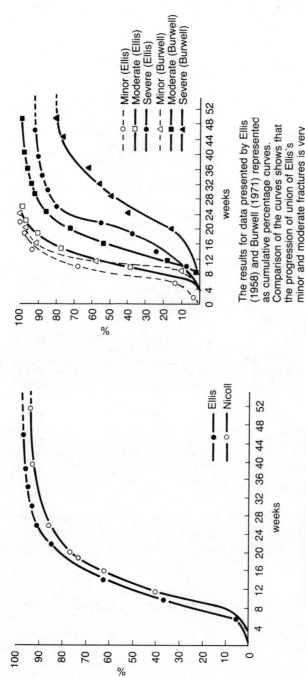

The results for data presented by Ellis (1958) and Burwell (1971) represented as cumulative percentage curves. Comparison of the curves shows that the progression of union of Ellis's minor and moderate fractures is very similar, also that class by class internally fixed fractures took longer to unite. The difference is more striking when severe fractures are considered and, in this group, the incidence of non-union is higher in internally fixed fractures

Cumulative percentage curves for the data presented by Ellis (1958) and Nicoll (1964). It is easy to compare the incidence of non-union in each series and the incidence of delayed union can be read off directly for any stated definition

Figure 22.1 Cumulative percentage curves for healing time. (Taken from Austin, 1977)

definition of 'normal' union to include the majority of fractures and so reflect a wide range of normality.

By contrast, the incidence of non-union is not time dependent, since this is usually diagnosed on the basis of specific radiological criteria (e.g. hypertrophic or atrophic non-union). Consequently the reported incidence of non-union is less variable, but in Keller's study still ranged in varying reports from 0% to 35% (Keller, 1983).

The decision whether a fracture has soundly united is based on a combination of clinical and radiological evidence. Various workers (e.g. Hammer et al., 1985) have clearly shown that on the whole, clinical and radiological tests of union are insensitive, invalid and unreliable, and it is therefore of some importance that more objective methods of assessing union are developed. In this regard, strength of union, bone imaging, ultrasonography, resonant frequency measurement, MRI and tests of fracture stiffness may ultimately provide more objective means of assessing tibial and femoral fracture union. At present, most of these techniques are, at best, research tools, and must be developed further before they will be suitable for routine clinical use.

Complication rates (see also Chapter 12)

By reporting complication rates, various authors have attempted to use these variables as measures of outcome. The sensitivity of using complication rates as a measure of outcome depends upon the variables included under this heading and the criteria used to establish their presence or absence. For example, Kempf et al. (1985) tried to compare four studies on the basis of incidence rates for pulmonary embolism, fat embolism, sepsis and aseptic non-union amongst other criteria. Other authors have made frequent reference to the incidence of infection in different series of patients.

Unfortunately, like fracture classification, there is no standard way for reporting complication rates, some authors being more comprehensive than others. Just because a particular complication is not mentioned in a report does not mean that it can be assumed to have not occurred. For example, Jensen et al. (1977) comprehensively distinguished between general and local postoperative complications in their series of patients treated for diaphyseal femoral fractures using either medullary nailing or compression plates. Winquist et al. (1984), in what is regarded as a classic article, reported on closed medullary nailing for femoral fractures, but in their report combined clinical complications and deformity under one heading. The list of complications reported in this publication was less comprehensive than that reported by Jensen et al. (1977). In comparing these two articles, it is therefore not possible to ascertain whether the omissions in reporting specific complications in the latter paper are indicative of trouble-free recovery, or whether it simple means that these particular complications were not noted. Certain events, such as death or amputation, may appear to be unequivocal outcomes, but others such as re-fracture or the need for a secondary operation are imprecise and require further explanation.

Complication rates may not always be valid tests of success of treatment. Some complications may arise irrespective of the treatment given, and it is probably appropriate that only secondary complications should be considered as dependent variables. Complications attributable to the

---

Table 22.3 Complications of fractures of the lower limb

Bone and fracture site
   Deep infection
   Acute
   Chronic osteitis, drainage or osteomyelitis
   Bone loss
   Delayed union
   Non-union
   Malunion
   Loss of alignment in cast or brace
   Fixation problems
      Failure of hardware
      Failure of bone
   Refracture

Skin and subcutanous tissue
   Wound slough
   Wound infection (superficial)
   Pressure score

Nerve
   Direct injury
   Pressure from cast or brace
   Ischaemic damage (compartment syndrome)
   Reflex sympathetic dystrophy

Vascular
   Arterial occlusion
   Venous insufficiency
   Deep venous thrombosis
   Compartment syndrome

Joint motion
   Associated joint surface fracture
   Contracture
      Hip
      Knee
      Ankle
      Subtalar
      Foot and toe
   Late arthritis (secondary to deformity)
   Fatigue fracture distally
   Heterotopic ossification

Function
   Pain
   Disability (temporary vs permanent)
      Objective
      Muscle strength
      Endurance
      Subjective
         Activities of daily living
         Work
         Sport

Cosmesis

injury itself must be viewed as independent or intervening variables. To give an example of this, the development of the fat embolism syndrome following femoral shaft fractures should be regarded as a clinical complication of the fracture itself rather than a consequence of treatment.

A list of complications which might result from either positive or negative action following a femoral or tibial fracture, thereby constituting potential outcome measures, is shown in Table 22.3. In order that the reported complication rates using these variables might be regarded as reliable, explicit instructions for data collection should be closely adherent to, and these methods clearly reported in order to help with validation of these variables.

Malunion

Angular and rotational deformity together with shortening of a femoral or tibial shaft fracture may give rise to malunion. Clinical and radiological examination are usually utilised to assess the degree of malunion, but the sensitivity of the measurement techniques employed and their reliability remain, for the most part, unknown. In general, in those publications where malunion has actually been reported (and, sadly, many do not), angulatory or rotational deformity are usually measured in degrees and shortening usually in centimetres. Frequently, these data are then summarised using an ordinal scale. For example, Nicoll (1964) considered anterior or posterior angulation, varus or valgus, rotational deformity and multiple deformity (occurring in two planes) as four separate variables which he scaled accordingly:

1. Functionally insignificant (less than 10 degrees).
2. Moderate deformity (10–20 degrees).
3. Severe deformity (over 20 degrees).

Geist and Laros (1979) recommended that, in the reporting of results following treatment of femoral shaft fractures, angulation should be reported as less than or greater than 10 degrees and limb shortening measured on a 3-point ordinal scale, namely:

1. < 10 mm.
2. 10–20 mm.
3. > 20 mm.

Despite these reports, the significance of these measurements remains uncertain. Some workers have reported that there has been a failure to show a threshold of deformity beyond which late results are compromised (Kristensen et al., 1989; Merchant and Dietz, 1989), whereas others support the well-accepted concept that excessive angulation ultimately gives rise to problems of joint dysfunction above and below the previous fracture site (Horster, 1985; Kettelkamp et al., 1988; Puno et al., 1991).

Joint stiffness

In most clinical studies, the measurement of joint range of motion is usually performed using a goniometer. There is no doubt, however, that clinical goniometric measurement is unreliable (Boone *et al.*, 1978; Pandya *et al.*, 1985). It follows, therefore, that the reliability of this technique should be tested in each study, and the sensitivity of assessing joint movement will depend on the error of measurement detected. In addition, there is considerable variability in which joint movement data following tibial and femoral fractures is reported. Kempf *et al.* (1985) reported restoration of hip and knee movement following femoral fractures at 6 months, but reported these movements in degrees without reference to a standard. Batten *et al.* (1978) expressed ankle range of movement following internal fixation of tibial fractures as a percentage of normal, and used an ordinal scale to summarise results. McMaster (1976) expressed the range of movement of the hind foot as a fraction of that measured in the opposite leg, thereby creating an interval scale based upon severity of limitation. This latter method has much to commend it, since this instrument does not use population norms which are best avoided when assessing return of movement, due to the large variance.

The time at which results are assessed following fractures is also important. For example, mobility of the hind foot after a tibial fracture, treated conservatively, may be limited a year after injury, but has often improved by 2 years. It is also unclear how long it takes for results to become final, especially with regard to function. Digby *et al.* (1983) studied function after cast brace treatment of a group of predominantly low energy tibial fractures. After a mean follow-up of 47 weeks (range 26–98 weeks), 27% of these patients had not recovered the ability to run.

In those reports where joint function has been studied following lower limb fractures, established joint scoring systems (e.g. Iowa Knee Evaluation, Hospital for Special Surgery Score) have been utilised to produce an objective score of outcome. A number of such systems are available (Pynsent *et al.*, 1993). These systems have been used predominantly for measuring outcome following joint replacement, and have only rarely been applied to joint assessment following fracture. Occasionally, authors have devised their own scoring systems. Merchant and Dietz (1989) used the Iowa Knee Evaluation, together with their own ankle evaluation system, when studying joint function after long-term follow-up of tibial and fibular shaft fractures.

Rehabilitation measures of outcome

Since most patients perceive recovery in terms of the restoration of function and the resumption of activities performed prior to injury, it is appropriate to consider rehabilitation measures as potential instruments for assessing outcome following femoral or tibial shaft fractures. In fact, since rehabilitation spans a number of health care disciplines, a wide range of tests have been developed, orthopaedic surgeons usually tending to assess functional outcome by devising their own unique instruments. In reality, most rehabilitation measures have been developed for specific purposes and are not necessarily directly applicable to measuring outcome following lower limb fractures.

Socioeconomic outcome

Individuals disabled as a result of lower limb fracture, on the whole, strive to become as normal as possible, as quickly as possible, in order to regain their former social and economic status. The measurement of 'normality' has therefore previously been expressed in terms of return to work, return to social commitments and to sports activities, at standards matching those displayed prior to the injury. There are a number of validated, reliable scales and indices to measure activities of daily living (ADL – Katz *et al.*, 1963; Granger *et al.*, 1979; Durham *et al.*, 1985). Unfortunately, ADL scales which consider ability to perform such tasks as toileting, dressing and bathing are insensitive tests of outcome for use in those recovering from lower limb fractures. There is, therefore, a need to select and/or create activity indices which fulfil the specific goals required in any studies of these injuries.

Dependent socioeconomic variables which have been used in studies of lower limb fracture include return to work (Edwards, 1965; Rokkanen *et al.*, 1969; Hutchins, 1981; Chan *et al.*, 1984; Hooper *et al.*, 1991), length of hospital stay (Haines *et al.*, 1984; Bondurant *et al.*, 1988; den Outer *et al.*, 1990), loss of earnings (Hutchins, 1981) and inpatient hospital costs (Bondurant *et al.*, 1988). Once again, the validity of length of hospital stay and return to work measures is also questionable since the whim of the treating surgeon or the routine practice of the ward might ultimately determine the length of time a patient stays in hospital or remains off work. Work itself is also a complex outcome, since the actual type of job undertaken will influence the time at which employment is resumed. Unemployment further complicates this issue.

Psychological outcome

This type of outcome measurement has seldom been used in the past for research relating to rehabilitation following lower limb fractures. The psychological experience of pain is of questionable value, particularly since the absence of pain is a prerequisite for standard clinical tests of fracture healing. Although pain scales and questionnaires have been thoroughly tested, these have been used infrequently in this context. The measurement of patient satisfaction, and attitudes of well-being, especially in relation to work (Warr *et al.*, 1979) are two other psychological measures which may be potentially useful in patients with lower limb fractures. However, to date, the psychological tests have not been used widely.

Functional outcome

The assessment of functional end-result of fracture treatment has been attempted by a number of authors, who have devised their own measurement instruments. Batten *et al.* (1978) devised a scoring system whereby marks were subtracted from 10 for the presence of the following:

1. Limited knee flexion.
2. Tenderness or warmth at the fracture site.

3. Bad scar.
4. Limited tip-toe walking.
5. Flat hop.
6. Any unsatisfactory sign of X-ray.
7. Limited midtarsal or subtalar movement.

The authors made no attempt to assess reliability using this scoring system and its usefulness must be questioned as an acceptable functional outcome measure, particularly since the score combined functional activities with diagnostic signs and symptoms.

Other authors have, unfortunately, adopted a similar approach. Geist and Laros (1979) recommended a standard method for reported results following femoral fracture (Table 22.4). This combines data relating to

Table 22.4 Geist and Laros' recommendations for reporting of results following femoral fractures

Classification groups, based on:
Age
Location of fracture
Fracture type
Open or closed fractures
Concomitant injuries

Results: 1. Hospitalisation, e.g.
      0–14 days
      15–30 days
      31–60 days
      > 60 days
2. Rehospitalisations
3. Re-operations
4. Ambulation, i.e. return to full unaided weight bearing (no stick, crutch, walker)
      0–30 days
      31–60 days
      61–120 days
      121–240 days
      241–360 days
      > 360 days
5. Return to work (no. and %)
      0–30 days
      31–60 days
      61–120 days
      121–240 days
      241–360 days
      > 360 days
6. Limb shortening
      < 10 mm
      10–20 mm
      > 20 mm
7. Angulation
      < 10 degrees
      > 10 degrees
8. Knee motion
      > 125 degrees – able to squat, carry out most normal activities
      110–124 degrees – permit shoe tying
      100–109 degrees – stair handling, sit comfortably
      < 100 degrees – difficulty sitting

deformity, joint range of movement and socioeconomic outcome measures. Their grading of knee motion into four categories was based on the work of Laubenthal and others (Laubenthal *et al.*, 1972) who made recommendations for the average ranges of motion required for normal daily activities such as sitting, stair climbing, tying shoelaces or squatting to lift an object. Edwards (1965) classified final results using eight different parameters, plus non-union, osteomyelitis and amputation, to classify results (Table 22.5). His system considers pain, ability to work, gait, sports activity, motion of knee, ankle and foot, and leg swelling. Notably absent in this scheme is any reference to deformity.

Johner and Wruhs (1983) used a four-level scale for classifying results of tibial fractures (Table 22.6). They included deformity, which is often omitted, but otherwise their assessment was similar to that of Edwards. The 'excellent' and 'good' categories of Johner and Wruhs correspond fairly well to Edwards' 'good' category, while 'poor' has essentially the same criteria in both studies.

Finally, certain tests of physical fitness and exercise tolerance, such as the 12-minute walking test for assessing disability (Macnicol *et al.*, 1980), have been evaluated, and may prove useful ultimately in the assessment of tibial and femoral shaft fractures. Objective gait analysis is gaining acceptance as a clinical tool, particularly in the field of neuromuscular handicap, but its potential for assessment of outcome following lower extremity fractures remains, for the most part, unexplored.

Occupational assessments (Crewe and Athelston, 1981; Watson, 1987) have also been developed, based upon basic movements and function such as walking uphill, bending and kneeling, as opposed to activity of daily living (ADL) tasks. Each item is scaled according to the person's ability to perform it. Watson (1988) performed an extremely thorough longitudinal study in a series of patients with tibial fractures, and standardised, tested and selected instruments for measurement of outcome, including occupational assessment criteria. From this study, three instruments most capable of measuring outcome following lower limb fracture were identified, namely time to union, time to return to work and the ability to kneel, 38 weeks following injury.

Conclusions

There is no set way to measure outcome following a tibial or femoral shaft fracture. Clinical measures have attempted to quantify outcome in terms of time to union, complication rates and the incidence of limitations and deformities. Unfortunately, the variables on which these instruments depend have been based to a large extent upon subjective, non-standardised criteria. The best comparison between treatments is usually made by well-designed prospective randomised studies. Few of these have been presented for either femoral or tibial fractures, but there are notable exceptions (Owen *et al.*, 1967; Van Der Linden and Larsson, 1979; Spiegel *et al.*, 1988; Bach and Hansen, 1989; Holbrook *et al.*, 1989; Hooper *et al.*, 1991). Hopefully, the future will see carefully executed prospective studies for femoral and tibial fracture treatment, so that

Table 22.5 Edward's Classification System for results following tibial fracture treatment

	Good	Fair	Poor*
1. Pain	Little or none	Slight	Severe
2. Work capacity	Normal	Difficulty or inability to do heavy work	Markedly decreased; light seated work only
3. Limp	None	Slight with or after severe exercise	Constant
4. Sports activity	Normal	Decreased ability	Short walks only
5. Knee motion	Stable; full extension; loss of flexion < 20 degrees	Stable; full extension flexion to at least 90 degrees	Lack of full extension; flexion to < 90 degrees
6. Ankle motion	< 10 degrees loss of dorsiflexion; < 20 degrees loss of plantar flexion	Dorsiflexion > 90 degrees; < 30 degrees loss of plantar flexion	Dorsiflexion < 90 degrees; > 30 degrees loss of plantar flexion
7. Foot motion	< 25% decrease of pro- and supination	Moderately decreased	Severely decreased
8. Swelling of lower leg	Slight, only after exercise	Slight	Constant

Reproduced from Edwards, 1965.
*Poor results also include: amputation; osteomyelitis with recurrent drainage; pseudarthrosis.

Table 22.6 Johner and Wruh's criteria for evaluation of final results after tibial shaft fracture

	Excellent (left = right)	Good	Fair	Poor
Non-union, osteitis, amputation	None	None	None	Yes
Neurovascular disturbances	None	Minimal	Moderate	Severe
Deformity				
Varus/valgus (degrees)	None	2–5	6–10	> 10
Anteversion/recurvation (degrees)	0–5	6–10	11–20	> 20
Rotation (degrees)	0–5	6–10	11–20	> 20
Shortening (mm)	0–5	6–10	11–20	> 20
Mobility (%)				
Knee	Normal	> 80	> 75	< 75
Ankle	Normal	> 75	> 50	< 50
Subtalar joint	Normal	> 75	> 50	< 50
Pain	None	Occasional	Moderate	Severe
Gait	Normal	Normal	Insignificant limp	Significant limp
Strenuous activities	Possible	Limited	Severely limited	Impossible

Reproduced from Johner and Wruhs, 1983, with permission.

anecdote and clinical impression can be replaced by reliable, scientific data.

Group discussion

Femoral fractures

The AO classification was recommended for uniformity of communication only. The classification itself was purely descriptive and has not been validated in terms of outcome.

It was felt that the best classification should take into account modern treatment methods. In femoral shaft fractures particularly, interlocking nailing had now become orthodox practice in adult fractures, replacing virtually all other forms of treatment for midshaft injuries other than severe open fractures and multiple injuries in polytrauma where plating or external fixation might be used.

It was felt that soft tissue injuries could only be implied from bony fragmentation and displacement.

Technical satisfaction of treatment

The assumption was made that the results from closed interlocking nail were sufficiently advantageous that this was now widely and increasingly adopted and that the technical satisfaction should relate to the integrity of the nail–screw–bone construct, although there were technical problems with a prominent nail in the greater trochanter and pain around the screws in the trochanteric and distal femoral region. There were also fractures of implants which should be noted.

Outcome should be assessed in terms of function, union and deformity. Function should be related purely to the femoral shaft fracture and particularly in high violent injuries, knee ligament disruption should be excluded both after fixation and late.

Radiological union

It was felt that attempting to quantify various degrees of callus crossing a fracture line with implanted metal already *in situ* was flawed and not reproducible, although an increasing gap between bone ends was definable as progressing non-union. Consolidated union could probably be recognised. The time to union is usually recorded as a mean value, even though it has been measured at intervals of weeks or months. It was felt that very frequent X-ray examination of fractures was unjustified in terms of radiation exposure and not particularly helpful in assessing outcome. Rather, the patient should be examined and the fractures X-rayed every 6 weeks and the proportion of patients achieving full weight bearing without a limp and without bone resorption at the fracture site should be recorded. The complications in Table 22.3 should address 'degree of' and 'time to' resolution. Complications specific to intervention should be recorded.

The functional outcome should be based in principle on that described by Edwards and Johner and Wruhs but there needed to be an extra category as treatment had improved, a proportion of patients were quite indistinguishable from normal with modern treatment and this should be recognised. There was considerable reservation at the arbitrary downgrading of results on clinical measurements based on goniometric measurement. Work capacity, likewise, elicited reservations as it was considered that the demands of heavy manual and clerical work were different and that unemployment further compromised this index of outcome.

It was considered that length of admission should take into account the more rapid discharge prevalent at present and be measured in days rather than weeks.

Future research

The group felt research was required to establish the relative merits of reamed versus unreamed nailing, techniques to improve distal locking, particularly with the new translucent drill, and refinements in nail design. The systemic effects of femoral nailing and the validation of fracture classification scoring systems were also required.

Tibial fractures

Again the group felt that the AO classification enhanced uniformity of reporting but lacked the important aspect of displacement identified by Nicoll. Fractures should be identified as 'closed' or 'open', but high violence closed injuries requiring fasciotomies were rendered open by procedure and, therefore, should be classified within this group.

Open fractures should be classified according to Gustilo. It was considered that there was a need to classify soft tissue injuries and skin loss, particularly in relation to the plastic surgery procedures now available. The time taken to such interventions and the time to stable skin cover thereafter should be recorded in assessing outcome of open tibial fractures.

Functional and radiological union all suffered from the same problems as femoral shaft fractures and it was felt that these should be addressed in the same manner.

Future research

It was felt that a validated classification was necessary as the last one in which treatment was uniform was that published by Nicoll almost 30 years ago. The practicalities of randomising fractures of similar complexity was considered to be beyond any one centre and the most sensible approach to improving information on this subject was a prospective review with simple outcome measures from a number of centres in which treatment was based on the preference of the surgeon in charge of the case. In addition to this particular approach the long-term psychological effects of open tibial fractures or below-knee amputation and comparative effects of energy consumption and gait should be assessed.

References

Austin RT (1977) Fracture of the tibial shaft: is medical audit possible? *Injury*; **9**: 93–101

Bach AW, Hansen ST Jr (1989) Plates versus external fixation in severe open tibial shaft fractures. A randomised trial. *Clin. Orthop. Rel. Res.*; **241**: 89–94

Batten RL, Donaldson LJ, Aldridge MJ (1978) Experience with the AO method in the treatment of 142 cases of fresh fracture of the tibial shaft treated in the UK. *Injury*; **10**: 108–114

Bauer GCH, Edwards P, Widmark PH (1962) Shaft fractures of the tibia: etiology of poor results in a consecutive series of 173 fractures. *Acta. Chir. Scand.*; **124**: 386–395

Bondurant FJ, Cotler HB, Buckle R, Miller-Crotchett P (1988) The medical and economic impact of severely injured lower extremities. *J. Trauma*; **28**: 1270–1273

Boone DC, Azen SP, Lin CM, Spence C, Barron C, Lee L (1978) Reliability of goniometric measurements. *Phys. Ther.*; **58**: 1355–1560

Burwell HN (1971) Plate fixation of tibial shaft fractures: a survey of 181 injuries. *J. Bone Joint Surg.*; **53B**: 258–271

Chan KM, Tse PJT, Chow JJN, Leung PC (1984) Closed medullary nailing for fractured shaft of the femur – a comparison between Kuntscher and AO techniques. *Injury*; **15**: 381–387

Court-Brown CM, Wheelwright EF, Christie J, McQueen MM (1990) External fixation for type III open tibial fractures. *J. Bone Joint Surg.*; **72B**: 801–804

Crawford-Adams J (1983) *Outline of Fractures*. Edinburgh: Churchill Livingstone

Crewe NM, Athleston GT (1981) Functional assessment in vocational rehabilitation. A systematic approach to diagnosis and goal setting. *Arch. Phys. Med. Rehabil.*; **62**: 299–305

den Outer AJ, Meeuwis JD, Hermans J, Zwaveling A (1990) Conservative versus operative treatment of displaced noncomminuted tibial shaft fractures. A retrospective comparative study. *Clin. Orthop. Rel. Res.*; **252**: 231–237

Digby JM, Holloway GMN, Webb JK (1983) A study of function after tibial cast bracing. *Injury*; **14**: 432–439

Durham J, MacNeish A, Rooney PJ, Rooney K, Hart LE, Norman G (1985) The MDR index of function in rheumatoid arthritis. *Clin. Exp. Rheumatol.*; **3**: 297–302

Edwards P (1965) Fractures of the shaft of the tibia: 492 consecutive cases in adults. Importance of soft tissue injury. *Acta. Orthop. Scand. Suppl.*; **76**: 1–83

Ellis H (1958) The speed of healing after fracture of the tibial shaft. *J. Bone Joint Surg.*; **40B**: 42–46

Geist RW, Laros G (1979) Symposium. Rigid internal fixation of fractures. Femoral shaft fractures: editorial comment and comparative results. *Clin. Orthop. Rel. Res.*; **138**: 5–9

Granger CV, Albrecht GL, Hamilton BB (1979) Outcome of comprehensive medical rehabilitation. A measurement of PULSES profile and the Barthel Index. *Arch. Phys. Med. Rehabil.*; **60**: 145–154

Gregory RT, Gould RJ, Peclet M, Wager JS, Gilbert DA, Wheeler JR, Synder SO, Gayle RG, Schwab CW (1985) The Mangled Extremity Syndrome (MES): a severity grading system for multisystem injury of the extremity. *J. Trauma*; **25**: 1147–1150

Gustilo RB, Anderson JT (1976) Prevention of infection in the treatment of one thousand and twenty five open fractures of the long bones. *J. Bone Joint Surg.*; **58A**: 453–458

Gustilo RB, Mendoza RM, Williams DN (1984) Problems in the management of type III (severe) open fractures: a new classification of type III open fractures. *J. Trauma*; **24**: 742–746

Haines JF, Williams EA, Hargadon EJ, Davies DRA (1984) Is conservative treatment of displaced tibial shaft fractures justified? *J. Bone Joint Surg.*; **66B**: 84–88

Hammer RRR, Hammerby S, Lindholm B (1985) Accuracy of radiologic assessment of tibial shaft fracture union in humans. *Clin. Orthop. Rel. Res.*; **199**: 233–238

Hansen ST Jr (1987) The type-IIIC tibial fracture: a salvage or amputation (Editorial). *J. Bone Joint Surg.*; **69A**: 799–800

Helfet DL, Howey T, Sanders R, Johansen K (1990) Limb salvage versus amputation. Preliminary results of the Mangled Extremity Severity Score. *Clin. Orthop. Rel. Res.*; **256**: 80–86

Henley MB (1989) Intramedullary devices for tibial fracture stabilisation. *Clin. Orthop. Rel. Res.*; **240**: 87–96

Holbrook JL, Swiontkowski MF, Sanders R (1989) Treatment of open fractures of the tibial shaft: Ender nailing versus external fixation. A randomised, prospective comparison. *J. Bone Joint Surg.*; **71A**: 1231–1238

Hooper GJ, Keddell RG, Penny ID (1991) Conservative management or closed nailing for tibial shaft fractures. A randomised prospective trial. *J. Bone Joint Surg.*; **73B**: 83–85

Horster G (1985) Principles of the surgical correction of post-traumatic deformities of the lower extremities. In Hierholzer G, Muller KH (eds) *Corrective Osteotomies of the Lower Extremity after Trauma*. Berlin: Springer-Verlag, pp. 59–62

Hutchins PM (1981) The outcome of severe tibial injury. *Injury*; **13**: 216–219

Jensen JS, Johansen J, Morch A (1977) Middle third femoral fractures treated with medullary nailing or AO compression plates. *Injury*; **8**: 174–181

Johner R, Wruhs O (1983) Classification of tibial shaft fractures and correlation with results after rigid internal fixation. *Clin. Orthop. Rel. Res.*; **178**: 7–25

Katz S, Ford AB, Moskowitz RW, Jackson BA, Jaffe MW (1963) Studies of illness in the aged. The index of ADL: a standardised measure of biological and psychological function. *JAMA*; **85**: 914–919

Keller CS (1983) The principles of treatment of tibial shaft fractures. A review of 10 146 cases from the literature. *Orthopaedics*; **6**: 993–1006

Kempf I, Gross A, Beck G (1985) Closed locked intramedullary nailing: its application to comminuted fractures of the femur. *J. Bone Joint Surg.*; **67A**: 709–720

Kettelkamp DB, Hillberry BM, Murrish DE, Heck DA (1988) Degenerative arthritis of the knee secondary to fracture malunion. *Clin. Orthop. Rel. Res.*; **234**: 159–169

Kristensen KD, Kiaer T, Blicher J (1989) No arthrosis of the ankle 20 years after malaligned tibial shaft fractures. *Acta Orthop. Scand.*; **60**: 208–209

Lange RH, Bach AW, Hansen ST Jr, Johansen KH (1985) Open tibial shaft fractures with associated vascular injuries: prognosis for limb salvage. *J. Trauma*; **25**: 203–208

Laubenthal RN, Smidt GL, Kettelkamp DB (1972) A quantitative analysis of knee motion during activities of daily living. *Phys. Ther.*; **52**: 34

McMaster M (1976) Disability of the hindfoot after fracture of the tibial shaft. *J. Bone Joint Surg.*; **58B**: 90–93

Macnicol MF, McHardy R, Chalmers J (1980) Exercise testing before and after hip arthroplasty. *J. Bone Joint Surg.*; **62B**: 326–331

Merchant TC, Dietz FR (1989) Long-term follow-up after fractures of the tibial and fibular shafts. *J. Bone Joint Surg.*; **71A**: 599–606

Muller ME, Nazarian S, Koch P, Schatzker J (1990) *The Comprehensive Classification of Fractures of Long Bones*. New York: Springer-Verlag

Nicoll EA (1964) Fractures of the tibial shaft. *J. Bone Joint Surg.*; **46B**: 373–387

Oestern H-J, Tscherne H (1984) Pathophysiology and classification of soft tissue injuries associated with fractures. In: Tscherne H, Gotzen L (eds) *Fractures with Soft Tissue Injuries*. Berlin: Springer-Verlag, pp. 1–9

Oni OO, Hui A, Gregg PJ (1988) The healing of closed tibial shaft fractures. The natural history of union with closed treatment. *J. Bone Joint Surg.*; **70B**: 787–790

Owen C, Covin JJ, Kang LW (1967) Fractures of the shaft of the tibia and fibula. *J. Bone Joint Surg.*; **49A**: 194

Pandya S, Florence JM, King WM, Robison JD, Oxman M, Province MA (1985) Reliability of goniometric measurements in patients with Duchenne Muscular dystrophy. *Phys. Ther.*; **65**: 1339–1342

Puno RM, Vaughan JJ, Stetten ML, Johnson JR (1991) Long-term effects of tibial angular malunion on the knee and ankle joints. *J. Orthop. Trauma*; **5**: 247–254

Pynsent PB, Fairbank JCT, Carr AJ (1993) *Outcome Measures in Orthopaedics*. Oxford: Butterworth-Heinemann

Rokkanen P, Slatis P, Vankka E (1969) Closed or open intramedullary nailing of femoral shaft fractures? *J. Bone Joint Surg.*; **51B**: 313–323

Spiegel J, Bray T, Chapman M, Swanson T (1988) The Lottes nail versus AO external fixation in the treatment of open tibial fractures. *Orthop. Trans.*; **12**: 656

Van Der Linden W, Larsson K (1979) Plate fixation versus conservative treatment for tibial shaft fractures: a randomised trial. *J. Bone Joint Surg.*; **61A**: 873–878

Warr P, Cook J, Wall T (1979) Scales for the measurement of some work attitudes and aspects of psychological well-being. *J. Occup. Psychol.*; **52**: 129–148

Watson HJ (1987) Occupational assessment: the Activity Matching Ability System (AMAS). *J. Int Disabil. Studies*; **9**: 71–74

Watson HJ (1988) Longitudinal Study of Recovery Following Diaphyseal Fracture of the Tibia or Femur. PhD Thesis, University of Edinburgh

Winquist RA, Hansen T, Clawson DK (1984) Closed intramedullary nailing of femoral fractures. A report of 520 cases. *J. Bone Joint Surg.*; **66A**: 529–539

Chapter 23

The knee

D. R. Bickerstaff

Soft tissue trauma

Instruments used to measure the outcome of soft tissue trauma of the knee are principally devoted to ligament injury and have been dealt with in detail in the preceding book in this series (Miller and Carr, 1993). Outcome measure of meniscal trauma is less well defined and further confused by its common association with ligamentous injury. Therefore, the results of meniscal surgery cannot easily be differentiated from those of ligament surgery, particularly with reference to clinical measurements of impairment and function. For this reason the precise pathology and exact treatment of meniscus or ligament injury must be clearly defined in studies of soft tissue knee trauma.

Potentially ligament repair will restore function, prevent further meniscal and possible articular cartilage damage and, by restoring normal biomechanics, it may prevent or delay the development of osteoarthritis. There is good evidence that an anterior cruciate ligament (ACL) deficiency predisposes to further meniscal damage (Irvine and Glasgow, 1992), though there is no convincing evidence that ACL reconstruction prevents this risk (Bray *et al.*, 1988).

The deleterious effect of meniscectomy on the knee joint was highlighted by Fairbank in 1948. He demonstrated the degenerative changes that took place subsequent to meniscectomy. These changes have been well documented in further studies (Johnson *et al.*, 1974; Dandy and Jackson, 1975a, 1975b; Jones *et al.*, 1978) and appear to be accelerated in ACL-deficient knees (Lynch *et al.*, 1983; Henning and Lynch, 1985). This has led to the concept of repairing meniscus tears either with open or arthroscopic surgery. Although there is evidence of meniscal healing 3–5 years after repair, there is no substantive evidence that this prevents the late degenerative changes. In addition, there is increasing interest in allograft replacement of menisci to prevent the deleterious effects of meniscectomy.

In view of the above trends in meniscal surgery, it is important to design accurate and reproducible methods of assessing the outcome of surgical techniques that will be universally applicable. In designing these measurements, allowance must be made in the clinical assessment of associated ligamentous instability when applicable.

Assessment of results

The results of both ligament and meniscal surgery are dependent upon the patient, the precise pathology, the surgical procedure and post-operative care. These must all be clearly defined.

Initial assessment

An assessment in isolation cannot be used as a measurement of outcome but the difference in assessment before and after surgery can be used to measure improvement. Unfortunately, unlike elective surgery, the unexpected nature of trauma makes this form of measurement difficult. Details of initial pathology are crucial in assessing change and every effort should be made to clearly record them.

The use of arthroscopy as a measure of outcome will be discussed later, but its rôle in defining the initial pathology should be emphasised. The side and description of site and type of meniscal tear must be recorded. Dandy (1990) produced a comprehensive description of types of meniscal tears. Henning *et al.* (1990) in their study of meniscal suture provided a simpler description (Figure 23.1) which, for the purpose of observing the outcome of meniscal repair, is more applicable. In addition, the distance of the tear from the periphery, proximity of the tear to the posterior horn and the length and depth of tear should be recorded. Any articular cartilage pathology should be defined using the Noyes and Stabler (1989) classification for grading articular cartilage damage (Table 23.1).

In view of the variety of meniscal surgery available, a clear account of techniques used should be made, including the method and extent of resection, open or closed meniscal suture, type of suture material used and technique used to augment vascular ingrowth. Either a clear operative description should be made or the technique adequately referenced.

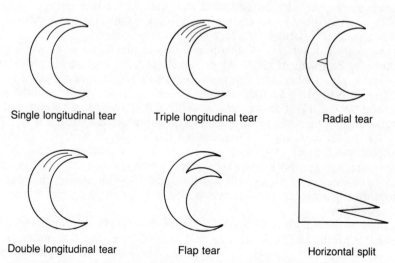

Single longitudinal tear   Triple longitudinal tear   Radial tear

Double longitudinal tear   Flap tear   Horizontal split

Figure 23.1 Different descriptions of meniscal tears. (After Henning *et al.*, 1990, with permission)

If ligament surgery is undertaken, information on the type of graft used, implantation technique, graft orientation, tensioning and fixation should be provided. It is also important to record postoperative care, such as the period of non-weight bearing after meniscal suture and the time until return to work.

Knee evaluation

In evaluating the results of knee trauma, consideration must be given to the presence of symptoms related to meniscal tear, ligament instability and the presence of degenerative changes which may be the result of one or both of the former. The methods used to assess ligament instability overlap with those of meniscal pathology, and it is therefore theoretically possible to use the accepted knee scoring systems with the addition of factors more specifically referable to soft tissue injury. However, instruments specifically designed and validated for this purpose are preferable.

The evaluation is divided into five parts:

1. Functional level.
2. Symptoms and impairment.
3. Clinical examination.
4. Imaging techniques comprising radiography and MRI.
5. Ancillary tests.

FUNCTION

Treatment of soft tissue injuries of the knee should result in the patient regaining the level of activity he or she possessed before surgery.

Ideally, the assessment of knee function should record the regular maximum performance the knee is capable of. If the injury is repaired acutely, then performance at two time points can be measured; preinjury (retrospectively) and postrepair. In a chronic injury an extra measure of performance, prerepair, can be added. The difference in the assessments is a measure of the patient's functional outcome following treatment.

The patient's functional level should be carefully defined. A top class athlete may well have an apparently poor outcome compared with a recreational athlete as a result of the differing demands and expectations. A comparison of outcome in these two examples is, therefore, not valid. In assessing function it is important to measure the activity level, intensity level and exposure level (frequency of participation). An example of such a scale is given in Table 23.2.

Two or more of these function levels have been incorporated into one scale (Noyes et al., 1984; Tegner and Lysholm, 1985). However, it is probably best to document the three aspects of function separately (Daniel et al., 1990).

In assessing the change in functional level it is important to recognise that some patients decrease their activity level by choice rather than because of problems associated with their ligament or meniscal repair. For example, changing the level of sport participation with age. This change in activity should be differentiated from that due to persisting knee symptoms.

Table 23.1 Grading system for articular cartilage lesions

Surface description	Extent of involvement	Diameter	Location	Degree of knee flexion

1. Cartilage intact	A. Define softening with some resilience remaining
	 B. Extensive softening with loss of resilience (deformation)
		< 10 mm
		 < 15 mm
		 < 20 mm
		 < 25 mm
		 > 25 mm
			Patella
			 A. prox third
			   middle third
			   distal third
			 B. odd facet
			   medial facet
			   lateral facet
				Degree of knee flexion where the lesion is in weight-bearing contact (20–40 degrees)

2. Cartilage surface damaged: cracks, fissures, fibrillation, or fragmentation	A. Less than half of the thickness B. Greater than half of the thickness		Trochlea Medial femoral condyle a. anterior third b. middle third c. posterior third	
3. Bone exposed	A. Bone surface intact B. Bone surface cavitation		Lateral femoral condyle a. anterior third b. middle third c. posterior third Medial tibial condyle a. anterior third b. middle third c. posterior third Lateral tibial condyle a. anterior third b. middle third c. posterior third	

Reproduced from Noyes and Stabler, 1989, with permission.

Table 23.2 Determining the patient's functional level

Activity level	I Activities of daily living
	II Straight running, sports that do not involve lower limb agility activities or occupations that do not involve heavy lifting
	III Activities that require lower limb agility but not jumping, hard turning or pivoting
	IV Activities that involve jumping hard turning or pivoting
Intensity	I Work related or occupational
	II Light recreational
	III Vigorous recreational
	IV Competitive
Exposure	Number of hours per year participation at any given functional level and intensity

SYMPTOMS AND IMPAIRMENTS

Symptoms related to meniscal damage are not specific enough to differentiate meniscal from ligamentous or articular cartilage lesions. Therefore, care must be taken in attributing the failure of a procedure to one component of the surgery (e.g. meniscal versus ACL repair) unless the specific cause can be confirmed by further investigations such as second-look arthroscopy or arthrography.

The difficulty in recording symptoms is that they are highly subjective. In addition, minor symptoms during intense activity are common in the normal population and should not necessarily downgrade the result of a procedure.

A semiquantitative method of assessing symptoms is to relate them to the four levels of activity described in Table 23.2. This is the basis of the symptomatic assessment in the recently proposed assessment format form from the International Knee Documentation Committee (IKDC) (Figure 23.2). The committee recommend that pain, swelling, partial giving-way and full giving-way are recorded. Although they are not included in the IKDC evaluation, further symptoms such as locking and catching, or impairments to turning and jumping can be recorded. A patient must be able to participate at an activity level for a minimum of 50 hours per year (approximately 1 hour per week) before it can be stated that there are no symptoms or impairments at that level.

CLINICAL EXAMINATION

Three of the seven groups in the IKDC evaluation form concern examination. As with the assessment of symptoms, the physical signs are graded into four groups to give a semiquantitative measurement. There are no adequately described studies of the reliability of these measures.

Range of movement is recorded on the injured and uninjured side. Loss of flexion and extension on the injured side are graded depending upon the degree of impairment.

Ligament examination includes the Lachman test (including an estimation as to whether the end-point was soft or firm), anterior draw, posterior draw, medial and lateral joint opening, pivot and reversed pivot

The Seven Groups	The Four Grades				Group Grades (see footnotes)
1. PATIENT SUBJECTIVE ASSESSMENT	A: normal	B: nearly normal	C: abnormal	D: sev. abnorm	A B C D
On a scale of 0 to 3 how did you rate your pre-injury activity level?	☐ 0	☐ 1	☐ 2	☐ 3	
On a scale of 0 to 3 how did you rate your current activity level?	☐ 0	☐ 1	☐ 2	☐ 3	
If your normal knee performs 100%. What percentage does your operated knee perform?	_____ %				☐☐☐☐
2. SYMPTOMS (Grade at highest activity level known by patient)	I Strenuous Activities	II Moderate Activities	III ADL/Light Activities	IV ADL Problems	
Pain	☐	☐	☐	☐	
Swelling	☐	☐	☐	☐	
Partial giving way	☐	☐	☐	☐	
Full giving way	☐	☐	☐	☐	☐☐☐☐
3. RANGE OF MOTION Flex/Ext: / / Index side: / / Opposite side: / /					
Lack of extension (from zero degrees)	☐ <3°	☐ 3–5°	☐ 6–10°	☐ >10°	
△ Lack of flexion	☐ 0–5°	☐ 6–15°	☐ 16–25°	☐ >25°	☐☐☐☐
4. LIGAMENT EXAMINATION					
△ Lachman (25° flex.)	☐ 1 to 2 mm	☐ 3 to 5 mm	☐ 6 to 10 mm	☐ > 10 mm	
(manual, instrumented, x-ray)					
Endpoint: ☐ firm ☐ soft	☐ firm		☐ soft		
△ Total a.p. transl. (70° flex)	☐ 0 to 2 mm	☐ 3 to 5 mm	☐ 6 to 10 mm	☐ > 10 mm	
△ Post. sag in 70° flex	☐ 0 to 2 mm	☐ 3 to 5 mm	☐ 6 to 10 mm	☐ > 10 mm	
△ Med. joint opening (valgus rotation)	☐ 0 to 2 mm	☐ 3 to 5 mm	☐ 6 to 10 mm	☐ > 10 mm	
△ Lat. joint opening (varus rotation)	☐ 0 to 2 mm	☐ 3 to 5 mm	☐ 6 to 10 mm	☐ > 10 mm	
Pivot shift	☐ neg.	☐ + (glide)	☐ ++ (clunk)	☐ +++ (gross)	
Reversed pivot shift	☐ equal	☐ glide	☐ marked	☐ gross	☐☐☐☐
5. COMPARTMENTAL FINDINGS					
Crepitus patellofemoral	☐ none		☐ moderate	☐ severe	
Crepitus medial compartment	☐ none		☐ moderate	☐ severe	
Crepitus lateral compartment	☐ none		☐ moderate	☐ severe (palpable & audible)	☐☐☐☐
6. X-RAY FINDINGS					
Med joint space narrowing	☐ none		☐ <50 %	☐ >50 %	
Lat joint space narrowing	☐ none		☐ <50 %	☐ >50 %	
Patellofemoral joint space narrowing	☐ none		☐ <50 %	☐ >50 %	☐☐☐☐
7. FUNCTIONAL TEST					
△ One leg hop (% of opposite side)	☐ 100–90%	☐ 90–76%	☐ 75–50%	☐ <50%	☐☐☐☐
FINAL EVALUATION					☐☐☐☐

Footnotes: ○ Group Grade: The lowest grade within a group determines the group grade.
○ Final evaluation: The worst group determines the final evaluation.
○ In a final evaluation all 7 groups are to be evaluated, for a quick knee profile the evaluation of groups 1–4 are sufficient.
○ IKDC = International Knee Documentation Committee
Members of the Committee:
AOSSM: Anderson, A, Clancy, WG, Daniel, D, DeHaven, KE, Fowler, PJ, Feagin, J, Grood, ES Noyes, FR, Terry, GC, Torzilli, P, Warren, RF.
ESKA: Chambat, P, Eriksson, E, Giliquist, J, Hefti, F, Huiskes, R, Jakob, RP, Moyen, B, Mueller, W, Staeubli, H, VanKampton, A.

Figure 23.2 The International Knee Documentation Committee's assessment form

shift. With the exception of the last two tests, they are placed into four gradings dependant upon the degree of translation or opening elicited (Gurtler *et al.*, 1987).

Compartmental findings record crepitation in the patellofemoral, lateral and medial compartments.

In addition to this clinical examination is a functional test, the one-leg hop test (Daniel *et al.*, 1982, Tegner *et al.*, 1986). Joint tenderness and the results of the McMurray test could be recorded as more specific tests for meniscal pathology, these are not included in the IKDC form. The disadvantage of these two signs is that they provide a measurement in binary form which is of less value in comparative studies.

The IKDC evaluation form was presented to the International Knee Society meeting in Toronto, Canada, in May 1992. The committee which recommended this form of evaluation was formed jointly from the American Orthopaedic Society for Sports Medicine (AOSSM) and the European Society of Sports Traumatology, Knee Surgery and Arthroscopy (ESSKA). Their brief was to produce an evaluation form for knee pathology (anterior cruciate injury) which would, it is hoped, be universally accepted. It has not yet been validated by full clinical trials.

ARTHROSCOPY

The accuracy of arthroscopic diagnosis has been demonstrated in several studies (Jackson and Abe, 1972; Henry, 1977). It might be proposed that arthroscopy should be used to assess the results of meniscal surgery. However, arthroscopy is an invasive procedure with a small but recognised morbidity and doubts have been cast on the ability to assess the posteromedial corner of the knee (Ireland *et al.*, 1980). The adequacy of healing, assessed by arthroscopy, is subjective but can be classified as healed (stable bonding at the repair site without evidence of any residual defect on the surface), incompletely healed (stable bonding at the repair site but with evidence of some partial-thickness defect of the surface) or not healed (no evidence of bonding at the repair site, with a full-thickness defect present) (Scott *et al.*, 1986). Henning *et al.* (1990) classified healing as complete (90–100% of the vertical height healed), incomplete (50–90%) and failed (less than 50%). The timing of the second-look arthroscopy is largely empirical but Henning *et al.* (1990) reported 88% of lateral meniscal repairs healed or incompletely healed at 4 months after surgery.

Second-look arthroscopy can be used to assess the site, extent and degree of articular cartilage damage using Noyes' classification (Figure 23.1) and the appearance of an ACL graft.

IMAGING TECHNIQUES

Plain radiography
This should be a routine part of the evaluation of the knee both at the initial assessment and at the time of review to allow comparison in the assessment of early degenerate change.

Arthrography
Double-contrast arthrography is a less invasive procedure than second-look arthroscopy and has a high reported accuracy in diagnosing tears of the medial meniscus (Nicholas *et al.*, 1970; Gillies and Seligson, 1979; Tegtmeyer *et al.*, 1979). The main drawback of arthrography is the difficulty in identifying tears of the posterior third of the lateral meniscus as compared with arthroscopy. Ireland *et al.* (1980) recommended that arthroscopy and arthrography were complimentary investigations for the diagnosis of different meniscal problems. Scott *et al.* (1986) in their review of 178 meniscal repairs used arthrography to assess the healing rates of medial meniscal tears and arthroscopy under local anaesthesia to assess lateral repair.

Magnetic resonance imaging (MRI)
There are many reports on the use of MRI in diagnosing meniscal tears but there are increasing doubts concerning its overdiagnosis of these lesions. It does, however, have a high negative predictive value approaching 100% and is, therefore, of use in the initial assessment of a patient as a negative result is most likely to be correct (Boeve *et al.*, 1991). Doubt has also been cast on its ability to diagnose healing following meniscal repair. Bronstein *et al.* (1992) found MRI was unable to differentiate between the scar tissue of a healed meniscal repair and a fresh meniscal tear. They concluded that MRI was not a useful diagnostic tool in evaluating healing or re-injury following meniscal tear. Spiers *et al.* (1993) made a prospective study of 58 patients undergoing arthroscopy and MRI of the knee. The preoperative clinical assessment was found to have a diagnostic sensitivity of 77% and a specificity of 43% compared with 100% and 63% respectively for MRI. Comparison of MRI and arthroscopy confirmed the accuracy of MRI in the diagnosis of internal derangement but the results for articular cartilage lesions were less good with a sensitivity of only 18% but a specificity of 100%.

ANCILLARY TESTS

These include tests of knee function to assess stability, strength and gait.

Instrumented knee testing
One indication of successful ligament repair or reconstruction is the re-establishment of normal knee stability. Instrumented knee testing involves positioning the limb in a specified manner, applying a known disciplinary force and measuring the displacement (Edixhoven *et al.*, 1987). Instrumented knee testing is more accurate in determining motion limits than clinical assessment. The equipment is expensive and requires training to use it efficiently (Daniel *et al.*, 1985). There is concern about the sensitivity, specificity and reliability of these tests.

Strength tests
These compare the muscle power of the affected limb against the un-affected limb. Due to the doubtful accuracy of such a measurement in a clinical setting, machines have been developed to assess strength both statically and dynamically (Gurtler *et al.*, 1987). As yet, the data from this equipment has not been included in the major evaluation systems.

Gait laboratory studies
These studies appear to be of little benefit in assessing outcome (Marans *et al.*, 1989), although there is a lack of published material in this field.

Intra-articular fractures

Treatment goals

The aim in treating intra-articular fractures of the knee is to return the patient to his or her previous full function with no impairment, such as loss of movement, in a normally aligned limb with congruent articular surfaces to decrease the risk of late traumatic osteoarthritis. This is a rigorous end-point which is impossible to achieve with certain fractures but provides a measure against which results can be compared.

Methods of assessment

The difficulty in devising adequate instruments for measuring outcome in intra-articular fractures of the knee is the huge variability in the type and site of the fracture and also, unlike soft tissue injuries, the increased incidence of such fractures in the elderly who have different functional expectations.

Although not a measure of outcome, the classification of fractures is an important component to any study. It should convey the type and degree of injuries being treated and allows a more exact comparison of treatment options. More importantly, classification provides a basis for comparing studies in different centres. There are numerous classification systems for distal femoral, patella and tibial plateau fractures. The Association for the Study of Internal Fixation of Fractures (ASIF) classification is comprehensive and universally recognised but is based solely on the radiographic appearance. There are moves, however, within the organisation to extend this classification to include soft tissue trauma. It would seem prudent to standardise the classification of fractures in reported series and such a plea has been made for the ASIF system (Colton, 1991).

The two main facets in measuring the outcome of a procedure are the clinical and radiographic assessments.

Clinical assessment

Patient function should be differentiated from knee function in long-term studies. Deteriorating function may reflect the patient becoming older and having different demands on the knee, or be secondary to other disease processes which affect function, such as osteoarthritis and stroke. This deterioration in function may occur despite no change in the knee. It is, therefore, pertinent to assess patient and knee function separately.

KNEE FUNCTION

This should include an assessment of symptoms, principally pain, and clinical examination.

Symptoms

The measurement of pain is highly subjective though attempts have been made to quantify its measurement using visual analogue scales. Too often pain is reported as mild, moderate or severe with no guidelines as to how the differentiations have been made (Schatzker and Lambert, 1979; Siliski et al., 1989; Volpin et al., 1990). A better system is to relate the pain to different activity levels as in the IKDC evaluation form (Figure 23.2). Other symptoms such as giving way, stiffness or locking may also be important.

Examination

Examination of the knee should address limb alignment, range of move-ment and stability. The assessment of alignment, particularly following distal femoral fractures, is important as loss of alignment is a major factor in precipitating a poor result. It may predispose to non-union or implant failure in the short term and is a factor in the development of osteoarthritis in the long term. A clinical estimation of the difference in the mechanical or anatomical axis, compared with the uninjured side, should be made with the patient weight-bearing. Radiographic assessment of alignment may be more reproducible. The assessment of range of movement should include the presence of a flexion deformity and any extensor lag.

Stability should be assessed as in the IKDC format testing AP translation and varus/valgus displacement. Soft tissue injury can be a major component of skeletal knee trauma and if not addressed will result in a poor function, despite an excellent skeletal reconstruction.

PATIENT FUNCTION

Many reports on the outcome following intra-articular fracture of the knee use assessments designed for the measurement of outcome of knee osteotomy or arthroplasty (Siliski *et al.*, 1989; Lachiewicz and Funcik, 1990; Volpin *et al.*, 1990). The principal drawback of this type of assessment is that the functional tasks are only relevant to an elderly population and not applicable to a young person who sustains a knee fracture. Function is often measured in terms of the patient's ability to climb stairs, their walking distance and use of walking aids (Insall *et al.*, 1989). A young person may be able to score highly with this system and yet feel they have poor function as they cannot play sport to their expected ability or perform strenuous activity at work such as climbing ladders or scaffolding. A compromise for the younger patient would be to include an assessment of function as detailed in the IKDC knee ligament evaluation chart (Figure 23.2). This assesses their activity levels before and after surgery.

A second facet to consider is the patient's own assessment of their function. This was included in the BOA knee function chart (Aichroth *et al.*, 1978) but is open to considerable patient and investigator bias. For this reason this subjective assessment is not included in more recent assessment formats (Insall *et al.*, 1989).

Radiographic outcome

The most frequent reason for long-term failure following intra-articular fractures is the development of degenerative changes. In the short term, therefore, postoperative radiographs should be examined to identify features that predispose to degenerative changes such as limb alignment and joint congruity. In the long term, the site and degree of degenerative changes should be assessed.

Radiographic grading of osteoarthritis of the knee was carefully described by Ahlbäck in 1968. This grading system has been modified by a number of authors (Keyes et al., 1992). It is based in its early stages on assessing the degree of loss of articular cartilage and subsequently on the amount of bony erosion evident on anteroposterior radiographs. Separate scores can be used for the medial and lateral tibiofemoral compartments.

In addition, a comment on the adequacy of reduction is needed. Schatzker and Lambert (1979) demonstrated a significant difference in outcome if patients were divided into two groups depending upon whether the supracondylar fracture had been managed strictly adhering to the ASIF 'principles'. Consequently, indifferent results may arise not only from inappropriate treatment but also inappropriately executed treatment.

Standardised evaluation formats

There are some systems which are designed for specific fractures (e.g. supracondylar fractures, Neer et al., 1967) but none to assess all fractures. Although some fractures cause particular problems, it would seem sensible to rationalise the measurement of outcome using one standard format to assess knee function and the degree to which this affects overall patient function.

In the absence of a system specifically for measuring the outcome of knee fracture management, formats which were designed to assess the results of arthritis surgery are commonly used (Hospital for Special Surgery Knee Rating Score – Insall et al., 1976; BOA knee function assessment chart – Aichroth et al., 1978). Both the above assessments include a functional assessment which may measure a deterioration as the patient becomes older, although the knee remains unchanged. This has led to a rationalisation of the HSS chart by the American Knee Society (Insall et al., 1989), altering the weighting of certain functions, increasing the number of points deducted for impairments and critically assessing function separately (Table 23.3). The disadvantage of this system for use in fracture management is that the functional assessment is aimed at the elderly patient.

Group discussion

The outcome measures for ligament disorders have been previously described by Miller and Carr (1993) and thus not rigorously investigated in this chapter.

The group recommended the International Knee Documentation Committee's (IKDC) evaluation form for ligament and meniscal injuries but found several deficiencies:

1. Subjective assessment might be improved by the use of a visual analogue score.
2. Difficulty in grading or assessing pain.
3. The range of movement – small losses may not be related to function and they are difficult to observe.

Table 23.3 The American Knee Society's assessment system

A. Unilateral or bilateral (opposite knee successfully replaced)
B. Unilateral, other knee symptomatic
C. Multiple arthritis or medical infirmity

Pain	*Points*	*Function*	*Points*
None	50	Walking	50
Mild or occasional	45	Unlimited	40
Stairs only	40	> 10 blocks	30
Walking and stairs	30	5–10 blocks	20
Moderate		< 5 blocks	10
Occasional	20	Housebound	0
Continual	10	Unable	
Severe	0	Stairs	
		Normal up and down	50
Range of motion		Normal up; down with rail	40
(5 degrees = 1 point)	25	Up and down with rail	30
		Up with rail; unable down	15
Stability (maximum movement		Unable	0
in any position)		Subtotal	—
Anteroposterior (mm)			
< 5	10		
5–10	5	*Deductions (minus)*	
10	0	Cane	5
Mediolateral (degrees)		Two canes	10
< 5	15	Crutches or walker	20
6–9	10		
10–14	5	Total deductions	—
15	0		
Subtotal	—	Function score	—

Deductions (minus)	
Flexion contracture (degrees)	
5–10	2
10–15	5
16–20	10
> 20	15
Extension lag (degrees)	
< 10	5
10–20	10
> 20	15
Alignment (degrees)	
5–10	0
0–4	3 points each degree
11–15	3 points each degree
Other	20
Total deductions	—
Knee score	—
(If total is a minus number, score is 0)	

4. Ligament laxity is difficult to quantify, particularly for the Lachman test. The draw test is of little value. The pivot shift test is crucial to the outcome but difficult to grade and to compare.
5. X-rays are becoming less relevant as the use of MRI increases.

A combination of the first half of the IKDC form and the whole of the HSS form was considered the best instrument for measuring fracture outcome.

More information is needed about the natural history of these disorders before optimal timings for applying the instruments can be chosen and, therefore, an annual assessment is recommended until this is known.

It was felt that the HSS score would be poor for measuring function in those aged under 50 years. The interobserver error has not been measured but the group felt that it was likely to be unacceptably high for both clinical and radiographic assessment. There is no ideal instrument.

References

Ahlbäck S (1968) Osteoarthritis of the knee. A radiographic investigation. *Acta. Radiol Diagn. Stockh.* (Suppl. 277): 7–72

Aichroth PM, Freeman MAR, Smillie IS, Souter WA (1978) A knee function assessment chart. *J. Bone Joint Surg.*; **60B**: 308–309

Boeve BJ, Davidson RA, Staab EV (1991) Magnetic resonance imaging in the evaluation of knee injuries. *South Med. J.*; **84**: 1123–1127

Bray RC, Flanagan JP, Dandy DJ (1988) Reconstruction for chronic anterior cruciate instability. *J. Bone Joint Surg.*; **70B**: 100–105

Bronstein R, Kirk P, Hurley J (1992) The usefulness of MRI in evaluating menisci after meniscal repair. *Orthopaedics*; **15**: 1149–1152

Colton C (1991) Telling the bones. *J. Bone Joint Surg.*; **73B**: 362–364

Dandy DJ (1990) The arthroscopic anatomy of symptomatic meniscal lesions. *J. Bone Joint Surg.*; **72B**: 628–633

Dandy DJ, Jackson RW (1975a) The diagnosis of problems after meniscectomy. *J. Bone Joint Surg.*; **57B**: 349–352

Dandy DJ, Jackson RW (1975b) Meniscectomy and chondromalacia of the femoral condyle. *J. Bone Joint Surg.*; **57A**: 1116–1119

Daniel DM, Malcolm L, Stone ML, Peth H, Morgan J, Riehl B (1982) Quantification of knee stability and function. *Contemp. Orthop.*; **5**: 83–91

Daniel DM, Stone ML, Sachs R, Malcolm L (1985) Measurement of anterior laxity in patients with acute anterior cruciate ligament disruption. *Am. J. Sports Med.*; **13**: 401–407

Daniel DM, Acheson N. O'Connor JJ (1990) *The Knee Ligaments*. New York: Raven

Edixhoven P, Huiskes R, DeGraf P, van Pens TJ, Scoof TJ (1987) Accuracy and reproducibility of instrumented knee drawer tests. *J. Orthop. Res.*; **5**: 378–387

Fairbank TJ (1948) Knee joint changes after meniscectomy. *J. Bone Joint Surg.*; **30B**: 664–670

Gillies H, Seligson D (1979) Precision in the diagnosis of meniscal lesions: a comparison of clinical evaluation, arthrography and arthroscopy. *J. Bone Joint Surg.*; **61A**: 343–346

Gurtler RA, Stine R, Torg JS (1987) Lachman test evaluated. *Clin. Orthop. Rel. Res.*; **216**: 141–150

Henning CE, Lynch MA (1985) Current concepts of meniscal function in pathology. *Clin. Sports Med.*; **4**: 259–265

Henning CE, Lynch MA, Yearout PT, Vequist SW, Stallbaumer RJ, Decker KA (1990) Arthroscopic meniscal repair using an exogenous fibrin clot. *Clin. Orthop. Rel. Res.*; **252**: 64–72

Henry AN (1977) Arthroscopy in practice. *Br. Med. J.*; **1**: 87–88

Insall JN, Ranawat CS, Aglietti P, Shine J (1976) A comparison of four models of total knee replacement models. *J. Bone Joint Surg.*; **58A**: 754–765

Insall JN, Dorr LD, Scott RD, Scott WN (1989) Rationale of the Knee Society clinical rating system. *Clin. Orthop. Rel. Res.*; **248**: 13–14

Ireland J, Trickey EL, Stoker DJ (1980) Arthroscopy and arthrography of the knee. *J. Bone Joint Surg.*; **2B**: 3–6

Irvine GB, Glasgow MMS (1992) The natural history of the meniscus in anterior cruciate insufficiency: arthroscopic analysis. *J. Bone Joint Surg.*; **74B**: 403–405

Jackson RW, Abe I (1972) The role of arthroscopy in the management of disorders of the knee. An analysis of 200 consecutive examinations. *J. Bone Joint Surg.*; **54B**: 310–322

Johnson RJ, Kettlekamp DB, Clark W, Leaverton P (1974) Factors affecting late results after menisectomy. *J. Bone Joint Surg.*; **56A**: 719–729

Jones R, Smith EC, Reisch JS (1978) Effects of medial meniscectomy in patients older than forty years. *J. Bone Joint Surg.*; **60A**: 783–786

Keyes GW, Carr AJ, Miller RK, Goodfellow JW (1992) The radiographic classification of medial gonarthrosis. *Acta Orthop. Scand.*; **63**: 497–501

Lachiewicz PF, Funcik T (1990) Factors influencing the results of open reduction and internal fixation of tibial plateau fractures. *Clin. Orthop. Rel. Res.*; **259**: 210–215

Lynch MA, Henning CE, Glick KR (1983) Knee joint surface changes, long-term follow-up meniscus tear treatment in stable anterior cruciate reconstructions. *Clin. Orthop. Rel. Res.*; **172**: 148–153

Marans HJ, Jackson RW, Glossop ND, Young MC (1989) Anterior cruciate ligament insufficiency: a dynamic three dimensional motion analysis. *Am. J. Sports Med.*; **17**: 325–332

Miller RK, Carr AJ (1993) The knee. In: *Outcome Measures in Orthopaedics*. Oxford: Butterworth Heinemann, pp. 228–244

Neer CS, Granthan SA, Shelton ML (1967) Supracondylar fractures of the adult femur. A study of one hundred and ten cases. *J. Bone Joint Surg.*; **49A**: 591–613

Nicholas JA, Freiberger RH, Killoran PJ (1970) Double contrast arthrography of the knee. Its value in the management of two hundred and twenty-five knee derangements. *J. Bone Joint Surg.*; **52A**: 203–220

Noyes FR, Stabler CL (1989) A system of grading articular cartilage lesions at arthroscopy. *Am. J. Sports Med.*; **17**: 505–513

Noyes FR, McGinnis GH, Modar LA (1984) Functional disability in the anterior cruciate insufficient knee syndrome: a review of knee rating systems and projected risk factors in determining treatment. *Am. J. Sports Med.*; **1**: 278–302

Schatzker J, Lambert DC (1979) Supracondylar fractures of the femur. *Clin. Orthop. Rel. Res.*; **138**: 77–83

Scott GA, Jolly BL, Henning CE (1986) Combined posterior incision and arthroscopic intra-articular repair of the meniscus. An examination of factors affecting healing. *J. Bone Joint Surg.*; **68A**: 847–861

Siliski JM, Mahring M, Hofer HP (1989) Supracondylar and intercondylar fractures of the femur treated by internal fixation. *J. Bone Joint Surg.*; **71A**: 95–104

Spiers ASD, Meaguer T, Ostlere SJ, Wilson DJ, Dodd CAF (1993) Can MRI of the knee affect arthroscopic practice? *J. Bone Joint Surg.*; **75B**: 49–52

Tegner Y, Lysholm J (1985) Rating systems in the evaluation of knee ligament injuries. *Clin. Orthop. Rel. Res.*; **198**: 43–49

Tegner Y, Lysholm J, Lysholm M, Gillquist J (1986) A performance test to monitor rehabilitation and evaluate anterior cruciate ligament injuries. *Am. J. Sports Med.*; **14**: 156–159

Tegtmeyer CJ, McCue FC, Higgins SM, Ball DW (1979) Arthography of the knee: a comparative study of the accuracy of single and double contrast techniques. *Radiology*; **132**: 37–41

Volpin G, Dowd GSE, Stein H, Bentley G (1990) Degenerative arthritis after intra-articular fractures of the knee. Long-term results. *J. Bone Joint Surg.*; **72B**: 634–638

Chapter 24

The ankle

A. H. R. W. Simpson

What the outcome instruments of ankle trauma need to measure

Ankle fractures vary in the amount of displacement, the amount of damage to the articular surface and the amount of disruption of the ligamentous structures, therefore the optimum treatment depends on the whole injury complex. Various systems exist for classifying ankle trauma; the most commonly used are the ASIF and Lauge-Hansen systems. The final result, however, depends mainly on the position of the fracture after treatment.

The consequences of the injury will vary according to the patient; for instance the risk of complications in women over the age of 50 is thought to be greater than in younger male patients (Beauchamp *et al.*, 1983). Therefore, the best treatment option for an elderly woman with a low functional demand may be non-operative whereas for a young male it may be surgical. Thus the optimum type of treatment must depend on the patient and not on the ankle injury alone and any evaluation should take this into account.

When a patient sustains an injury, we would like to know both the early result and the late result of the treatment of this patient. The patient's assessment of health status could be considered under the three D's; discomfort, disability and dissatisfaction (White, 1967). The last of these is mainly determined by the patient, the clinician and the patient–clinician interaction rather than the procedure itself. Methods for measuring this are discussed by Fitzpatrick (1993). Discomfort (pain) and Disability (function) may be considered according to the schema shown in Figure 24.1. Early is used here to refer to the result at the end of treatment, i.e. within 6 months of injury. Late is used to refer to the result several years later when function and pain scores may have deteriorated due to post-traumatic osteoarthritis.

Ideally a patient should be assessed for the rest of their life (Figure 24.2). However, this is not feasible so instead the result should be 'sampled' at various stages.

The minimum number of sample points that define the result and the times postoperative depend on the pattern of deterioration with time. Different patients may have different patterns of deterioration

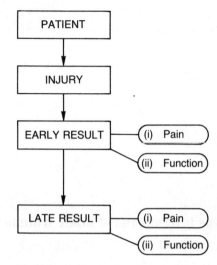

Figure 24.1 Schema for assessing discomfort and disability

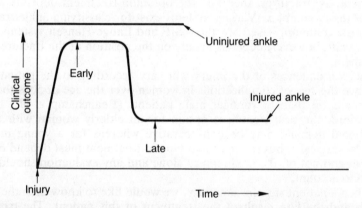

Figure 24.2 Hypothetical picture of how the clinical outcome may change with time from injury

(Figure 24.3); it would be useful to know whether the results have a plateau or whether they continue to deteriorate and also whether the function and pain scores run in parallel.

It would also be useful to know how a particular complication will alter the pain and functional outcomes and the risk of this complication occurring (Figure 24.4).

There is debate about whether the measures of pain and function should be objective or subjective. Historically clinicians (without any sound rationale) have struggled to find objective measures of pain and function, in the belief that these measures were more reliable and a better indicator of the quality of the procedure. If the means of measuring the objective result is unreliable it is better to measure the subjective result directly in each patient. For this reason there is now a move to place

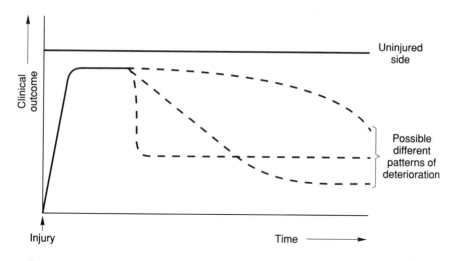

Figure 24.3 Different patients may have different patterns of deterioration of their outcome scores. In addition, the component scores may be affected at different rates

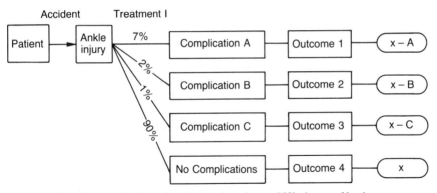

Figure 24.4 In this example the patient is thought to have a 90% chance of having no complications and a 7, 2 and 1% chance of having complications A, B and C respectively. The complications A, B and C have each been found to reduce the outcome score by a, b and c respectively from the 'complication free' score of x

more emphasis on good subjective instruments which measure the results of pain and function more directly (Wright and Feinstein, 1992).

The outcome measures that have been used and are currently commonly used for assessing the result of treatment of ankle injuries

The outcome measures used for pain and function will be considered under the subheadings subjective and objective.

A. Pain

Subjective

Magnusson (1944) used a 3-point scale, asking the patients whether the pain was constant, intermittent or absent. Brooks *et al.* (1981) gave 3 points out of a score of 15 for 'subjective pain', they then added this to scores for each of the following: pain on stressing the ankle (presumably in inversion); plantar flexion; swelling and bruising. The majority of studies, however, have used a 'semiobjective' system relating the pain to activity or analgesic use.

More recently, much work has been done on other instruments, such as the McGill Pain Questionnaire and visual analogue scales (cf. Chapter 2). Melzack's McGill Pain Questionnaire has been tested for reliability and validity extensively, but not in the context of ankle injury. There are several different ways of scoring the questionnaire, some of which are laborious, however it is considered by some authors (e.g. McDowell and Newell, 1987) to be the leading instrument for describing the various dimensions of pain. Visual analogue or numerical scales have the advantage that they are quick and simple to apply. The visual analogue scales were tested for reliability and repeatability in rheumatology patients (again not specifically for the ankle) by Scott and Huskisson (1979). They found good reliability with a correlation of 0.99 for the scores from horizontal and vertical scales of patients. For validity, they compared the scores to a descriptive pain rating scale of slight, moderate, severe or agonising and found correlations of 0.71 to 0.78*.

Objective

The majority of studies attempt to make the assessment of pain 'semi-objective' by asking the relationship between pain and activity. The majority of the studies in the literature (e.g. Magnusson, 1944; Burwell and Charnley, 1965) only assess pain on a 3-point scale of good, fair and poor. This is known to be insensitive and unreliable (Olerud and Molander, 1984), especially as patients have a desire to please their surgeon. Joy *et al.* (1974) and Olerud and Molander (1984) have increased this to a 5-point scale and specified the categories more clearly (Tables 24.1, 24.2). Phillips *et al.* (1985) and Mazur *et al.* (1979) are two of the few studies that provide a more comprehensive assessment of pain. They relate this to activity on a 50-point scale, although there are really still only six categories (Table 24.3, Figure 24.5). The second method of 'semiobjective' assessment is to try and quantify the amount and strength of analgesia used (Table 24.3). However, Phillips *et al.* (1985) attribute 50 points out of 54 for pain after activity and 4 out of the 54 points for the need for analgesic medication. The scores for these two techniques are simply added, thus there is a relative weighting of the former method of

---

* Editors' note: The correlation statistic indicates an association and is not an appropriate test for validity.

Table 24.1 Scoring system of subjective clinical evaluation

Score	Subjective clinical result
4	No pain; normal ankle
3	Pain is noted only after severe and prolonged stress; participation in sports and ability to walk or work not limited
2	Pain is moderately incapacitating, but no cane or other walking aid is used; mild analgesics are occasionally required; walking is restricted, but patient is able to walk more than five blocks; patient may have changed occupations due to painful ankle but works full-time and has had no reduction in pay
1	Pain is severe and may require use of a brace or cane and daily analgesics; walking is restricted to less than five blocks; patient is unemployable on a full-time basis due to the ankle but is able to care for himself
0	Pain is constant and incapacitating; patient is unable to walk sufficiently to care for himself and desires fusion of the ankle

Reproduced from Joy *et al.*, 1974.

Table 24.2 The Olerud and Molander scoring system

Parameter	Degree	Score
I. Pain	None	25
	While walking on uneven surface	20
	While walking on even surface outdoors	10
	While walking indoors	5
	Constant and severe	0
II. Stiffness	None	10
	Stiffness	0
III. Swelling	None	10
	Only evenings	5
	Constant	0
IV. Stair-climbing	No problems	10
	Impaired	5
	Impossible	0
V. Running	Possible	5
	Impossible	0
VI. Jumping	Possible	5
	Impossible	0
VII. Squatting	No problems	5
	Impossible	0
VIII. Supports	None	10
	Taping, wrapping	5
	Stick or crutch	0
IX. Work, activities of daily life	Same as before injury	20
	Loss of tempo	15
	Change to a simpler job/part-time work	10
	Severely impaired work capacity	0

Table 24.3 Clinical scoring system

Subjective (80 points)
Pain (54 points)
    Always alter any activity ... 0
    Prolonged after mild activity ... 10
    Transient after mild activity ... 20
    Prolonged after heavy activity ... 35
    Transient after heavy activity ... 40
    None ... 50
    Requires medication for pain regularly ... 0
    Requires medication occasionally ... 2
    Requires no medication ... 4
Function (26 points)
    Unable to climb stairs ... 0
    Uses normal foot first ... 1
    Requires aid of banister ... 2
    Climbs normally ... 3
    Unable to descend stairs ... 0
    Uses normal foot first ... 1
    Requires aid of banister ... 2
    Descends normally ... 3
    Walks < 1 block ... 0
    Walks < 5 blocks ... 2
    Walks < 10 blocks ... 3
    Walks > 10 blocks ... 5
    Walks unlimited distances ... 6
    Recreational activities limited ... 0
    No activities limited ... 3
    Requires walker ... 0
    Requires crutches ... 1
    Requires one crutch ... 2
    Requires cane ... 4
    Requires no aids ... 8
    Dissatisfied ... 0
    Moderately satisfied ... 2
    Very satisfied ... 3
Objective (20 points)
Gait (6 points)
    Antalgic limp ... 0
    External rotation gait ... 3
    Normal gait ... 6
Range of motion: difference from normal side (14 points)
    Dorsiflexion
        Difference > 20 degrees ... 0
        Difference 10–20 degrees ... 2
        Difference < 10 degrees ... 4
        No difference ... 7
    Plantar flexion
        Difference > 20 degrees ... 0
        Difference < 20 degrees ... 2
        No difference ... 3
    Supination
        Difference > 0 degrees ... 0
        No difference ... 2
    Pronation
        Difference > 0 degrees ... 0
        No difference ... 2

Reproduced from Phillips *et al.*, 1985.

Pain
    None, or patient ignores it 50
    Slight when going up or down stairs or
        walking long distances (no restriction
        of activities of daily living) 45
    Moderate when going up or down
        stairs or walking long distances;
        none during level gait; occassional
        non-narcotic medication needed 40
    During level gait, with more pain on
        stairs; none at rest; daily medication
        used 25
    At rest or at night in addition to during
        walking; narcotic medication required 10
    Continuous, regardless of activity 0
    Disabled because of pain 0

                                            Total ———

Function
    Limp, antalgic
        None 6
        Slight 4
        Moderate 2
        Marked 0

                                            Total ———

    Distance
        Unlimited 6
        4–6 blocks 4
        1–3 blocks 2
        Indoors only 1
        Bed-chair 0
        Unable to walk 0

                                            Total ———

    Support
        None 6
        Cane, long walks only 5
        Cane, full time 3
        2 canes or crutches 1
        Walker required or unable to walk 0

                                            Total ———

Hills (up)
    Climbs normally 3
    Climbs with foot externally rotated 2
    Climbs on toes or by side-stepping 1
    Unable to climb hills 0

                                            Total ———

Hills (down)
    Descends normally 3
    Descends with foot externally rotated 2
    Descends on toes or by side-stepping 1
    Unable to descend 0

                                            Total ———

Stairs (up)
    Climbs normally 3
    Needs banister 2
    Steps up with normal foot only 1
    Unable to climb stairs 0

                                            Total ———

Stairs (down)
    Descends normally 3
    Needs banister 2
    Steps down with normal foot only 1
    Unable to descend stairs 0

                                            Total ———

Ability to rise on toes (stability)
    Able to rise on toes × 10 repetitions 5
    Able to rise on toes × 5 repetitions 3
    Able to rise on toes × 1 repetition 1
    Unable to rise on toes 0

                                            Total ———

Running
    Able to run as much as desired 5
    Able to run but limited 3
    Unable to run 0

                                            Total ———

Range of motion
    Dorsiflexion beyond neutral 5
        40 degrees 4
        30 degrees 3
        20 degrees 2
        10 degrees 1
        5 degrees 0
        0 degrees

                                            Total ———

Plantar flexion
    40 degrees 5
    30 degrees 4
    20 degrees 3
    10 degrees 2
    5 degrees 1
    0 degrees 0

                                            Total ———

Figure 24.5 An ankle grading system. (Reproduced from Mazur *et al.*, 1979)

$50/4 = 12.5$. Whether this is a suitable weighting is not validated. If linear scales were being used and the extremes of the scale were the same, i.e. if the regular narcotic analgesia was thought to equate with constant severe pain, then it would be more logical to give the methods of scoring equal weighting. (The patients were assessed by questionnaire on one occasion at a variable time after operation. This may also have affected the outcome.) However, their analysis of pain is superior to many other ankle studies.

Late versus early scores

Most of the studies quoted test for pain (and function) on one occasion (exceptions to this are Finsen *et al.* (1989) and Brooks *et al.* (1981)). These studies assume a normal ankle prior to injury, which seems reasonable unless there is any history to contradict this. The period of follow-up, even within a single study, varies widely, e.g. 1–7.5 years in the Joy *et al.*, (1974) study. Most of the trials do not test early and late and, therefore, the measures have not been tested for their responsiveness, i.e. their sensitivity in detecting a change between tests on different occasions.

B. Functional outcome

The majority of the early studies used a system for 'objective' assessment. Some of the more recent studies use a more subjective functionally related assessment.

Subjective instruments

As Olerud and Molander (1984) state: 'what really counts, however, is the total clinical end result, which is more difficult to describe as relevant functional aspects have to be included. These subjective symptoms seem to be a major problem as regards recording them in a reproducible way.'

Beauchamp *et al.* (1983) simply asked their patients whether they were satisfied or not, and Burwell and Charnley (1965) simply divided them into: Good, Fair and Poor, as follows:

Good   Complete recovery apart from slight aching after use.
Fair   Aching during use, slight stiffness (not enough to interfere with work). Ability to walk not seriously* impaired.
Poor   Any serious impairment of ability to work or walk. Pain.

Many patients with ankle fractures are young and wish to return to sporting activities. There is no mention of these in these analyses nor is there any consideration of the more mundane but important activities of driving, cycling or even climbing stairs.

Phillips *et al.* (1985) in their study include questions on the ability to climb stairs and to do sport, as well as on the length of time the patients can walk. Also, the need for any ambulatory aids is questioned. Only 3 of the 26 points are allocated to recreational activities. For some patients this may be a critical part of their functional demand of their ankle. For these patients this scoring system will not be sensitive enough to detect a deterioration in this aspect. Indeed, as the authors themselves admit, the assignment of numerical values to their scores was an arbitrary process.

The difficulty with these questionnaires is knowing what weighting to give to each of these activities. For instance, Olerud and Molander (1984) give 5 points for running, 5 for squatting and 5 for jumping out of 55 points for function, whereas Phillips *et al.* (1985) gave 3 points out of 26 for recreational activities. Therefore, the weightings are: $15/55 = 0.3$ and $3/26 = 0.1$. The problem is that the relative importance of recreational

---

* What 'serious' entails is not defined

activities such as running will differ for different patients and hence the relative weighting will vary from patient to patient. An assessment based on the relative importance of these activities is therefore required, and is being evaluated by Davis (1993).

'Objective' instruments

All of the following objective measures of function have been used at variable times after injury.

RANGE OF MOVEMENT (ROM)

A few studies have taken measures of ROM independently.

The ankle joint

Lindsjo et al. (1985) describe a simple method for measuring loaded ankle dorsiflexion, which they used in 317 patients who had had ankle fractures. They state that it was found to give more reproducible results than with unloaded measurements, but unfortunately the evidence of reliability is not given. The range of dorsiflexion and plantar flexion has been used by other authors (Zenker and Nerlich, 1982; Rowley et al., 1983) and said to correlate well with function. Ahl et al. (1988) also used this outcome and give estimates of error of 5% for loaded dorsiflexion and 6% for loaded plantar flexion. Clapper and Wolf (1988) diligently examined the reliability of a standard goniometer and an 'orthoranger' pendulum device. They found reasonable reliability for both techniques (Intraclass Correlation Coefficients 0.8–0.96).

The various inaccuracies of measurement of ankle ROM must be analysed when considering using this as an outcome measure as summarised by O'Doherty (1993). Intraobserver reliability is considerably better than interobserver reliability (Elveru et al., 1988) and, therefore, the same observer should make all the measurements in the study. The ability of other joints, e.g. the subtalar joint/midtarsal joint, in the foot to compensate for a reduced range of ankle motion (Mazur et al., 1979) must be borne in mind for two reasons:

1. The perceived ROM of the ankle will be increased.
2. Compensating movements at other joints may mean that there is no overall loss of function.

In addition, because the range of normal ankle movement is variable (American Academy of Orthopaedic Surgeons, 1965), it is standard practice to give the results as a percentage of the uninjured side. Although at first sight this appears reasonable, it does not necessarily follow that the percentage of ROM compared to the opposite side will correlate better with function than the actual value in degrees for the ROM. For instance if 10 degrees of dorsiflexion was needed for normal gait (Lindsjo, 1985), then a person who normally has ankle dorsiflexion of 20 degrees will have an impaired gait after a 50% reduction in ROM, whereas a hyperlax individual with a normal range of dorsiflexion of 35 degrees will have an impaired gait only after they have lost more than 70% of their normal dorsiflexion.

For the present both the percentage compared to the opposite side and the actual ROM should be recorded (both with estimates of reliability).

Subtalar and midtarsal joints

The ROM at the subtalar and midtarsal joints may have a major bearing on function. These are notoriously hard to measure accurately. Rowley *et al.* (1983) have described a system for the subtalar joint utilising the angle of progression of the foot. Some results for the reliability of this technique are given (Rowley, 1985). They do, however, attempt to correlate their results with pain severity.

SWELLING

Most of the studies quoted have not recorded whether the swelling was subjectively or objectively measured. This is essential, as Lindsjo (1985) has found that there was no correlation between these two assessments. Rarely have investigations attempted to measure swelling. Until swelling is shown to be related to pain or function its use as an outcome measure will remain limited. However, Drabu (1987) does point out that swelling may cause discomfort with footwear. He then goes on to describe and test a system for assessing swelling based on the soft tissue thickness, measured from X-rays, over the malleoli on the injured and uninjured sides. Unfortunately, he gives no figures for the reliability of this technique.

MUSCLE BULK

Magnusson (1944) in his study just comments on whether muscle wasting was present or not. Klossner (1962) used a 1-cm difference of calf circumference as the cut off for deciding whether muscle wasting was present or not. The accuracy of his measurement technique is not given, nor is the justification for the 1-cm limit. Ahl *et al.* (1988) also measured the calf circumference. Their technique is not given but the standard deviation of their measurements was 2%.

As the muscle bulk reflects the overall usage of the limb compared to the other side, the bulk may actually give an effective 'integration' of the true use of the limb. However, this may be confounded by: swelling due to a deep vein thrombosis; or by bilateral wasting because the patient's level of activity has decreased; or when the patient's level of activity may be maintained by performing more work with the uninjured ankle. Despite these problems, this may be a measure that would be useful to assess for reliability and validity in future studies.

PASSIVE STIFFNESS

Patients sometimes complain of stiffness after ankle injuries, however only recently has this been measured objectively. A system has been described for measuring ankle stiffness which has been evaluated on the normal population and found to have a reliability of 0.77–0.94 (Chesworth and Vandervoort, 1989; Chesworth et al., 1991; Vandervoort *et al.*,

1992). Chesworth and Vandervoort are currently evaluating their system for patients recovering from ankle fractures.

INSTABILITY

Stiehl *et al.* (1989) describe a system for biomechanically testing the effects of syndesmosis screws on ankle stability in cadaveric specimens. In patients, stress radiographs, ankle arthrograms and peroneal tenography have all been used to try to assess the degree of disruption of the lateral ligament complex. However, as relatively few ankle ligament injuries are operated upon acutely there is no good evidence for the degree of correlation of the radiographic technique with the anatomical disruption. The validity of these radiographic tests has also been questioned by Cass and Morrey (1984) as the values correlate poorly with symptoms of instability. However, after reconstruction Karlsson *et al.* (1988) report that their results of stress radiographs do correlate with symptoms. They standardised their measurement technique by using 'TELOS' equipment which applies a standard force of 150 N to the ankle. The clinical results have been assessed on a 4-point scale (Sefton *et al.*, 1979; St Pierre *et al.*, 1982):

Excellent	Full activity, including strenuous sports. No pain, swelling or giving-way.
Good	Occasional aching, only after strenuous exercise. No giving-way or feeling of apprehension
Fair	Some residual instability and remaining apprehension, although less than before operation.
Poor	Recurrent instability and giving-way in normal activities with episodes of pain and swelling. Need for re-operation.

The agreement between the clinical and radiographic measures is not given.

However, it is possible that the most important aspect of instability is the actual 'functional' instability. The functional instability in patients with inversion ligament injuries has been assessed by Konradsen and Ravn (1990) who used a specially constructed jig to measure peroneal reaction time.

GAIT ANALYSIS

As previously mentioned, Rowley *et al.* (1986) have described a simple form of gait analysis. If an outcome instrument for measuring the range of subtalar joint movement is needed, then their technique should be evaluated further for reliability and validity. However, at present, the need for any more detailed gait analysis than this is difficult to justify until the simpler and cheaper methods of assessment have been properly evaluated for reliability and validity.

Mazur *et al.* (1979) measured their patients both with and without footwear. They demonstrated that the gait after ankle arthrodesis is closer to normal when the patients are assessed whilst wearing shoes, which indicates that suitable footwear may improve a patient's function.

RADIOGRAPHIC

The quoted studies use X-rays for two reasons:

1. The assessment of fracture reduction.
2. To assess post-traumatic arthritis.

The assessment of fracture reduction
Many earlier studies used relatively inexact methods of internal fixation such as circlage wires and even chromic catgut (Klossner, 1962). The grades of reduction (Joy *et al.*, 1974) are fairly generous:

Good
- Normal or up to 2 mm of anterior, posterior or distal displacement of the medial malleolar fragment, if fracture is less than 3 mm distal to the plafond.
- Up to 2 mm* of anterior, posterior, or distal displacement of the medial malleolar fragment, if fracture is more than 3 mm distal to the plafond.
- Up to 2 mm* of displacement of the lateral malleolar fragment in any direction.
- Displacement of the posterior malleolar fragment not more than 2 mm in any direction.
- 0.5 mm of tilt of the talus or less. Other displacement of the talus of less than 0.5 mm.

Fair
- Anterior, posterior or distal displacement of the medial malleolar fragment of 2–5 mm, if fracture is less than 3 mm distal to the plafond; or displacement greater than 5 mm, if fracture is more than 3 mm distal to the plafond.
- Displacement of the lateral malleolar fragment of 2–5 mm.
- Medial, lateral, anterior or posterior shift of the talus of up to 1 mm.
- Minimum or questionable joint damage noted on the roentgenogram or at the time of surgery.

Poor
- Any value worse than the above.
- Any lateral tilt or shift of the medial malleolar fragment; definite axial rotation of the medial malleolar fragment; severe joint damage; any shift of the talus of more than 1 mm as measured by the weight-bearing line or medial clear space; any tilt of the talus greater than 0.5 mm.

Joy *et al.* (1974) assessed the accuracy of their technique to be only to within 1 mm. This was quite an achievement as their radiographs were performed while the patients were still in plaster. However, as Ramsey and Hamilton (1976) have shown even 1 mm of lateral shift of the talus leads to a 40% loss of contact surface area, this suggests that the measurement technique was not accurate enough.

The scales differ in different studies. For instance Klossner (1962), Burwell and Charnley (1965) and Beauchamp *et al.* (1983) used many different sets of criteria. Overall, as reductions have become more accur-

---

* The original article states 5 mm. However, it would seem likely that the authors intended 2 mm.

ate the trend has been for more accurate and stricter criteria of reduction. However this does make comparison between the studies more difficult.

There is a low correlation between these radiographic measures and the objective and subjective measures of function (Magnusson, 1944; Lindsjo, 1985). Although Klossner (1962) and Wheelhouse and Rosenthal (1980) consider this less of a problem, their objective and subjective measures have not been correlated. Joy et al. (1974), Sarkisian and Cody (1976) and Pettrone et al. (1983) tried to find other radiographic measures that correlated better with function. Sarkisian and Cody (1976) and Phillips et al. (1985) suggest that the talocrural angle is significantly correlated with the overall outcome score. However, the scores used in each of these studies have not been validated with function or pain and therefore the talocrural angle as a useful measure of reduction needs to be further evaluated.

To assess post-traumatic osteoarthritis

Some of the studies have tried to assess the wear in the ankle joint by taking measurements on late postoperative X-rays. For instance Klossner (1962) uses the score:

+++ Joint space completely or almost completely absent.

++ Joint space about half of that of the uninjured ankle. Osteophytic changes rather distinct. Sclerosis present.

+ Joint space barely decreased. Distinct moderately plentiful osteophytic excrescences at the edges of the joint space.

(+) A few yet distinct osteophytic excrescences at the edges of the joint space.

0 Normal radiographic appearance

These early postoperative radiographic measures do seem to have some ability to predict which patients will later develop radiographic degeneration of the ankle joint. For instance from Burwell and Charnley's paper (1965) the results shown in Table 24.4 can be deduced (i.e. the worse the reduction, the greater the risk of osteoarthritis on X-ray, but there is a low correlation between the patients with painful osteoarthritis and radiographic signs of osteoarthritis). Overall in this study 50 patients had X-ray signs of osteoarthritis: 22 had symptoms and 28 did not.

The assessment of X-ray evidence of osteoarthritis was ill defined but said to be on the basis of any diminution in joint space, irregularities of

Table 24.4 Postoperative radiographic measures and subsequent review results (Burwell and Charnley, 1965)

	Postoperative	At review	
	Quality of reduction	Total patients with radiographic signs of osteoarthritis (no.)	Patients with radiographic signs of osteoarthritis and pain (no.)
Anatomical	104	26	9
Fair	22	16	7
Poor	8	8	6

the articular surface and evidence of ossification at the joint margins. Burwell and Charnley (1965) and Klossner (1962) included marginal osteophytic changes in their arthritis scores even though they considered that they are not associated with a progressive arthritis.

Phillips *et al.* (1985) used a 3-point scale on the basis of the X-ray appearance related to osteophytes, joint space narrowing or periarticular cysts. There are also points arbitrarily given according to the presence of non-union, synostosis or osteoporosis. The rationale for these being included in the arthritis score is not given. The X-rays were rated by two observers and the worst score taken. Unfortunately the interobserver variability was not given.

The joint space narrowing (either the absolute value or in comparison with the opposite side) may be the most useful measure if: (i) it can be measured accurately and (ii) it is shown to be related to the level of symptoms or time to onset of symptoms. CT may improve the accuracy of this assessment (Magid *et al.*, 1990). The measurement may need to be done at one site to improve reliability, for instance the peak of the dome on the coronal plane. Secondly, the measurement may need to be taken with a standardised axial compressive load.

The situation with the joint space measurements seems to be similar to the ROM measurements: both quantities have a large degree of variation between individuals but far less so between the right and left sides. Once again it may well be more reliable to take the percentage of joint width compared to the uninjured side. However, it is possible that the absolute value will correlate more closely with the rate of onset (and possibly severity) of symptoms. If the joint space was narrower in elderly patients, (which is not a view held by Jonsson *et al.*, 1984), this would explain the higher incidence of symptomatic osteoarthritis in the older patients (Magnusson, 1944; Klossner, 1962; Burwell and Charnley, 1965).

There are several problems with these studies:

1. The relationship to symptoms.
2. The length of follow-up.

1. The relationship to symptoms
Klossner (1962) found that 'slight arthrosis did not seem to affect the patients subjective status to any degree, but severe arthrosis caused considerable inconvenience'. Using the same instrument, Magnusson (1944) and Burwell and Charnley (1965) found that the scores had a very low correlation with symptoms. More recently, Lindsjo (1985) confirmed this low correlation between the radiographic appearance and the symptoms. So to date, none of these arthritis scores has been shown to correlate well with the patients' symptoms.

2. The effect of length of follow-up
Klossner (1962) suggests the same fraction of patients have X-ray osteoarthritis in each of his groups (Table 24.5). Similarly Joy *et al.* (1974) found a similar fraction of patients with osteoarthritis in each of his follow-up groups (Table 24.6). However their criteria for reduction are such that those ankles that are destined to deteriorate may do so quickly and, therefore, any effect on increasing incidence of post-traumatic arth-

Table 24.5 X-ray osteoarthritis at follow-up: Klossner, 1962

Years of follow-up	Patients (no.)	Patients with osteoarthritis (no.)	% with osteoarthritis
2–3	72	23	32
3–7	65	15	23
> 7	45	13	29

Table 24.6 X-ray osteoarthritis at follow-up: Joy et al., 1974

Years of follow-up	Patients (no.)	Considered good (no.)	Fair/Poor (no.)
1–2	11	9	2
2–4	19	17	2
> 4	14	11	3

ritis with time may be hidden. Other authors (Yablon and Leach, 1989; Wright, 1990) suggest that post-traumatic arthritis may not become apparent until 5–10 years after injury.

The earlier series (Magnusson, 1944; Klossner, 1962; Burwell and Charnley, 1965) where criteria for reduction are less rigorous than current standards, should be disregarded as one would expect poorly reduced ankles to declare themselves much more rapidly. These studies, therefore, would not detect whether slight posterior displacement of the lateral or superior displacement of the posterior malleolus was relevant.

ANKLE JOINT FAILURE

As an alternative or a supplement to radiographic grading of osteoarthritis, the final failure (i.e. the need for arthrodesis) of the joint could be taken as an outcome measure. This is a good definitive end-point, however there are problems in using this because of its rarity (and therefore the need for a large, long-term study) and because the indications vary considerably according to the patient's demands, the risks of surgery and anaesthesia and surgeon preference.

COMBINED MEASURES

Klossner (1962) reviews 12 series of patients with ankle fractures between 1950 and 1961 that utilised a 3-point measure for the clinical result, dividing the results into 'good, fair or poor'. Burwell and Charnley (1965) also use a 3-point scale although it differs in the categories of ROM compared to the one used by Klossner (1962).

Burwell and Charnley's (1965) system divides the functional results into:

Good Ankle and foot ROM at least 75% normal, trivial swelling, normal gait.

Fair   Ankle and foot ROM at least normal, small amount of swelling, normal gait.

Poor   Ankle and foot ROM less than 50% normal, or swelling or limp.

There are several problems with this type of instrument:

1. It combines ROM, swelling, gait and limp in a fixed manner without any justification as to why the relative weighting of each should be as it is.
2. It does not specify what 'trivial' or 'small amount' refer to.
3. There is no justification as to whether the divisions for ROM relate to function.
4. There is no evidence that swelling affects function.

ANKLE TRAUMA SCORES

The majority of the papers, having measured a number of diverse items, give them various numbers, which in some studies is arbitrarily done (Phillips *et al.*, 1985). These numbers are then added to give an overall score. Very few of the studies (Joy *et al.*, 1974; Olerud and Molander, 1984) have tried to validate their scores with the clinical result. The study of Olerud and Molander has the most validation. However, their data are not interval and it may well be that the visual analogue scale on its own would have been as good an indicator of the overall clinical result.

At present the ankle trauma scores:

1. Do not appear to address the correct questions.
2. Have not been validated or tested for reliability.
3. Arbitrarily weight the different items chosen to be in the score.
4. Need to have different weighting for different patients but, at present, should keep the main components separate.

C. Complications

The recording of complications is variable in the different studies and the early and late outcome both for pain and function after a complication are not clearly recorded.

Thus, for instance, it is difficult to assess from the studies the additional morbidity of a wound infection and whether after treatment the late result was equivalent to other patients (cf. Chapter 12 of this volume and Frostick and Hunter, 1993).

The rationale for objective and subjective measures in evaluating ankle trauma

To answer the question: 'How has this particular patient faired after this ankle injury?', subjective instruments for both pain and function may be most appropriate, as shown in the schema in Figure 24.6.

However, to answer the question: 'For this patient, what is the optimum treatment for this injury?', we need to know how this patient

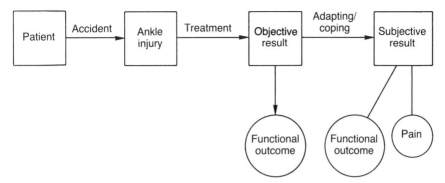

Figure 24.6 A schema to show the appropriateness of subjective instruments for both pain and function

differs from a 'standard' patient (for whom we should know the results of the various treatment options) in three ways:

1. How his/her functional demands are different?
2. How his/her response to pain differs?
3. How his/her relative risks of complications vary?

For this question both objective and subjective measures may have their role. The objective measures will be useful in building up a database for how the musculoskeletal system responds to injury and its treatment, which is more direct than measuring the final result which has been modulated by the patient's functional demands and ability to cope with pain and disability.

Research studies, it is hoped, will produce the baseline information of:

1. The expected objective result for each way of treating this type of injury.
2. The way in which the patient's functional demand and pain response (i.e. a patient profile) alter the subjective result for a given objective result (Figure 24.7).

So the combination of objective and subjective measures from previous studies as well as a profile of the patient's future requirements will help plan an individual's treatment.

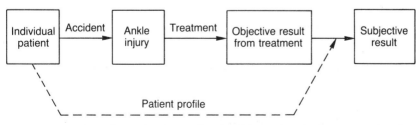

Figure 24.7 A schema illustrating the way functional demands and pain response alter the subjective result

Summary

1. The instruments used in studies on ankle trauma have not been adequately tested for reliability and validity.
2. There is a need for instruments to measure pain and function. At present there is no rationale for combining these components of health into a single index.
   Pain severity has been evaluated by relating its presence to activity levels and analgesic requirements. Linear analogue scales or McGill questionnaires have not been used to date for ankle injuries but may well be of value.
   Function: A number of objective measures, including ROM, muscle circumference, passive stiffness, joint width, have been made, but most have not been tested for reliability or validity. Olerud and Molander (1984) utilised a visual analogue score for subjective functional evaluation.
3. There may be a role for both objective and subjective measures and future studies should help us to understand the relationship between these two types of instrument.
4. The activity demands of patients have not been measured or controlled for in trials of treatment.

A number of the studies give overall clinical result scores. As already discussed the needs of each individual are different. For instance, whereas some patients may accept a minor amount of stiffness as long as the ankle is completely pain free, other patients may prefer to accept some mild discomfort in order to retain a full ROM. Therefore, the relative weighting put on discomfort and dysfunction by each patient differs. Simply to add a score for each of the components either with equal weighting or even with a fixed weighting may, therefore, be inappropriate.

Other abnormalities in the lower limb must also be taken into account.

Corollary

Several of the instruments for outcome assessment used in earlier studies exhibited a reasonable spread between categories (e.g. criteria of reduction). Nowadays, the vast majority of cases will lie in only one of the categories. This indicates that as treatments evolve, outcome instruments must also evolve so that they retain their sensitivity.

Group discussion

The chapter's summary was in agreement with the group's views. The group felt that Olerud and Molander's system was the best instrument but three shortcomings were highlighted, namely:

1. Weighting of the score.
2. Arbitrary numbers given for pain.
3. Too few points for function.

The group considered the optimum timing for an early assessment to be 1 year, and 10 years for a late assessment.

References

Ahl T, Dalen N, Selvik G (1988) Mobilisation after operation of ankle fractures. *Acta Orthop. Scand.*; **59**: 302–306

American Academy of Orthopaedic Surgeons (1965) *Joint Motion: method of measuring and recording.* Chicago: American Academy of Orthopaedic Surgeons

Beauchamp CG, Clay NR, Thexton PW (1983) Displaced ankle fractures in patients over 50 years of age. *J. Bone Joint Surg.*; **65B**: 329–332

Brooks SC, Potter BT, Rainey JB (1981) Treatment of partial tears of the lateral ligament of the ankle: a prospective trial. *Br. Med. J.*; **282**: 606–607

Burwell NH, Charnley DA (1965) The treatment of displaced fractures at the ankle by rigid internal fixation and early joint movement. *J. Bone Joint Surg.*; **47B**: 634–660

Cass JR, Morrey BF (1984) Ankle instability: current concepts, diagnosis, and treatment. *Mayo Clin. Proc.*; **59**: 165–170

Chesworth BM, Vandervoort AA (1989) Age and passive ankle stiffness in healthy women. *Phys. Ther.*; **69**: 217–224

Chesworth BM, Vandervoort AA, Koval JJ (1991) A pilot study to compare the subjective and objective evaluation of passive ankle joint stiffness. *Physiother. Can.*; **43**: 13–18

Clapper P, Wolf SL (1988) Comparison of the reliability of the Orthoranger and the standard goniometer for assessing active lower extremity range of motion. *Phys. Ther.*; **68**: 214–218

Davis A (1993) MSc Thesis, University of Toronto (in preparation)

Drabu KJ (1987) Soft-tissue swelling following fractures of the ankle. *Injury*; **18**: 401–403

Elveru RA, Rothstein JM, Lamb RL (1988) Goniometric reliability in a clinical setting. Subtalar and ankle joint measurements. *Phys. Ther.*; **68**: 672–677

Finsen V, Saetermo R, Kibsgaard L, Farran K, Engebretsen L, Bolz KD, Benum P (1989) Early postoperative weight-bearing and muscle activity in patients who have a fracture of the ankle. *J. Bone Joint Surg.*; **71A**: 2327

Fitzpatrick R (1993) Satisfaction and quality of life measures. In Pynsent PB, Fairbank JCT, Carr AJ (eds) *Outcome Measures in Orthopaedics.* Oxford: Butterworth-Heinemann, chap. 4, pp. 45–58

Frostick SP, Hunter JB (1993) Complications. In Pynsent PB, Fairbank JCT, Carr AJ (eds) *Outcome Measures in Orthopaedics.* Oxford: Butterworth-Heinemann, chap. 6, pp. 81–93

Jonsson K, Fredin HO, Cederlund CG, Bauer M (1984) Width of the normal ankle joint. *Acta Radiol. Diagn.*; **25**: 147–149

Joy G, Patzakis MJ, Harvey JP (1974) Precise evaluation of the reduction of severe ankle fractures. Technique and correlation with end results. *J. Bone Joint Surg.*; **56A**: 979–993

Karlsson J, Bergsten T, Lansinger O, Peterson L (1988) Lateral instability of the ankle treated by the Evans procedure. *J. Bone Joint Surg.*; **70B**: 476–480

Klossner O (1962) Late results of operative and non-operative treatment of severe ankle fractures. A clinical study. *Acta Chir. Scand. Suppl.*; **293**: 26–76

Konradsen L, Ravn JB (1990) Ankle instability caused by a prolonged peroneal reaction time. *Acta Orthop. Scand.*; **61**: 388–390

Lindsjo U (1985) Operative treatment of ankle fracture-dislocations. *Clin. Orthop. Rel. Res.*; **199**: 28–38

Lindsjo U, Danckwardt-Lilliest ROM G, Sahlstedt B (1985) Measurement of the motion range in the loaded ankle. *Clin. Orthop. Rel. Res.*; **199**: 68–71

McDowell I, Newell C (1987) *Measuring Health.* Oxford: Oxford University Press

Magid D, Michelson JD, Ney DR, Fishman EK (1990) Adult ankle fractures: comparison of plain films and three dimensional CT scans. *AJR*; **154**: 1017–1023

Magnusson R (1944) On the late results in non-operated cases of malleolar fractures. *Acta Chir. Scand. Suppl.*; 84

Mazur JM, Schwartz E, Simon SR (1979) Ankle arthrodesis: long term follow-up with gait analysis. *J. Bone Joint Surg.*; **61A**: 964–975

O'Doherty D (1993) The ankle and foot. In Pynsent PB, Fairbank JCT, Carr AJ (eds) *Outcome Measures in Orthopaedics.* Oxford: Butterworth-Heinemann, chap. 12, pp. 245–268

Olerud C, Molander H (1984) A scoring scale for symptom evaluation after ankle fracture. *Arch. Orthop. Trauma Surg.*; **103**: 190–194

Pettrone FA, Gail M, Pe D, Fitzpatrick T, Van Herpe LB (1983) Quantitative criteria for prediction of the results after displaced fracture of the ankle. *J. Bone Joint Surg.*; **65A**: 667–677

Phillips WA, Schwartz HS, Keller CS, Woodward HR, Rudd WS, Spiegel PG, Laros GS (1985) A prospective, randomised study of the management of severe ankle fractures. *J. Bone Joint Surg.*; **67A**: 67–78

Ramsey PL, Hamilton W (1976) Changes in tibio-talar area of contact caused by lateral talar shift. *J. Bone Joint Surg.*; **58A**: 346–357

Rowley DI (1985) An Investigation into the Mechanism of Injury and Treatment of Ankle Fractures. MD Thesis, University of Sheffield

Rowley DI, Norris SH, Duckworth T (1983) A simple method of gait analysis for the assessment of ankle fractures. *J. Bone Joint Surg.*; **65B**: 366

Rowley DI, Norris SH, Duckworth T (1986) A prospective trial comparing operative and manipulative treatment of ankle fractures. *J. Bone Joint Surg.*; **68B**: 610–613

St Pierre R, Allman F, Bassett FH, Goldner JL, Fleming LL (1982) A review of lateral ligamentous reconstructions. *Foot Ankle*; **3**: 114–123

Sarkisian JS, Cody GW (1976) Closed treatment of ankle fractures: a new criterion for evaluation – a review of 250 cases. *J. Trauma*; **16**: 323–326

Scott J, Huskisson EC (1979) Vertical or horizontal visual analogue scales. *Ann. Rheum. Dis.*; **38**: 560

Sefton GK, George J, Fitton JM, McMullen H (1979) Reconstruction of the anterior talofibular ligament for the treatment of the unstable ankle. *J. Bone Joint Surg.*; **61B**: 352–354

Stiehl JB, Needleman RR, Skrade DA (1989) The biomechanical effect of the syndesmotic screw on ankle motion. *AO/ASIF Dialogue*; **II**: 1–3

Vandervoort AA, Cheswort BM, Cunningham DA, Rechnitzer PA, Paterson DH, Koval JJ (1992) Age and sex effects on mobility of the human ankle *J. Gerontol. Med. Sci.*; **47**: 17–21

Wheelhouse WW, Rosenthal RE (1980) Unstable ankle fractures: comparison of closed versus open treatment. *South. Med. J.*; **73**: 45–50

White KL (1967) Improved medical care statistics and health services system. *Public Health Rep.*; **82**: 847–854

Wright JG, Feinstein AR (1992) Improving the reliability of orthopaedic measurements. *J. Bone Joint Surg.*; **74B**: 287–291

Wright V (1990) Post-traumatic osteoarthritis-a medico-legal minefield. *Br. J. Rheumatol.*; **29**: 474–478

Yablon IG, Leach RE (1989) Reconstruction of malunited fractures of the lateral malleolus. *J. Bone Joint Surg.*; **71A**: 521–527

Zenker H, Nerlich M (1982) Prognostic aspects in operated ankle fractures. *Orthop. Trauma Surg.*; **100**: 237–241

Chapter 25

The foot

D. O'Doherty

Introduction

The management of foot trauma is often less than ideal. Patient dissatis-faction may occur because of persistent symptoms or loss of function, which may delay or prevent return to work or sporting activities. In view of the extensive literature on the subject, it is surprising that there is little agreement on the classification of injuries (Perlman *et al.*, 1989) and their management. A number of reasons could account for this.

First, no acceptable definition exists for normality in the foot. Marked variations have been observed in healthy persons with asymptomatic feet, for shape (Staheli *et al.*, 1987; Steel *et al.*, 1980; Perlman *et al.*, 1989; Welton, 1992), joint range of motion (Oatis, 1988; Lundberg *et al.*, 1989a–c) and gait (Katoh *et al.*, 1983). In addition Roass and Anderson (1982) and Nigg *et al.* (1992) have demonstrated significant variations in the range of joint movement with age and sex. It seems illogical therefore to try and define the normal foot in anatomical terms. There is increasing evidence to suggest that a looser, more subjective, definition of normal is more appropriate (Steel *et al.*, 1980; Jahss, 1984; Myerson, 1989).

Secondly the anatomy and biomechanics of the foot are complex. Functionally the foot can be considered to act as a single unit in conjunc-tion with the ankle. The effects of injury to one part of the foot would therefore depend not only on the nature and severity of the injury, but also on the ability of the rest of the foot to compensate. Re-establishment of normal anatomy may not be necessary for a return of normal function in the foot following injury (Aitken, 1963). Once again this emphasises the importance of function, and suggests that more attention should be paid to what the foot can do, rather than its appearance when evaluating outcome.

Finally, the natural history of many of these injuries are not fully understood. Most reported studies are of small numbers of patients, studied retrospectively and with only a short period of follow-up. Out-come is seldom defined adequately in these studies and the methods of outcome evaluation vary from study to study. Interpretation of such data is next to impossible. In consequence, many different treatments have been described for these injuries but whether they offer a true benefit remains uncertain.

In order to determine the value of a specific treatment regimen for particular injuries, we need to be able to study patients prospectively in properly controlled trials. Injuries should be adequately classified and the appropriate outcome measures applied. Two themes recur throughout this chapter. The first is that the foot is a functional unit, and the major thrust of evaluation should be to examine its function as a whole rather than in its parts. The second is that objective measurements, which are the mainstay of many orthopaedic evaluations, have only a limited place in the assessment of the foot.

What should be measured?

In the final analysis the patient recovering from an injury is most concerned by what the foot is able to do. Evaluating the degree of residual disability is difficult (Burton and Wright, 1983). The ideal outcome measure should fulfil certain criteria: it should look as though it is measuring something useful (face validity); it should actually measure what it is claiming to (content validity); it should be accurate and reproducible (criterion validity); it should be sensitive to change (discriminatory validity); and it should correlate with an acceptable 'gold standard' of outcome. Unfortunately few of these criteria are fulfilled by outcome measures used in foot trauma, and there is no gold standard to aim for.

Objective data, such as ranges of joint motion, are commonly reported, because they are readily quantifiable and appear, superficially at least, to add the prestige of science to the study (Boring, 1961). However, their relation to function remains uncertain, and there are few studies of validity or reliability. Such data are probably less reliable than we would like to think (Feinstein, 1977) and their value overstated.

By contrast, subjective data, such as pain and disability, are traditionally held to be unreliable, implying that the data are somehow inherently bad (Jette, 1989). There is now a great weight of evidence to suggest that this is not so (Fries, 1983; Wood-Dauphinee and Troidl, 1986). In retrospect it is surprising that we can accept a patient's description of their symptoms for clinical decision-making but find the same descriptions suspect when describing the outcome of treatment. The fallacy of this is being increasingly recognised and there is growing awareness that the measurement of discomfort, functional limitation and dissatisfaction provide better measures of outcome than do most of the commonly used objective measurements.

Two further points need making. First, in any study the clinician must be aware of potential sources of measurement error, and attempt to minimise them. Three distinct sources have been identified from which measurement error can arise: the examiner, the examined and the examination itself. Common sources of error include: the inappropriate application of a clinical test, together with variations in the expertise of the examiner(s) in both applying and interpreting the test (the examiner); regression of extreme values towards the mean, effects of biological variability (the examined); the environment, relationship between the patient and clinician, and the instrument itself (the examination).

Secondly one should be aware that individual patients may react quite differently to apparently similar levels of physical impairment. This implies that one should be cautious not to overinterpret results.

Subjective evaluation of the foot and ankle

A consistent and recurring theme, in all studies into foot trauma and pathology, is the limited number of ways in which abnormality may be expressed clinically. Thus, significant deviation from normal tends to present, primarily, as pain, loss of function, swelling and stiffness. This implies that a painfree, supple foot which functions as it did prior to injury and is not swollen, might be a useful working definition of normal for the individual patient. This approach is advocated by Steel *et al.* (1980) who defined the normal foot as being painless, with no history of significant pain, disability, musculoskeletal disease or surgery, and without skin or soft tissue lesions. Indeed they preferred the term 'painless' rather than 'normal' foot. Further support comes from Jahss (1984), who felt that the rôle of surgery in the foot was to produce a flexible plantigrade foot with painless metatarsal head weight bearing, and Myerson (1989), who felt that the aim of treatment after injuries to the Lisfranc joint complex was to produce functionally painless weight bearing. It should be noted that each of these definitions is deliberately loose and does not necessarily imply the presence of 'normal' anatomy. Indirect support for lowering the emphasis on anatomy comes from the observations that some deformities, such as flexible flat feet, are very well tolerated (Staheli *et al.*, 1987), and that anatomical reduction of fractures does not always correlate with the functional outcome of treatment (Aitken, 1963).

Discomfort, disability and dissatisfaction are the subjective components of the assessment of health status described by White (1967). Although difficult to measure these variables are being increasingly advocated as criteria of successful treatment.

Measuring pain (see also Chapter 2)

Pain is a highly subjective sensory modality that is subject to various mechanisms which alter its perception by the patient. Thus the degree of disability associated with a given painful stimulus varies from individual to individual, and what may be incapacitating for one individual may be barely noticeable in another. This suggests that in addition to trying to measure pain intensity we need to know to what extent it affects function.

No objective methods for directly quantitating pain have been described, although dolorimetry which measures pain thresholds has been found useful in the assessment of algodystrophy (Bryan *et al.*, 1991; Sarangi *et al.*, 1991). In contrast, a number of subjective methods for evaluating pain have been reported.

The McGill Pain Questionnaire (MPQ) remains the 'gold standard' by which other methods of pain evaluation should be compared. This questionnaire measures the sensory and affective components of pain, in addition to its intensity. Three scores derive from this questionnaire: the Pain Rating Index; the total number of descriptive words chosen; and the Present Pain Intensity Index (PPI). It has proven validity and reliability (Reading, 1983), but is cumbersome and time-consuming, taking approximately 10 minutes to complete. This restricts its value both in the clinical and research setting. A shorter variation (Short Form McGill Pain Questionnaire – SFMPQ), which can be completed in approximately two minutes, has been described (Melzack, 1987). Validation studies suggest that this may be an acceptable alternative to completion of the entire questionnaire. Neither the MPQ nor the SFMPQ have been used in the evaluation of the traumatised foot and, in addition, they have not been used to validate any of the treatment alternatives employed.

Visual analogue scales (VAS) for pain have been widely used throughout medicine (Scott and Huskisson, 1976). Erdmann et al. (1992) used a VAS to assess pain following fractures of the os calcis but, in general, this method of evaluating pain has been ignored by clinicians interested in the foot. There are no clear reasons for this but it may reflect the retrospective nature of much of the literature on clinical disorders of the foot and ankle.

In the majority of studies on foot trauma pain has been evaluated using categorical scales, based on whether the pain was mild, moderate or severe (Rowe et al., 1963; Hawkins, 1970; Kenwright and Taylor, 1970; Wilson, 1972; Hardcastle et al., 1982; Flick and Gould, 1985; Szyszkowitz et al., 1985). In these scales assignation of the patient to a particular group was made by the clinician. The reliability of such methods is low, because of differences in clinicians' perceptions of patients' symptoms. Myerson et al. (1986) and Crosby and Fitzgibbons (1990) introduced more categories for pain, the latter study also distinguishing between the severity of pain on activity and at rest. The use of more categories has been shown to improve intraobserver reliability (Streiner and Norman, 1989) but, unfortunately, only at the expense of a reduction in interobserver reliability (Hutchinson et al., 1979). This suggests that scales of this type may be useful for individual clinicians in day-to-day practice, but their value in the research setting is very limited as they will not allow valid comparisons between studies.

For elective procedures on the foot some authors have tried to improve reliability by relating pain to functional activities (Mazur et al., 1979; McKay, 1983; Olerud and Molander, 1984; Bray et al., 1989; Lau et al., 1989; Merchant and Dietz, 1989; Karlsson and Peterson, 1991). Such scales might be expected to have improved interobserver reliability, in particular because they are more patient than clinician dependent, but as yet this has not been tested. La Tourette et al. (1980), Spector et al. (1984), Myerson et al. (1986), Brunet and Wiley (1987) and Crosby and Fitzgibbons (1990) have used such scales for foot trauma but only in limited numbers of patients. The value of this sort of scale therefore remains uncertain, although it appears promising.

In summary, none of the pain scales used for the assessment of the injured foot have been adequately tested. In the design of new scales, testing against the McGill Pain Questionnaire should be mandatory. The most promising avenues appear to be either the use of the Short Form McGill Pain Questionnaire or of scales that relate pain to function.

Measuring functional disability

Injuries that result in pain, stiffness or weakness in the foot or ankle will be likely to interfere with the normal function of the foot. This will have effects on all aspects of a patient's life, including the ability to work and play sport, together with activities of daily living. Documenting functional status would appear therefore to be a useful method for measuring outcome, as it provides indirect evidence of foot function.

The difficulty lies in knowing which are the important components to measure (Table 25.1). Useful data comes from a number of long-term follow-up reports on foot trauma, which although retrospective provide detail of the symptoms noted by patients (Essex-Lopresti, 1952; Lance et al., 1963; Nade and Monahan, 1973; Wilson, 1972; Bach Christensen et al., 1977; Lorentzen et al., 1977; Peterson et al., 1977; Sneppen et al., 1977; Canale and Kelly, 1978; Norgrave Penny and Davis, 1980; Hardcastle et al., 1982; Pozo et al., 1984; May et al., 1985; Brunet and Wiley, 1987; Myerson et al., 1986; Millstein et al., 1988; Myerson, 1991; Sangeorzan et al., 1990). The various components documented in these studies are listed in Table 25.1. Reviewing the measurement of outcome at the foot and ankle, O'Doherty (1993) noted six criteria of function that appeared to be in common usage: limitation at work; limitation of walking, running and sporting activities; ability to climb stairs; use of a support; presence of stiffness or a limp; and feelings of instability. These are similar criteria to those developed by Paley and Hall (1989) for a prospective study of os calcis fractures, and by the Painful Foot Centre at the University of Maryland (Myerson et al., 1986). Each of these criteria has face validity, appear to be easy to apply and to be clinically suitable.

Table 25.1 Commonly reported criteria of function in long-term follow-up studies in foot trauma: the specific criteria used have varied considerably from study to study

Time to return to work
Time to maximum recovery
Ability to return to work
Walking ability on different surfaces
Sport and recreational activity level
Activities of daily living
Use of support
Limp
Stiffness
Swelling
Stability
Shoe-wear
Cosmesis
Tiredness
Walking distance

Although it is recognised that this list may not be complete, these six criteria seem to cover the most important consequences of disability and should be the minimum information obtained in any functional assessment.

Measuring patient satisfaction

In contrast to the situation in elective foot surgery, overall patient satisfaction with treatment has not been widely reported after injury. The categorical scales used in elective surgery are meaningless because, in most instances, the foot is asymptomatic prior to injury, and these scales measure how a patient's symptoms have improved with treatment. Many factors will have a bearing on the level of patient satisfaction, including the patient's understanding of the severity of the initial injury, the patient and the patient–clinician interaction, in addition to the level of residual symptoms at the end of treatment. The method of questioning used and who the question is administered by also affect the answer received. The degree of patient satisfaction does not necessarily correlate with the relief of symptoms. On balance, therefore, no case can be made for the use of this index as an outcome measure in foot trauma.

Objective assessment

Many authors place great emphasis on foot shape, the presence or absence of deformity (as determined clinically or radiographically) and the ranges of motion of the various joints in the foot, for measuring outcome after injury. Indeed most reports on foot trauma document at least some objective measurements, most usually ankle and subtalar joint range of motion and the degree of osteoarthrosis. The popularity of these indices lies in the ease with which they can be measured and the prevailing belief that such data are accurate, meaningful and reliable. For the foot and ankle, the available data do not support such a faith in measurement and these data do not stand up well under scrutiny.

Only for patients with unilateral injuries do objective measures seem to be of use. A number of studies have demonstrated the remarkable similarity between the right and left feet, in terms of shape and range of motion (Thoren, 1964; Boone and Azen, 1979; Steel et al., 1980; Roass and Anderson, 1982; Jonsson et al., 1984; Backer and Kofoed, 1989; Perlman et al., 1989). This suggests that where only one foot has been injured the unaffected foot can act as a measure of normality.

Measuring ranges of movement

Measurement of joint ranges of motion are considered an acceptable clinical technique for evaluating disability, and are widely used in orthopaedic surgery (Boone and Azen, 1979). For a number of reasons, however, this acceptance may not be valid for the foot and ankle.

First, stiffness at a joint may reflect either loss of range of motion or a difficulty in getting the joint moving until it has 'loosened up'. This is an important distinction. A common complaint after foot trauma is of an intermittent limp but some of these patients may have regained their full range of motion. On the other hand, because of the foot's tremendous capacity to compensate, loss of range of motion may not have any functional effects and indeed, on occasion, may not have been noticed by the patient. While it seems reasonable to measure joint range of motion at the foot one should not overemphasise its importance.

Secondly, the available data on the accuracy and reliability of the measured joint ranges in the foot and ankle are a source of considerable concern. There is clear evidence that the reliability of measurement varies according to the joint under consideration (Low, 1976) and also that reliability is reduced with increasing complexity of joint movement (Gadjosik and Bohannon, 1987). Because the bones of the foot are small and irregular in shape, their axes are short and may be difficult to define accurately and reproducibly. In addition, the ranges of motion to be measured are usually small, which increases the magnitude of any measurement error.

Thirdly, there are few 'normal' data for ranges of motion at the foot and ankle. The available data suggest a great variability in what could be considered normal at each joint (Oatis, 1988). Range of motion in general appears to be greater in females and to vary with age (Nigg et al., 1992). This makes it important to detail the population from which range of motion measurements are being obtained.

Finally, the statistical methods used in studies on the reliability of joint range of motion have varied and may not have always been appropriate (Stratford et al., 1984). Most studies report reliability in terms of intraclass correlation coefficients (ICC) and/or Pearson product–moment coefficients. Each has associated strengths and weaknesses with the ICC being better at demonstrating systematic bias, but other tests may be better at examining the degree of agreement (Bland and Altman, 1986). In general, reliability coefficients of greater than 0.8 are considered good, and between 0.7 and 0.8 acceptable, but values less than 0.7 suggest that the test is unreliable.

Terminology

The movements of the ankle and foot are complex and three dimensional. For descriptive purposes, movements are described with reference to the cardinal planes of the trunk, that is sagittal (or median), coronal (or frontal) and transverse (or horizontal). These movements are considered to occur around theoretical axes passing perpendicularly to these planes and are respectively described as dorsiflexion/plantar flexion, eversion/inversion and abduction/adduction (Kirkup, 1988; Alexander, 1990). Combinations of plantar flexion, adduction and inversion produce supination, whereas dorsiflexion, eversion and abduction produce pronation. The true mechanical axes of movement of the various joints do not, however, pass through these theoretical axes, and indeed for a given joint may vary in position throughout the range of movement (Lundberg et al.,

1989a). In consequence movements in the ankle–foot complex have vectors in all three cardinal planes, although in any one particular joint one vector tends to predominate (Oatis, 1988; Lundberg et al., 1989b–d). For ease of measurement, it is usual to make the assumption that motion at a given joint is uniplanar but it should be recognised that this is at best a convenient approximation of the true situation and may be a source of error in the presence of gross joint malalignment.

Ankle joint

The predominant vector of motion at the ankle joint is in the sagittal plane and it is a reasonable assumption to use dorsiflexion and plantar flexion as measures of ankle motion, at least during the stance phase of gait (Scott and Winter, 1991). Clearly, however, in the presence of gross ankle malalignment sagittal motion will not necessarily be due to ankle dorsiflexion and plantar flexion and, under these circumstances, data should be interpreted with caution. In addition, although a fixed axis is assumed for convenience, the true axis of motion appears to vary slightly throughout the range of movement (Lundberg et al., 1989a).

There remains no clear consensus regarding the best way to measure ankle motion. Some authors measure passive range of motion (Backer and Kofoed, 1989; Porter et al., 1990;), some active (Boone and Azen, 1979) and still others recommend that the range of motion in the weight-bearing ankle be measured (Rowley et al., 1986; Olerud and Molander, 1984). There is also debate as to whether the knee should be extended or flexed at the time of measurement (Roass and Anderson, 1982; Olerud and Molander, 1984; Rowley et al., 1986). All of these clinical methods of measurement may be subject to error due to difficulty in isolating tibio-talar movement, and in detecting the axes of motion (Backer and Kofoed, 1989). Indeed, up to 40% of plantar flexion occurs in the arch of the foot (Lundberg et al., 1989b), and this can be a cause of significant error for the unwary. Radiographic measurement of ankle range of motion is more accurate but is difficult to justify for routine usage (Backer and Kofoed, 1989).

Intraobserver reliability is high for active (Clapper and Wolf, 1988 – dorsiflexion ICC = 0.92 and plantar flexion ICC = 0.96) and passive (Elveru et al., 1988 – dorsiflexion ICC = 0.9 and plantar flexion ICC = 0.86) ankle range of motion. For passive ankle motion the reliability of measurement between observers was less good, that for dorsiflexion being unacceptably low (Elveru et al., 1988 – dorsiflexion ICC = 0.5 and plantar flexion ICC = 0.72). No data are available for active ankle motion, but experience at other joints suggests that interobserver reliability may be higher for active rather than passive movements (Gadjosik and Bohannon, 1987).

Some authors have recognised the difficulties with measurement of joint range of motion and have tried to record loss of motion by comparison with the unaffected ankle. Clearly these methods are only of use if the uninjured ankle joint is normal. Loss of motion has been described either as mild, moderate or severe (Hawkins, 1970; Martin et al., 1989) or as a percentage reduction compared with the normal ankle joint (Flick and Gould, 1985; Bray *et al.*, 1989). No reliability data are available for these methods.

The subtalar joint

Motion at the subtalar joint is also clearly triplanar, with the predominant vector in the coronal plane, producing inversion and eversion. The axis of movement varies considerably from individual to individual (Inman, 1976), so that it comes as no surprise to find even greater variations in the reported normal ranges than have been observed for the ankle joint. Inman (1976) observed that the total range of movement of the subtalar joint could vary from 10 to 65 degrees (mean 40 degrees); measurement was made using a special goniometer designed to measure triplanar motion. Elveru *et al.* (1988) found intertester reliability to be poor, both for inversion (ICC = 0.32) and eversion (ICC = 0.17). However, intratester reliability was acceptable (ICC = 0.75 for eversion and ICC = 0.74 for inversion). They commented that using the subtalar joint neutral position as the starting point for measuring motion, as recommended by some authors (Alexander, 1990), consistently reduced reliability.

As with measurement of ankle joint motion, a number of authors have tried to overcome these difficulties by comparing overall range of subtalar motion to the unaffected foot, either qualitatively (Hawkins, 1970; Lau *et al.*, 1989; Kitaoka, 1991) or as a percentage change (Crosby and Fitzgibbons, 1990; Leicht and Kofoed, 1992). Leicht and Kofoed (1992) scored subtalar motion as a fraction of the range in the unaffected foot but did not find the method to be reproducible. No other reliability data are available for these methods.

Other joints in the foot

The anatomical complexity and the number of articulations in the midfoot mean that movements can be only grossly assessed (Alexander, 1990). No method has been described to clinically measure the motion of these joints individually, although Lundberg *et al.* (1989b–d) have studied the joints using stereophotogrammetric techniques. In the absence of objective data attempted quantitation of motion at these joints is inadvisable.

The metatarsophalangeal joints allow motion in the sagittal and transverse planes, whereas the interphalangeal joints allow motion only in the sagittal plane. The reported normal ranges are variable, which may be related, at least in part, to differences in measurement techniques (Norkin and White, 1985; Alexander, 1990). No reliability data are available.

Normal ranges of motion

For the foot and ankle there are few 'normal' data on which to base reference ranges of joint motion, much of this derives from inadequately described populations (American Academy of Orthopaedic Surgeons, 1965). Most of the available data are for the ankle joint, some data are also available for the subtalar and toe joints (Boone and Azen, 1979;

Roass and Andersson, 1982; Backer and Kofoed, 1987; Oatis, 1988; Backer and Kofoed, 1989). At each site, the range of normal values is large and there are significant differences between different measurement techniques. In addition, joint range varies with age and sex (Thoren, 1964; Nigg *et al.*, 1992). This marked heterogeneity, together with the questionable reliability of measurement, suggests that, at the foot and ankle, ranges of motion should not be compared to reference ranges. In all of the studies reported no difference was observed for values in the right and left feet, thus, for unilateral pathology, comparison against the opposite limb is valid.

Guidelines

Clearly there are significant difficulties with the measurement of joint range of motion in the foot and ankle, and this must be taken into consideration when trying to interpret such data. Because loss of mobility in the foot and ankle is a common complaint following injury, there is no doubt that it would be useful to be able to quantitate this loss when measuring outcome. The major problem lies with the reliability of measurement – there is clear evidence that this can be improved using simple guidelines.

Reliability is increased by the use of standard methods for examination (Ekstrand *et al.*, 1982), suggesting that protocols should be used. This appears to be more important than the particular measurement technique employed. The use of the neutral zero position, which represents the normal anatomical position of the body, is widely recommended as the starting point for the measurement of joint movements (American Academy of Orthopaedic Surgeons, 1965; Debrunner, 1982; Stratford *et al.*, 1984). Measurers should also be aware of end-digit preference and expectation bias. When studies are being reported the measurement technique used and the reliability of the measurements should be recorded.

In all reported studies intraobserver error is consistently lower than interobserver error. Thus, in serial studies the same investigator should perform all the measurements. This also implies that data from different studies cannot be directly compared.

There is general acceptance that visual inspection is an unreliable method for measuring joint movement (Hellebrandt *et al.*, 1949). Goniometric measurement is likely to be more reliable (Low, 1976) but as goniometers are accurate only to 5 degrees they will be subject to major inconsistency when measuring small ranges of movement. Unfortunately few of the investigators who have studied the reliability of goniometric measurement have used the same study design, making it difficult to draw firm conclusions. Nevertheless there is consensus in several areas. First, the use of different goniometers does not seem to affect reliability, so long as the goniometers are of appropriate size for the joint examined (Rothstein *et al.*, 1983; Stratford *et al.*, 1984). Secondly, the reliability of goniometric measurement varies from joint to joint, being least acceptable in small joints, such as those of the foot, where it is difficult to accurately identify the centre of motion, the axes of movement and consistent surface landmarks. Stratford *et al.* (1984) comment that reliability of goniometric measurement is improved when only one arm of the goniometer is moved.

More sophisticated measuring devices have been employed by some authors in attempts to improve accuracy and reliability. Electrogoniometers have been used in some laboratories to measure joint angles during walking. The accuracy of these devices, particularly those based on potentiometers, has been questioned (Whittle, 1991). Pendulum goniometers have also been used but their accuracy in the foot and ankle does not appear to be as good as simple goniometry (Clapper and Wolf, 1988).

With consistent positioning of the foot the most accurate method for measuring joint motion is from radiographs, as it isolates the joint concerned thus removing error due to the use of surface landmarks (Backer and Kofoed, 1989; Bohannon *et al.*, 1989). Backer and Kofoed (1989) have demonstrated that with rigorous conditions the dose of radiation can be very small but nevertheless found radiography difficult to justify for routine usage.

In summary, the reliability of measurements of joint range of motion at the foot and ankle are suspect. Intertester reliability in particular is low, suggesting that direct comparisons of data between studies are not valid (Boone and Azen, 1979; Stratford *et al.*, 1984; Gadjosik and Bohannon, 1987; Elveru *et al.*, 1988a). Intratester reliability is general acceptable implying that serial measurements should be made by the same tester for a given study. It should be mandatory to document the measurement techniques used, and the reliability of these measurements must be stated. The demographics of the patients under study should also be recorded because of the observed variations in joint range with age and sex. Comparisons against nebulous 'normal ranges' should not be employed, but comparison to the unaffected limb is acceptable (Boone and Azen, 1979; Backer and Kofoed, 1989).

Measuring deformity

The same difficulties that apply to the measurement of joint range also apply to the measurement of deformity. Again the main problem lies in trying to describe in two dimensions events that are triplanar. Fixed deformity can only be measured with the foot non-weight-bearing as the posture taken up by the weight-bearing foot reflects the compensatory actions of all the other joints in the foot (Oatis, 1988). Clinical measurement is difficult, for the reasons already described, and for this reason radiographic measurements are widely reported. But are these measurements valid? The difficulty once again lies in defining what is normal.

Steel *et al.* (1980) studied the feet of 41 asymptomatic female volunteers in the age range 40–60 years, demonstrating that many of the commonly used radiographic measurements appear to have reference ranges that are either too narrow or are inaccurate. The findings of this study, which remains the most comprehensive of its kind, should nevertheless be interpreted cautiously. First, the population under study was a select group. Secondly no data is given on intra- and interobserver reliability. Thirdly, the population under study was small, as shown by the non-Gaussian distributions observed for some variables. Nevertheless, this paper clearly demonstrates the heterogeneous structure of the foot, and despite its shortcomings its conclusions seem valid. The authors observed little difference between sides for all measurements and felt that comparison to the normal contralateral was meaningful. However, attempts to compare radiographs with a nebulous 'normal range' are not to be recommended.

Objective measures of function

Few authors have reported on simple objective measurements of function, even though many are routinely used in clinical practice. Reported measures include the measurement of calf girth (Thoren, 1964; Pozo et al., 1984; Flick and Gould, 1985), the detection of a limping gait (Hawkins, 1970; Wilson, 1972; Hardcastle et al., 1982; Paley and Hall, 1989), the detection of joint stiffness (Essex-Lopresti, 1952; De Lee and Curtis, 1982; Brunet and Wiley, 1987), an assessment of the ability to stand on heels and/or toes (Thoren, 1964; Hardcastle et al., 1982; Pozo et al., 1984; Brunet and Wiley, 1987) and to hop (Pozo et al., 1984) and the measurement of heel height and width (Thoren, 1964; Harding and Waddell, 1985). It would seem logical to carry out simple measures of function, if for no other reason than to confirm the subjective statements of the patient. Most of these measures have face and content validity, but the accuracy and reproducibility of measurement have not been ascertained. This would appear to be a neglected area of evaluation.

Gait analysis

Clinical gait analysis is defined as the systematic measurement, description and assessment of those quantities thought to characterise human locomotion (Davis, 1988). Normal reciprocating human gait consists of a series of complex but coordinated movements of the body and limbs. Failure of any of these mechanisms may produce a gait abnormality and it follows, therefore, that analysis of gait should provide an objective evaluation of the patient's function. In interpreting the data one should be aware that the observed gait pattern is not just the direct result of the underlying pathological process but, rather, the net result of the pathological process and the subject's attempts to compensate for it.

Simple visual inspection of gait is a routine part of orthopaedic practice but is unsystematic, entirely subjective and highly dependent on the skill of the observer (Whittle, 1991). Indeed even skilled observers may miss subtle gait changes and have difficulty quantifying simple gait parameters such as cadence, stride length and velocity (Saleh and Murdoch, 1985). Formal gait analysis attempts to rectify this situation. Enthusiasts claim that gait laboratory analysis provides a more stringent assessment of function than do either subjective analysis or clinical examination.

The use of gait analysis in measuring outcome after foot trauma has been very limited. Erdmann et al. (1992) measured walking distance on a treadmill, and weight-bearing under the heel in patients following os calcis fracture. Floyd et al. (1983) used the Harris-Beath mat to examine the foot–ground interface following the treatment of tendon lacerations in the foot, and May et al. (1985) used it, in conjunction with force-plate analysis, to examine outcome after surgery to extensive soft tissue defects in the foot. There are, therefore, virtually no data upon which to base value judgements of these methods in foot trauma. However, some comments can be inferred from data on other disorders of the foot (Kabada, 1988; O'Doherty, 1993). First, there are still few reliability data. Secondly, a comprehensive gait analysis produces such a large amount of data that analysis and interpretation can be difficult. In outcome studies statistical pattern recognition techniques may simplify the data analysis. For this reason interpreting the results of gait analysis remains an art rather than a science. These features suggest that gait analysis, in skilled hands may provide useful adjunctive information regarding function but, at present, cannot be considered useful for routine outcome measurement.

Osteoarthritis

The development of osteoarthritis is a recognised sequelae of foot trauma and a commonly recorded outcome measure (Canale and Kelly, 1978; Hardcastle et al., 1982; Pozo et al., 1984). However, use of a test is not justified purely on the grounds that it is in popular usage, and it is necessary to determine the validity of the measure (Wood, 1983). The rationale that significant joint disturbance will be associated with the development of osteoarthritis seems sound and is one of the reasons why reduction is advocated for displaced fractures in the foot (Wilson, 1972; Myerson et al., 1986; Mayo, 1987; Heckman and Champine, 1989; Crosby and Fitzgibbons, 1990; Sangeorzan et al., 1990). However, good outcomes can be achieved without exact anatomical reduction (Aitken, 1963) and, in addition, the clinical and radiological features of osteoarthritis correlate only poorly with symptoms (Goosens and De Stoop, 1983; Myerson et al., 1986; Brunet and Wiley, 1987; Bagge et al., 1991; Hart et al., 1991). This suggests that either clinical signs are a poor test for osteoarthritis or conversely that radiographs are a poor test for early osteoarthritis. At least some of the problems may lie with the radiographic scales. The scale devised by Kellgren and Lawrence is the most widely accepted radiographic scale but, together with its derivatives, places significant weight on the presence of osteophytes (Kellgren et al., 1963; Mazur et al., 1979; Hattrup and Johnson, 1988; Heim, 1989; Merchant and Dietz, 1989). This is now considered controversial and the criteria used in these scales may need to be more stringent to improve clinical relevance (Croft, 1990). The original aim of the scale of Kellgren and Lawrence was to define the grades of severity using standard radiographs of each joint so that surveys would be comparable if the same set of standard radiographs was used. Unfortunately, different studies use different sets of standards, making interpretation difficult and increasing interobserver error. In addition, there is difficulty in defining early or mild osteoarthritis.

At the knee joint scales based predominantly upon loss of joint space appear to be more reproducible than those based upon the presence of osteophytes (Dacre *et al.*, 1988; Cooper *et al.*, 1990) but this type of scale, although employed by Ahl *et al.* (1989) and Olerud and Molander (1984), has not been formally evaluated for the foot. Data on the width of the normal ankle joint has been provided for the ankle by Jonsson *et al.* (1984), but there are no data for other joints in the foot. The most important of their findings was the observation of no systematic difference between ankle joint width between the two sides, suggesting that the normal ankle could be used for comparison. The authors observed a significant difference in joint width for men and women, with no significant change with age. Using their data would give a reference range for men of 2.6–4.2 mm and for women of 2.1–3.7 mm. Values of 2.5 mm for men and 2.0 mm for women could, therefore, be considered abnormal. Wherever possible, however, comparisons should be made with the unaffected limb.

Reliability data for radiographic scales of osteoarthritis are scant. Both Wright and Acheson (1970) and Kellgren and Lawrence (1957) observed relatively poor intra- and interobserver reliability but do not give data for measurement of joint width alone.

The detection of osteoarthritis, and quantitation of its severity, has relevance as an outcome measure. Unfortunately, the radiographic scales in current usage are of dubious validity and their usefulness must be questioned. Scales based predominantly upon loss of joint width may have greater clinical relevance but have not, as yet, been adequately evaluated. Until an acceptable scale becomes available, it is suggested that data be interpreted cautiously.

Scoring systems

The concept of a global measure of outcome by which one could assess the overall response to treatment is attractive. Ideally such a scale would allow individual, as well as groups of patients to be monitored during follow-up to assess progress. In addition, it would offer the opportunity to compare different study groups in the assessment of treatments. Unfortunately, no scale has been devised that is universally acceptable for the foot.

Most reports on foot trauma categorise the results into excellent, good, fair or poor outcomes on the basis of various qualitative criteria, such as ability to work and severity of pain (Thoren, 1964; Kenwright and Taylor, 1970; Peterson *et al.*, 1977; Noble and McQuillan, 1979; Hardcastle *et al.*, 1982; Floyd *et al.*, 1983; Szyszkowitz *et al.*, 1985; Stephenson, 1987; Milstein *et al.*, 1988; Sangeorzan *et al.*, 1990). These scales were originally devised to deal with data that was collected retrospectively at a single point in time, and suffer from a number of flaws. They are not truly interval scales, usually each of the categories has several criteria, which tend to vary from study to study. In addition, the assignation of an individual to a particular category is based upon the clinician's perception of outcome, which has been demonstrated to be unreliable (Wood-Dauphinee and Troidl, 1986). Finally, there is a regrettable tendency to try to 'improve' data by combining the good and excellent results together. As most treatments might be expected to offer at least some benefit, this makes data interpretation very difficult. The only justification for the use of these scales is their popularity, and this should not be considered acceptable (Wood, 1983) as these scales are seriously flawed.

Recently there have been attempts to develop scoring systems for outcome which, potentially, offer increased discrimination between outcomes and better ability to compare data between studies. A number of different scales have been devised, for os calcis fractures (Rowe et al., 1963; Paley and Hall, 1989; Crosby and Fitzgibbon, 1990), talar fractures (Hawkins, 1970), tarsometatarsal fractures and dislocations (La Tourette et al., 1980; Myerson et al., 1986), metatarsal fractures (Spector et al., 1984) and soft tissues defects (Gidumal et al., 1986). Each of these scales has a similar basic design, with a proportion of the scale scoring pain and the remainder function. The main differences between the scales lie in the proportions of the scale given over to pain and function, and in the components of function that are considered important (Tables 25.2, 25.3). There are also strong similarities with other outcome scales in the foot and ankle, devised for ankle fractures (Joy et al., 1974; Olerud and Molander, 1984; Bray et al., 1989), ankle arthrodesis (Mazur et al., 1979; Kitaoka, 1991; Gruen and Mears, 1991), operative ankle arthroscopy (Martin et al., 1989), injuries to the lateral ligament of the ankle (St Pierre et al., 1982; Brunner and Gaechter, 1991; Karlsson and Peterson, 1991), osteochondritis of the talus (Flick and Gould, 1985), clubfoot surgery (Magone et al., 1989; Lau et al., 1989; McKay, 1983) and forefoot surgery (Kitaoka and Holliday, 1991). The fact that these scales are so similar suggests that most surgeons find the clinical expression of foot pathology to be remarkably consistent irrespective of its cause. It also suggests that, sooner or later, a consensus opinion will be reached to devise a general purpose outcome scale for the foot and ankle.

With the scales in current usage there are some obvious problems. First, old habits die hard, so that after scoring the outcome each of the scales described divides patients into excellent, good, fair and poor categories based on specific scores (Table 25.3). Because the final scores will be dependent upon the weighting applied to each of the scale's components, scores from different scales may not be completely comparable. There seems little merit, therefore, in artificially categorising the outcome scores. Secondly, because these scales are being used for foot trauma, the preinjury status of the foot can only be inferred. One should, therefore, be cautious when comparing data from different studies which use the same outcome scale. Thirdly, there remains some debate regarding which components of function should be tested. The three most widely used functional scoring systems for the foot and ankle (Mazur et al., 1979 – ankle arthrodesis; St Pierre et al., 1982 – lateral ligament injuries; Olerud and Molander, 1984 – ankle fractures) rely almost totally upon subjective data. In view of the difficulties described with objective measurements,

Table 25.2 Components of function recorded in outcome scales for foot trauma

Injury	Rowe et al. (1963) os calcis fractures	Crosby and Fitzgibbons (1990) os calcis fractures	Hawkins (1978) talar fractures	Myerson et al. (1986) tarsometatarsal fractures	La Tourette et al. (1980) tarsometatarsal fractures	Spector et al. (1984) metatarsal fractures	Gidumal et al. (1986) soft tissue defects
Use of appliances	x						
Limp	x		x	x			x
Work level	x	x					
Distance walked				x	x	x	x
Stability					x		
Shoe-wear		x		x			
Walking ability		x		x			x
Stair climbing				x			x
Cosmesis				x			
Swelling		x					
Level of activities					x	x	
Use of public transport							x
Ability to run							x
Ability to dress							x
Recreational ability							x

Table 25.3 Weightings applied in outcome scales for foot trauma

Author	Total score	Pain	Function	Objective
Rowe et al. (1963)	100	30	70	—
Crosby and Fitzgibbon (1990)	100	30	50	20
Hawkins (1978)	15	6	3	6
Myerson et al. (1986)	100	45	50	5
La Tourette et al. (1980)	70	10	40	20
Spector et al. (1984)	50	10	30	10
Gidumal et al. (1986)	100	50	50	—

Pain accounts for 14–45% of the total score, and function for 20–70%. Note the lack of emphasis on objective measurements.

this seems reasonable as it eliminates a major source of error. Finally, because there is no gold standard arbiter of outcome, it has not been possible to validate these scales and there are no reliability data.

Although little validation work has been done, scales such as those described appear to offer a meaningful way of assessing outcome. They have face validity, are easy to apply and appear clinically relevant. They allow individual patients to be evaluated throughout the course of treatment and also the comparison of patient groups receiving different treatment regimens. However, before these scores can be completely accepted by clinicians, a consensus on the weighting of the components are needed as are reliability data.

Complications

If two treatments for an injury achieve the same results, the one that causes the least inconvenience to the patient and is associated with the lowest morbidity is likely to be the one chosen. It is important therefore that when studies are reported, the nature, site and severity of any complications are noted. Although most studies report on complications, it should be recognised that they can only be truly studied in well designed prospective trials. The severity of a given complication should be assessed using available classification systems.

When to measure outcome

A major problem in the design of any study is the determination of what duration of follow-up is appropriate. The longer the duration of follow-up the more likely it is that late complications such as osteoarthritis will be detected (Yablon and Leach, 1989; Wright, 1990). However, this needs to be traded off against a greater likelihood of patient drop-out from the study. In the case of post-traumatic osteoarthritis, for instance, it is generally felt that degenerative changes may take up to 10 years to develop but most of the data are anecdotal or based on retrospective surveys (Wright, 1990). Clinically most injuries to the foot have stabilised within 3 years (Brunet and Wiley, 1987; Foy, 1990) and this should probably be the minimum recommended follow-up.

Conclusions

This chapter has examined some of the more widely used methods of outcome assessment in the foot. The theme of the chapter has been to emphasise the difficulties encountered with objective measurements, and to demonstrate the growing awareness among orthopaedic surgeons that the patient is the final arbiter of outcome. Although it is difficult to offer didactic recommendations some guidelines may be given:

1. There should be a move away from retrospective studies towards well-designed prospective trials, as this is the only way that treatment benefits can be adequately assessed. Statistical advice should be sought in the planning, rather than analysis, stage. For any outcome index used the reliability of measurement should be established.
2. For any study the demographics of the population under study should be stated, including the sex and ages of the patients, together with the duration of follow-up, which should be at least 3 years.
3. Subjective data should include an assessment of the severity of pain and the effects of disability on patient function. The assessment of function should include, as a minimum, an evaluation of the ability to work, walk, run, climb stairs and to continue sporting activities, the use of a support, the presence of a limp or stiffness and feelings of instability.
4. Objective tests of function which form part of daily clinical practice, such as the presence and severity of a limp, the ability to heel and toe walk and ability to stand on one leg, have face validity but have been seldom reported in the literature. This is one area where objective testing is likely to be reliable but needs formal evaluation.
5. Measurement of joint range of motion and foot shape by clinical or radiographic means appears to be reliable only when performed by a single observer using a standard protocol. The validity of these measurements is suspect except when compared to a normal un-affected foot.
6. Formal gait analysis does not appear, at present, to offer any significant benefit.
7. Outcome scores appear to be useful. A consensus opinion from surgeons with an interest in the foot is needed to develop a standard scoring system. Until this is available no one scale appears to offer significant benefit over the others, but that of Myerson et al. (1986) seems to cover most of the components of function that we wish to test.

Group discussion

The group was entirely in agreement with the author's summary and thought the score of Myerson et al. was probably the 'best buy' at present. The group emphasised the following deficiencies of the scoring system:

1. The score should have a separate scale for pain and function.
2. The range of movement should not be included.
3. The weighting is not validated yet.

The optimum times for assessment were not known, the group suggested 1 year for early assessment, 10 years for late assessment. However, in many instances the natural history of the disorders is not properly understood and in these cases annual assessment is recommended.

References

Ahl T, Dalen N, Selvik G (1989) Ankle fractures. *Clin. Orthop. Rel. Res.*; **245**: 246–255

Aitken AP (1963) Fractures of the os calcis – treatment by closed reduction. *Clin. Orthop. Rel. Res.*; **30**: 67–75

Alexander IA (1990) *The Foot: examination and diagnosis.* New York: Churchill Livingstone

American Academy of Orthopaedic Surgeons (1965) *Joint Motion: method of measuring and recording.* Chicago: American Academy of Orthopaedic Surgeons

Bach Christensen S, Lorentzen JE, Krogsoe O, Sneppen O (1977) Subtalar dislocation. *Acta Orthop. Scand.*; **48**: 707–711

Backer M, Kofoed H (1987) Weight bearing and non-weightbearing ankle joint mobility. *Med. Sci. Res.*; **15**: 1309–1310

Backer M, Kofoed H (1989) Passive ankle mobility: clinical measurement compared with radiography. *J. Bone Joint Surg.*; **71B**: 696–698

Bagge E, Bjelle A, Eden S, Svanborg A (1991) Osteoarthritis in the elderly: clinical and radiological findings in 79 and 85 year olds. *Ann. Rheum. Dis.*; **50**: 535–539

Bland M, Altman DG (1986) Statistical methods for assessing agreement between two methods of clinical measurement. *Lancet*; **i**: 307–310

Bohannon RW, Tiberio D, Zito M (1989) Selected measures of ankle dorsiflexion range of motion: differences and intercorrelations. *Foot Ankle*; **10**: 99–103

Boone DC, Azen SP (1979) Normal ranges of motion of joints in male subjects. *J. Bone Joint Surg.*; **61A**: 756–759

Boring EG (1961) The beginning and growth of measurement in psychology. In: Woolf H (ed) *Quantification; a history of the meaning of measurement in the natural and social sciences.* Indianapolis: The Bobbs-Merrill Co Ltd, pp. 108–127

Bray TJ, Endicott M, Capra SE (1989) Treatment of open ankle fractures: immediate internal fixation versus closed immobilisation and delayed fixation. *Clin. Orthop. Rel. Res.*; **240**: 47–52

Brunet JA, Wiley JJ (1987) The late results of tarsometatarsal joint injuries. *J. Bone Joint Surg.*; **69B**: 437–440

Brunner R, Gaechter A (1991) Repair of fibular ligaments: comparison of reconstructive techniques using plantaris and peroneal tendons. *Foot Ankle*; **11**: 359–367

Bryan AS, Klenerman L, Bowsher D (1991) The diagnosis of reflex sympathetic dystrophy using an algometer. *J. Bone Joint Surg.*; **73B**: 644–646

Burton KE, Wright V (1983) Functional assessment. *Br. J. Rheumatol.*; **22**: (Suppl) 44–47

Canale ST, Kelly FB (1978) Fractures of the neck of the talus: long-term evaluation of seventy-one cases. *J. Bone Joint Surg.*; **60A**: 143–156

Clapper MP, Wolf SL (1988) Comparison of the reliability of the Orthoranger and the standard goniometer for assessing active lower extremity range of motion. *Phys. Ther.*; **68**: 214–218

Cooper C, Cushnaghan J, Kirwan J, Rogers J, McAlindon T, McCrae F, Dieppe P (1990) Radiographic assessment of the knee joint in osteoarthritis. *Br. J. Rheumatol.*; **29**: (suppl 1) 19

Croft P (1990) Review of UK data on the rheumatic diseases – 3: Osteoarthritis. *Br. J. Rheumatol.*; **29**: 391–395

Crosby LA, Fitzgibbons T (1990) Computerised tomography scanning of acute intraarticular fractures of the calcaneus: a new classification system. *J. Bone Joint Surg.*; **72A**: 852–859

Dacre JE, Herbert KE, Perret D, Huskisson EC (1988) The use of digital image analysis for the assessment of radiographs in osteoarthritis. *Br. J. Rheumatol.*; **27**: (suppl 1) 46

Davis RB (1988) Clinical gait analysis. *IEEE Eng. Med. Biol. Mag.*; **September**: 35–40

Debrunner HU (1982) *Orthopaedic Diagnosis*. Stuttgart: Georg Thieme

De Lee JC, Curtis R (1982) Subtalar dislocation of the foot. *J. Bone Joint Surg.*; **64A**: 433–437

Ekstrand J, Witkorsson M, Oberg B, Gillquist J (1982) Lower extremity goniometry measurements: a study to determine their reliability. *Arch. Phys. Med. Rehabil.*; **63**: 171–175

Elveru RA, Rothstein JM, Lamb RL (1988) Goniometric reliability in a clinical setting: Subtalar and ankle joint measurements. *Phys. Ther.*; **68**: 672–677

Erdmann MWH, Richardson J, Templeton J (1992) Os calcis fractures: a randomised trial comparing conservative treatment with impulse compression of the foot. *Injury*; **23**: 305–307

Essex-Lopresti P (1952) The mechanism, reduction technique, and results in fractures of the os calcis. *Br. J. Surg.*; **39**: 395–419

Feinstein AR (1977) Clinical biostatistics XLVI. The purposes and functions of criteria. *Clin. Pharmacol. Ther.*; **22**: 485–498

Flick AB, Gould N (1985) Osteochondritis dissecans of the talus (transchondral fractures of talus): review of the literature and new surgical approach for medical dome lesions. *Foot Ankle*; **5**: 165–185

Floyd DW, Heckman JD, Rockwood CA Jr (1983) Tendon lacerations in the foot. *Foot Ankle*; **4**: 8–14

Foy MA (1990) The foot. In: Foy M, Fagg PS (eds) *Medicolegal Reporting in Orthopaedic Trauma*. Edinburgh: Churchill Livingstone, pp. 356–383

Fries JF (1983) The assessment of disability: from first to future principles. *Br. J. Rheumatol.*; **22**: (Suppl) 48–58

Gadjosik RL, Bohannon RW (1987) Clinical measurement of range of motion: review of goniometry emphasising reliability and validity. *Phys. Ther.*; **67**: 1867–1872

Gidumal R, Carl A, Evanski P, Shaw W, Waugh TR (1986) Functional evaluation of nonsensate free flaps to the sole of the foot. *Foot Ankle*; **7**: 118–123

Goossens M, De Stoop N (1983) Lisfranc's fracture-dislocations: etiology, radiology, and results of treatment – a review of 20 cases. *Clin. Orthop. Rel. Res.*; **176**: 154–162

Gruen GS, Mears DC (1991) Arthrodesis of the ankle and subtalar joints. *Clin. Orthop. Rel. Res.*; **268**: 15–20

Hardcastle PH, Reschauer R, Kutscha-Lissberg E, Schoffmann W (1982) Injuries to the tarsometatarsal joint: incidence, classification and treatment. *J. Bone Joint Surg.*; **64B**: 349–356

Harding D, Waddell JP (1985) Open reduction in depressed fractures of the os calcis. *Clin. Orthop. Rel. Res.*; **199**: 124–131

Hart DJ, Spector TD, Brown P, Wilson P, Doyle DV, Silman AJ (1991) Clinical signs of early osteoarthritis: reproducibility and relation to X-ray changes in 541 women in the general population. *Ann. Rheum. Dis.*; **50**: 467–470

Hattrup SJ, Johnson KA (1988) Subjective results of hallux rigidus following treatment with cheilectomy. *Clin. Orthop. Rel. Res.*; **226**: 182–191

Hawkins LG (1970) Fractures of the neck of the talus. *J. Bone Joint Surg.*; **52A**: 991–1002

Heckman JD, Champine MJ (1988) New techniques in the management of foot trauma. *Clin. Orthop. Rel. Res.*; **240**: 105–114

Heim UFA (1989) Trimalleolar fractures: late results after fixation of the posterior fragment. *Orthopaedics*; **12/8**: 1053–1059

Hellebrandt FA, Duvall EN, Moore ML (1949) The measurement of joint motion: Part III.
Reliability of goniometry. *Phys. Ther. Rev.*; **29**: 302–307

Hutchinson TA, Boyd NF, Feinstein AR, Gonda A, Hollomby D, Rowat B (1979) Scientific
problems in clinical scales as demonstrated in the Karnofsky index of performance status.
J. Chron. Dis.; **32**: 661–666

Inman VT (1976) *The Joints of the Ankle*. Baltimore: Williams and Wilkins

Jahss MH (1984) Editorial. *Foot Ankle*; **4**: 227–228

Jette AM (1989) Measuring subjective clinical outcomes. *Phys. Ther.*; **69**: 70–74

Jonsson K, Fredin HO, Cederlund CG, Bauer M (1984) Width of the normal ankle joint.
Acta Radiol. Diag.; **25**: 147–149

Joy G, Patzakis MJ, Harvey JP (1974) Precise evaluation of the reduction of severe ankle
fractures. *J. Bone Joint Surg.*; **56A**: 979–993

Kabada MP (1988) Comments on gait analysis. *IEEE Eng. Med. Biol. Mag.*; **September**: 34

Karlsson J, Peterson L (1991) Evaluation of ankle joint function: the use of a scoring scale.
Foot; **1**: 15–19

Katoh V, Chao EYS, Laughman RK, Schneider E, Morrey BF (1983) Biomechanical
analysis of foot function during gait and clinical applications. *Clin. Orthop. Rel. Res.*; **177**:
23–33

Kellgren JH, Lawrence JS (1957) Radiological assessment of osteoarthritis. *Ann. Rheum.
Dis.*; **16**: 494–502

Kellgren JH, Jeffrey MR, Ball J (1963) *The Epidemiology of Chronic Rheumatism*, vol. 2,
(*Atlas of standard radiographs*). Oxford: Blackwell Scientific Publications

Kenwright J, Taylor RG (1970) Major injuries of the talus. *J. Bone Joint Surg.*; **52B**: 36–48

Kirkup J (1988) Terminology. In Helal B, Wilson D (eds) *The Foot*. Edinburgh: Churchill
Livingstone, pp. 202–210

Kitaoka HB (1991) Salvage of nonunion following ankle arthrodesis for failed total ankle
arthroplasty. *Clin. Orthop. Rel. Res.*; **268**: 37–43

Kitaoka HB, Holliday AD (1991) Metatarsal head resection for bunionette: long-term
follow-up. *Foot Ankle*; **11**: 345–349

Lance EM, Carey EJ, Wade PA (1963) Fractures of the os calcis: treatment by early
mobilisation. *Clin. Orthop. Rel. Res.*; **30**: 76–90

La Tourette G, Perry J, Patzakis MJ, Moore TM, Harvey JP (1980) Fractures and dis-
locations of the tarsometatarsal joint. In Bateman JE, Trott AW (eds). *The Foot and
Ankle: a selection of papers from the American Orthopaedic Foot Society Meetings*. New
York: Brian C Decker, pp. 40–51

Lau JHK, Meyer LC, Lau HC (1989) Results of surgical treatment of talipes equinovarus
congenita. *Clin. Orthop. Rel. Res.*; **248**: 219–226

Leicht P, Kofoed H (1992) Subtalar arthrosis following ankle arthrodesis. *Foot*; **2**: 89–92

Lorentzen JE, Bach Christensen S, Krogsoe O, Sneppen O (1977) Fractures of the neck of
the talus. *Acta Orthop. Scand.*; **48**: 115–120

Low J (1976) Reliability of joint measurements. *Physiotherapy*; **62**: 227–229

Lundberg A, Svensson OK, Nemeth G, Selvik G (1989a) The axis of rotation of the ankle
joint. *J. Bone Joint Surg.*; **71B**: 94–99

Lundberg A, Goldie I, Kalin B, Selvik G (1989b) Kinematics of the ankle/foot complex:
plantarflexion and dorsiflexion. *Foot Ankle*; **9**: 194–200

Lundberg A, Svensson AK, Bylund C, Goldie I, Selvik G (1989c) Kinematics of the
ankle/foot complex – Part 2: pronation and supination. *Foot Ankle*; **9**: 248–253

Lundberg A, Svensson OK, Bylund C, Selvik G (1989d) Kinematics of the ankle/foot
complex – Part 3: influence of leg rotation. *Foot Ankle*; **9**: 304–309

Magone JB, Torch MA, Clark RN, Kean JR (1989) Comparative review of surgical treatment of the idiopathic clubfoot by three different procedures at Columbus Children's
Hospital. *J. Paediatr. Orthop.*; **9**: 49–58

Martin DF, Baker CL, Curl WW, Andrews JR, Robie DB, Haas AF (1989) Operative ankle arthroscopy: long-term followup. *Am. J. Sports Med.*; **17**: 16–23

May JW, Halls MJ, Simon SR (1985) Free microvascular muscle flaps with skin graft reconstruction of extensive defects of the foot: a clinical and gait analysis study. *Plast. Reconstr. Surg.*; **75**: 627–641

Mayo KA (1987) Fractures of the talus: principles of management and techniques of treatment. *Techn. Orthop.*; **2**: 42–54

Mazur JM, Schwartz E, Simon SR (1979) Ankle arthodesis: long-term follow-up with gait analysis. *J. Bone Joint Surg.*; **61A**: 964–975

McKay DW (1983) New concept of and approach to clubfoot treatment: Section III – evaluation and results. *J. Pediatr. Orthop.*; **3**: 141–148

Melzack R (1987) The short-form McGill Pain Questionnaire. *Pain*; **30**: 191–197

Merchant TC, Dietz FR (1989) Long-term follow-up after fractures of the tibial and fibular shafts. *J. Bone Joint Surg.*; **71A**: 599–606

Millstein SG, McCowan SA, Hunter GA (1988) Traumatic partial foot amputation in adults: a long term review. *J. Bone Joint Surg.*; **70B**: 251–254

Myerson M (1989) The diagnosis and treatment of injuries to the Lisfranc joint complex. *Orthop. Clin. North Am.*; **20**: 655–664

Myerson MS (1991) Management of compartment syndromes of the foot. *Clin. Orthop. Rel. Res.*; **271**: 239–248

Myerson MS, Fisher RT, Burgess AR, Kenzora JE (1986) Fracture dislocations of the tarsometatarsal joints: end results correlated with pathology and treatment. *Foot Ankle*; **6**: 225–242

Nade S, Monahan PRW (1973) Fractures of the calcaneum: a study of the long-term prognosis. *Injury*; **4**: 200–207

Nigg BM, Fisher V, Allinger TL, Ronsky JR, Engsberg JR (1992) Range of motion of the foot as a function of age. *Foot Ankle*; **13**: 336–343

Noble J, McQuillan WM (1979) Early posterior subtalar fusion in the treatment of fractures of the os calcis. *J. Bone Joint Surg.*; **61B**: 90–93

Norgrove Penny J, Davis LA (1980) Fractures and fracture-dislocations of the neck of the talus. *J. Trauma*; **20**: 1029–1037

Norkin CC, White DJ (1985) *Measurement of Joint Motion: a guide to goniometry*. Philadelphia: FA Davis

Oatis CA (1988) Biomechanics of the foot and ankle under static conditions. *Phys. Ther.*; **68**: 1815–1821

O'Doherty DP (1993) The Foot. In Pynsent PB, Fairbank JCT, Carr AJ (eds) *Outcome Measures in Trauma and Orthopaedics*. Oxford: Butterworth-Heinneman, pp. 245–268

Olerud C, Molander H (1984) A scoring scale for symptom evaluation after ankle fracture. *Arch. Orthop. Trauma Surg.*; **103**: 190–194

Paley D, Hall H (1989) Calcaneal fracture controversies: can we put Humpty Dumpty together again? *Orthop. Clin. North Am.*; **20**: 665–677

Perlman MD, Leveille D, Gale B (1989) Traumatic classifications of the foot and ankle. *J. Foot Surg.*; **28**: 551–585

Peterson L, Goldie IF, Irstam L (1977) Fracture of the neck of the talus. *Acta Orthop. Scand.*; **48**: 696–706

Porter RW, Roy A, Rippstein J (1990) Assessment in congenital talipes equinovarus. *Foot Ankle*; **11**: 16–21

Pozo JL, Kirwan EO'G, Jackson AM (1984) The long-term results of conservative management of severely displaced fractures of the calcaneus. *J. Bone Joint Surg.*; **66B**: 386–390

Reading AE (1983) The McGill Pain Questionnaire: an appraisal. In Melzack R (ed) *Pain Measurement and Assessment*. New York: Raven, pp. 55–61

Roass A, Andersson GBJ (1982) Normal range of motion of the hip, knee and ankle joints in male subjects, 30–40 years of age. *Acta Orthop. Scand.*; **53**: 205–208

Rothstein JM, Miller PJ, Roettger RF (1983) Goniometric reliability in a clinical setting: elbow and knee measurements. *Phys. Ther.*; **63**: 1611–1615

Rowe CR, Sakellarides HT, Freeman PA, Sorbie C (1963) Fractures of the os calcis: a long-term follow-up study of 146 patients. *JAMA*; **184**: 920–923

Rowley DI, Norris SH, Duckworth T (1986) A prospective trial comparing operative and manipulative treatment of ankle fractures. *J. Bone Joint Surg.*; **68B**: 610–613

Saleh M, Murdoch G. (1985) In defence of gait analysis. *J. Bone Joint Surg.*; **67B**: 237–241

Sangeorzan BJ, Veith RG, Hansen ST Jr (1990) Salvage of Lisfranc's tarsometatarsal joint by arthrodesis. *Foot Ankle*; **10**: 193–200

Sarangi PP, Ward AJ, Smith EJ, Atkins RM (1991) The use of dolorimetry in the assessment of post-traumatic algodystrophy of the foot. *Foot*; **1**: 157–163

Scott J, Huskisson EC (1976) Graphic representation of pain. *Pain*; **2**: 175–184

Scott SH, Winter DA (1991) Talocrural and talocalcaneal joint kinematics and kinetics during the stance phase of walking. *J. Biomech.*; **24**: 743–752

Sneppen O, Bach Christensen S, Krogsoe O, Lorentzen J (1977) Fractures of the body of the talus. *Acta Orthop. Scand.*; **48**: 317–324

Spector FC, Karlin JM, Scurran BL, Silvani SL (1984) Lesser metatarsal fractures: incidence, management and review. *J. Am. Podiatry Assoc.*; **74**: 259–264

Staheli LT, Chew DE, Corbett M (1987) The longitudinal arch: a survey of eight hundred and eighty-two feet in normal children and adults. *J. Bone Joint Surg.*; **69A**: 426–428

St Pierre R, Allman F, Bassett FH, Goldner JL, Fleming LL (1982) A review of lateral ankle ligamentous reconstructions. *Foot Ankle*; **3**: 114–123

Steel MW, Johnson KA, DeWitz MA, Ilstrup DM (1980) Radiographic measurements of the normal adult foot. *Foot Ankle*; **1**: 151–158

Stephenson JR (1987) Treatment of displaced intra-articular fractures of the calcaneus using medial and lateral approaches, internal fixation, and early motion. *J. Bone Joint Surg.*; **69A**: 115–130

Stratford P, Agostino V, Brazeau C, Gowitzke BA (1984) Reliability of joint angle measurement: a discussion of methodology issues. *Physiother. Can.*; **36**: 5–9

Streiner DL, Norman GR (1989) *Health Measurement Scales: a practical guide to their development and use*. Oxford: Oxford Medical Publications

Szyszkowitz R, Reschauer R, Seggl W (1985) Eighty-five talus fractures treated by ORIF with five to eight years of follow-up study of 69 patients. *Clin. Orthop. Rel. Res.*; **199**: 97–107

Thoren O (1964) Os calcis fractures. *Acta Orthop. Scand. Suppl.*; **70**: 1–116

Welton EA (1992) The Harris and Beath footprint: interpretation and clinical value. *Foot Ankle*; **13**: 462–468

White KA (1967) Improved medical care statistics and health services system. *Pub. Health Rep.*; **82**: 847–854

Whittle M (1991) *Gait Analysis: an introduction*. Oxford: Butterworth-Heinemann

Wilson DW (1972) Injuries of the tarso-metatarsal joints: etiology, classification and results of treatment. *J. Bone Joint Surg.*; **54B**: 677–686

Wood PHN (1983) Where are we now with radiographic assessment of rheumatoid arthritis? *Br. J. Rheumatol.*; **22**: Suppl 24–33

Wood-Dauphinee S, Troidl H (1986) Endpoints for clinical studies: conventional and innovative variables. In Troidl H, Sspitzer WO, McPeek B, Mulder DS, McKneally MF (eds) *Principles and Practice of Research: strategies for surgical investigators*, New York: Springer-Verlag, pp. 53–68

Wright EC, Acheson RM (1970) New Haven survey of joint diseases.xi: Observer variability in the assessment of x-rays for osteoarthrosis of the hands. *Am. J. Epidemiol.*; **91**: 378–392

Wright V (1990) Post-traumatic osteoarthritis – a medico-legal minefield. *Br. J. Rheumatol.*; **29**: 474–478

Yablon IG, Leach RE (1989) Reconstruction of malunited fractures of the lateral malleolus. *J. Bone Joint Surg.*; **71A**: 521–527

Index